BODYFUELING®
CHANGES PEOPLE'S LIVES

"BodyFueling has changed my energy and my life. I no longer assume that as I get older, I must get fatter. Also, eating *before* running altered my training—I couldn't *believe* the difference—I ran a fantastic marathon."
> **—Peg Miller,** physical therapist

"I already knew most of the information, and yet I had never put it all together. What BodyFueling did was put me in touch with my commitment to my fitness and health, so now I'm actually *using* the information."
> **—Mark Weeks,** water quality specialist/rock climber

"I had heard a lot of the stuff before—I was an aerobics instructor for fourteen years—but the authenticity and clarity really pulled it together for me. I've never seen this information presented so thoroughly."
> **—Susan Bennett,** teacher

"BodyFueling gave me the support and clarity I needed to make choices that are good for my body. I have worked out for years trying to get definition through body sculpting and aerobics. After BodyFueling, the visual difference was amazing even though I didn't change my workout a bit. I heartily endorse this very practical material!"
> **—Karen Tuff,** corporate facilitator

"I was eating a low-fat diet and exercising, but I was still having problems. . . . Knowing what, when, and how much to eat has helped me take two inches of fat off my waist. I have been enthusiastically recommending BodyFueling to my patients."
> **—Dr. Michael Kinnear**

"Since BodyFueling I've been fueling my body so much better, and believe it or not, I have already felt a *big* difference. I feel good, my head is clearer, and I have more energy for my three-year-old son. I have told everyone about BodyFueling."
> **—Cathryn Davis,** TV/film producer

Copies of these and other signed testimonials are on file and may be examined at Warner Books, 1271 Avenue of the Americas, New York, NY 10020.

BodyFueling®

Stop Watching Your Weight, Start Fueling Your Life

ROBYN LANDIS

FOREWORD BY KAAREN NICHOLS, M.D.

toExcel

San Jose   New York   Lincoln   Shanghai

BodyFueling
Stop Watching Your Weight, Start Fueling Your Life

Published by toExcel
an imprint of iUniverse.com, Inc.

For information address:
iUniverse.com, Inc.
620 North 48th Street
Suite 201
Lincoln, NE 68504-3467
www.iuniverse.com

ISBN: 0-595-00106-8

Printed in the United States of America

There is nothing more difficult to take in hand, more perilous to conduct or more uncertain in its success than to take the lead in the introduction of a new order of things.

—inscription on Machiavelli's tomb

The real act of discovery consists not in finding new lands but in seeing with new eyes.

—Marcel Proust

CONTENTS

ACKNOWLEDGMENTS

I dedicate this book with deepest gratitude to the following people:

To Marty and Doris Weisen, my parents; and Steven Weisen, my brother, for being so generous with their love and so vocal about their pride for so many years that I began to believe all the great stuff they said—making me bold, and confident that my voice counts.

To my husband, Robert, whose observations and views found their way into the book through innumerable animated conversations. Thanks for sharing with me the vision that sparked BodyFueling. You paved the path to the finish line, and along the way cleaned it, repaired it, lit it, and lined it with flowers. As corny as it may sound, I know being the wind beneath someone's wings is not easy. Perhaps most of all, you made those last sleepless, interminable hours of manuscript preparation not only possible but survivable.

To Grandma Rose, the pioneer who preceded me, whose legendary capacity to love, forgive, and persevere continues to set an example for me that will smooth the way for what I've set out to accomplish. I know you're beside me, guarding the torch you passed to me by your instinctive urging: "Eat, *eat!*"

To my editor, Jeanmarie LeMense, for whose skillful and sensitive guidance I feel exceptionally fortunate. Every author hopes for this kind of commitment, genuine enthusiasm, fairness, keen sense of direction, and painless tempering of criticism with appreciation. I'm grateful that you saw an important book beneath a wild-horse manuscript, and helped tame it without subduing its passion. And I'm honored that you have become a fluent and persuasive champion not only of the book, but of its messages.

To every BodyFueling® workshop participant and consulting client: My commitment to you, and to the next generation of "yous," fueled this book. Every person I have ever spoken with on this subject contributed something to it. Thanks especially to Dr. Ann McCombs, Dr. Kaaren Nichols, the Scherers, the de Leñas, Dr. Mike and Susan Kinnear, Marty Jordan, Amanda Bergson-Shilcock, and Mark Weeks for going out of your way to provide support and encouragement.

To Karta Purkh Singh Khalsa, with great appreciation for your patience with my millions of curious questions, and for the healing wisdom that not only helped keep me robust and flu-free during the 17-hour-a-day editing season, but whose role in the future of health holds promise I can't quite put into words yet.

And to our friends, for understanding when I essentially disappeared off the face of the earth for the duration of this project, and while I tended to be rather . . . shall we say *absorbed.*

Finally, I would like to thank H. Ross Perot. Regardless of what one thinks of him or his policies, his work during 1992 provided an uplifting example for anyone dedicated to the power of an informed, independent-thinking public and the elimination of dysfunctional establishments. He has proven the viability of raising American consciousness about grave and pressing issues—quickly. He set a worthy standard for doing so, bringing urgency to problems, upbeat reassurance to solutions, and logic to priorities. Unflappable in a world that often fights truth rather than welcomes it, he launched previously slippery concepts into political and public awareness—and made them stick. To me, this is inspiration to usher crazy aunts out of basements whenever we find them, and constantly renews my faith that the ones I found will be received.

FOREWORD

by Kaaren A. Nichols, M.D.

As a family medicine physician with a busy practice, I daily encounter patients with bothersome and often serious medical symptoms that are a direct result of the food they eat—or don't eat. National statistics on disease and diet bear out this observation.

Last summer a patient came to me complaining of constant abdominal pain. None of the appropriate tests showed a problem; the revelation was Kate's eventual confession that she was subsisting on 15 diet sodas daily. Imagine! A week after my suggestion that Kate stop the sodas and replace them with real nourishment, her pain had completely disappeared. She has been well since then, with no recurrence of pain.

It makes perfect sense that a daily diet limited to 15 sodas would cause discomfort—*but it wasn't obvious to Kate.* Time and time again I see this connection not being made, this lack of a sense that what we put into our bodies is of supreme and utmost importance. The image of Kate has stayed with me as an icon for how Americans treat their bodies—without much awareness about priorities or costs.

How many Americans try to get through each day by filling their bodies up with substances that provide no sustenance, no energy—no fuel? How many people displace quality food and liquid with ones that offer no value?

And how come the average American manages to miss the significance of that?

If your car ran out of gas, would you put sugar water in the tank? No way! Why do we so often treat our bodies much worse than our cars? Why is the average American at such a loss about how to treat it at all? Food is fuel to make our bodies run; why has it become everything *but* that?

These are good questions, questions I have asked myself—and I have never seen them posed, framed, and answered with such a unique blend of intuition, history, science, and personal passion as Robyn Landis has in her classes and now in her book *BodyFueling*.

This is an important and comprehensive education that teaches you to think, to see, and to understand—and then to act. Robyn's book brings an entirely new, positive, even transformational perspective to that education. Her way of seeing food, eating, and the body—and her insightful and compassionate sense of the culture's viewpoint—slices through the confusion to reveal those basics that everyone should have grown up knowing (and soon may, if Robyn has her way!).

Robyn's book shows you, step by step, how to feed your body so it can be in prime condition—but she also explains exactly why those steps work. Her gift for metaphor and vivid analogy makes an often technical and complex subject easy for anyone to digest (so to speak!). Her analogies are thoughtful, graphic, and memorable, making abstract science come alive. She made me see in a fresh new way the science I know so well.

Robyn courageously challenges the established thinking that let you get this far without becoming an "educated owner" of your body. But, as a physician who believes the individual is also responsible for his or her health, I also appreciate Robyn's persuasive case for you taking charge and becoming knowledgeable. Her message is not presented as a platitude to swallow whole and follow blindly.

Patients of mine have had their worrisome medical symptoms significantly reduced and often completely alleviated by "fueling." Fueling is fully consistent with the type of eating most recommended by health authorities today (with a few additional, frequently overlooked caveats)—but when Robyn presents it as fueling, you don't feel as though you're "following orders."

As any health-care provider knows, inspiring action and a sense of personal responsibility for self-care is a real challenge, and yet one that is emerging as the ultimate answer to health. My patients are unanimously ecstatic at how well they feel and how great they look. So am I! But I'm even more excited that they took action on what they learned.

For these reasons and more, Robyn's book is definitely not a "diet book."

I'm confident that, unlike many diet books, it will gain the respect of professionals everywhere, not only because it is scientifically sound but because it strikes a chord culturally. Rather than promote yet another diet, Robyn cuts to the quick of why the facts aren't getting through to people—and she does get through. In fact, if you're ready to move from dieting to eating and living your life, this is the book to buy.

Though this is not a "program" per se, you can certainly lose excess fat and redefine your body if you take action on the book's information and inspiration. And I am willing to bet "taking action" turns out to be very different (for the better!) than you might assume it's going to be before you start reading.

The fact is that the vast majority of overfat people have simply trained their bodies to respond that way—through the way they eat, and through the way they don't eat. The vast majority can also retrain the body—by feeding it in a way that works with how *it* works. It all starts with retraining your thinking, as well as with some education about the human machine. I am so pleased to have discovered a resource like this that makes such an education accessible to everyone.

Because of my academic training in physiology and biochemistry, as both a physician and teacher, I expected to be critical of at least some of Robyn's material. Not so! It is so thoroughly researched and exceptionally accurate, I was nothing but impressed. I myself can say I learned. No matter how advanced your education, you can always benefit from a perspective that stimulates you to *use* more of what you know . . . and to feel more like you have a choice.

I've never seen the formidable task of bringing America to a new food/body consciousness undertaken with such fierce intelligence, razor-sharp logic, and genuine personal commitment. The case for new thinking in health and fitness education has found a unique and powerful voice in Robyn Landis.

I would nominate *BodyFueling* as required reading for every woman and man, curriculum for every child, and a word to the wise for every educator, health professional, and coach. I recommend it to all my patients, friends, and colleagues. I know you'll learn from it, enjoy it, and reap a lifetime of benefits—both in mind and body.

Here's to a happy, healthy, well-fueled you!

—KAAREN A. NICHOLS, M.D.
Founder and Director,
Seattle Medical and Wellness Clinic

BodyFueling

INTRODUCTION:
Lies and Truths—
Your World Turned
Upside Down

Have you ever thought, or do you believe, any of the following?

▶ Eating less and exercising more is the way to get fit.
▶ Losing "weight" is synonymous with getting fit; it is always good to have lost weight; there is an ideal weight you should weigh.
▶ Fat people are fat because they eat way too much food.
▶ You need to make up for overeating or eating something "bad" by cutting back.
▶ It's bad to eat when you're angry, lonely, sad, bored, or frustrated.
▶ You can eat anything you want as long as you stay within a certain range of calories.
▶ If you stop eating fat, you'll lose fat.
▶ If you exercise, you can eat anything you want.
▶ If you cut out caffeine and sodium, and avoid pesticides and preservatives, you'll be much fitter and live longer.
▶ Being fit is a matter of control and willpower.

These assumptions represent just a small sampling of the prevailing wisdom about diet, health, and exercise.

Which of these are true?

The answer is *none*.

1

Do you know *why* they're not? Do you know what *is* true? Can you describe what kind of fuel your body runs on? Do you know what it needs, how much, how often, and in what proportions? Or do you just know how to watch your weight? Does it seem odd to you that you know how to count calories—but you don't know what a calorie *is*?

To say that the list of statements above are myths may seem dubious. After all, some of these you may "know" to be true. But think for a moment about your own experiences. You've tried eating less and exercising more, but you don't look and feel like you think you should. You've whittled down the fat in your diet, but you haven't seen any dramatic results. You eat lots of salads, vegetables, and juices, but you're puzzled by your lack of performance. You've even investigated the benefits of eating organic, all-natural food, but you just haven't reaped the rewards all those magazines and studies have promised you. You're doing everything that everyone knows is right, so why does it look and feel so wrong?

In this book you'll find simple, logical, undisputed data to explain what's nonsensical about each and every one of the myths on the previous page. You'll see why these "truths" have been peddled to you—and why the odds have been against your digging yourself out from under them. You'll see how not knowing enough about your own body has left you powerless to dismiss the myths and live a fit, satisfying life of good eating.

The human body is a marvelously sophisticated machine, and like most machines it has fuel requirements. But did you grow up knowing how to fuel your body purposefully, consistently, and precisely—the way you fuel your automobile? Probably not. As a culture, we don't even think about food or our bodies this way. Most Americans, even otherwise highly educated ones, know far more about fueling their cars or how their computers work than about feeding their bodies.

Yet our bodies are the most important resource we have to get us where we're going. It's the "vehicle" we'll rely on most throughout the course of our lives. For the longevity, appearance, strength, and performance of that machine—your body—its needs don't get much more primary than fuel.

Food is our fuel, but food's been made the enemy. As a result, Americans are overfat largely because they *under* fuel (not overeat) in a misguided effort that stems from a basic ignorance of our own biology. It is both dangerous and frustrating to mess around with technology you don't understand. But you do this with your body all the time. Determined to be "thin" and fit, you labor at all the wrong things—things you've been assured are the answers. When it doesn't work, you think *you're* the problem.

We've all heard that diets don't work. What you don't hear much about is why. Teaching my BodyFueling® workshops, I've seen that while Americans are coming to some consensus about what not to do, the average person is at a loss about what to do instead, and why and how to do it. Everybody's saying it, but it's not inspiring any positive action.

At the same time, the one thing you still hear more about and do more of than any other is "losing weight." While "dieting" may be losing its luster, "weight"—rooted in the same misguided thinking as dieting—remains the centerpiece issue. Our so-called "fitness" efforts have been oriented around weight for generations, yet your weight is not relevant to how you look or feel or how long you live. There is no such thing as a "weight problem," "overweight," or "ideal weight." Rather than sell you yet another way to lose weight, *BodyFueling* unravels the premises that make weight an issue, so you can see it's nothing but a limiting, unhealthy, and counterproductive diversion.

Weight doesn't matter? My problem is undereating? While these may sound like radical assertions, they're just the beginning of many happy surprises you'll find substantiated here. You'll be enlightened about how "weight," "overeating," and other decoy issues have derailed the so-called "fitness revolution"—and how they've personally affected your efforts. Then you'll learn what to do about it.

As you'll see, "losing weight" as we currently pursue it is a process not only biologically determined to fail, but one that compounds the original problems. Yet more that half of all Americans are trying to do it. Why are we flocking down the wrong tunnel in droves? Why have you been led to believe what you believe? How have those beliefs managed to persist when basic science shatters their every premise? And how can you learn to think—and act—more effectively?

Stop parroting the cliché "diets don't work" and other trendy catchphrases that don't get at the heart of the matter. Start by becoming an educated owner of your body. Dependable information gets you halfway to the ultimate goal: informed choice. Armed with the most essential, substantiated facts about your body's requirements, you're in a position to make the healthiest choices possible.

Informed choice also means you know these choices are yours to make. Without information (or with misinformation) your commitment is constantly tested by the frustration of seeing no reward for your efforts. On the other hand, information without an authentic experience of choice also backfires. Don't you know things and not act on them? Isn't it grueling when you act strictly out of grim resolve?

Don't be hard on yourself if *have to, ought to, should,* and *must* haven't inspired a wholesale turnaround in your habits. The prevailing strategy of media and educators is to wag a finger at you, the naughty child who *should* eat better and *shouldn't* eat *bad* foods. Once informed, you're automatically supposed to do what works. There's no choice—and that doesn't work. Just look around you.

I'll treat you like the intelligent adult you are—someone who can understand and make responsible choices about your body. You'll see for yourself what will work—not what I think you "should" do. And you'll be encouraged to explore, in a positive, new way, why you *want* to fuel yourself—not be made to feel that you have to.

Informed choice means knowing what you want, knowing how to get it, and *choosing* whether or not to. To bring you to the position of informed choice—your most powerful tool for building a life of lasting fitness—this book offers four solid pillars as a foundation:

INSPIRATION—A BREAKTHROUGH IN THE CHALLENGE OF "MOTIVATION"

There's a vast difference between fueling your future and trying to fix your body (or "weight"). Rather than try to get you to fuel, I'll guide you in consideration of fueling as an investment in your body, an expression of your long-term commitment to your life.

INSIGHT—DIET THINKING DOESN'T WORK

It's not merely diets that are doomed to fail; the deeper problem is the entire way of thinking that gave birth to diets. Start recognizing the vague, negative, biased language and thinking that sustains an environment of rampant fallacy about eating and exercise. You'll see how groundless assumptions are made about fitness and fat loss, even by professionals—and why this misleading belief system has gone relatively unchallenged until now.

INFORMATION—WHAT DOES WORK AND WHY

Discover why poor fueling—not food—is the enemy! You'll understand the design of the human body, the relationship between food assimilation and energy, and how ways of eating you may think are "right" are actually counterproductive. You'll develop a frame of reference for navigating the information explosion and setting logical priorities. No magical theories, fads, or miracles—just solid explanations for the way your body actually works with food.

INTEGRATION—A HOW-TO STRUCTURE THAT MAKES IT EASY

Practical guidance will show you just how simple and enjoyable "fueling" is, and will help you make fueling a natural part of daily living—not "a diet."

Like you may be, I was once frustrated and confused about eating. I did everything "they" tell us to, but I didn't have the body my "healthy" habits were supposed to give me. I decided to take the matter into my own hands, making an in-depth study of basic science—biology, human physiology— and applying what I learned to my eating. The results were outstanding, and the utter backwardness of how we've approached "healthy eating" became obvious to me in the process.

Common assumptions about eating are clearly dispelled by the most fundamental facts. Fat loss and fitness have stunningly little to do with all those methods we never thought to question. Those popular practices have almost nothing to do with how your body works, are physiologically wired for failure, require deprivation, and are a source of suffering for countless people. It is unconscionable to me that the facts I have assembled here for you are not widely or completely circulated to the lay public.

As you'll see in the following pages, I have a few things to say about the media that promote what I call diet thinking, and the health/science professionals and educators who should know better. This book is a grassroots effort to provide and promote a bottom-line education that, in both content and form, has been kept from you until now. The physical and psychological rewards of such education are tremendous. I don't think people should have to go out of their way to get it, as I did.

Turn the page and leave behind the tired mentality that has crippled your past efforts. You'll be taking a critical step beyond traditional diet thinking into a provocative inquiry about your future and the relevance of what you eat. *BodyFueling* won't merely change the way you eat—*it will transform the way you think about eating and your life*. It isn't just about "changing your diet"—it's about fueling your future, working with your body to create the life you want, and caring for and respecting the marvelous machine that will get you there.

I'll make you a promise: *BodyFueling* will free you from the dismal sentence of denial and control you've been handed as the only path to fitness. You can develop an efficient, fun, and satisfying way of eating—and thinking—that offers high energy, reduced body fat, ease, and convenience at less expense. You'll find yourself eating in the ways most widely urged by health authorities—not only without suffering, but with joy and purpose.

What do you really want? If it's not only to look good, but to feel good, live long, and have food be a source of pleasure and power instead of a problem, then *BodyFueling* is for you. For once, it's really good news—so read, eat, and enjoy!

1

FUELING YOUR FUTURE:
A Breakthrough in Motivation

THINK OF FOOD AS FUEL

Food is the fuel that runs your body all the time. That's why, to start with, I call eating "fueling." When you think about food as fuel, it's hard to think of food as the enemy.

Thinking of the body as a machine with fuel requirements makes sense. It's a powerful way of looking at and thinking about food. It allows for analogies that even little kids can grasp. (What do we say to toddlers and their toys? "Vroom, vroom! Make the car go!")

If food fuels the body's functions, then "eating healthy," for starters, must involve eating. Obvious? You'd be amazed how many people overlook this. Look around you: People are *resisting eating* more than they are eating. And that's not just because they're dieting. Efforts at "healthier lifestyles" in general focus on cutting things out. Even when what's being limited is appropriate—such as dietary fat—people tend to cut total food volume along with it, which is unnecessary.

When you're looking at food choices from the nearsighted perspective of "weight loss/diet," your concerns are very narrow. Choices are based on "Is this 'allowed' on my 'diet'? Will it help me lose weight?" When you see food as fuel for your body, your questions become more thoughtful, intelligent, and direct: "Will this fuel my body? Is it good fuel?" This chapter begins the path to a completely new perspective. It will take you from "trying to fix your eating and your body" to "fueling your life."

That's why we start with *what you want*. We need to know what you want before we can talk about how to get it. So what you need, even before you know how to fuel, is why to fuel—a powerful, compelling purpose for fueling yourself optimally. Not because what works is hard; I bet that as you read this book, you'll find that what is biologically most efficient for the human body is easier, more convenient, more fun, more food, better tasting, and less expensive than you think it'll be or than what you do now. But change—for the better or not—is still change. And as you've probably noticed, it doesn't "just happen."

Fueling your body really starts with looking at your life, your future, your commitments and desires—something that initially has nothing to do with nutrition. But it's not off the subject. It's all connected. If whatever you embark upon fitness-wise doesn't have to do with your life, what does it have to do with? And why bother?

That's a very good question.

A NEW WAY OF THINKING ABOUT "MOTIVATION"

When people talk about motivation—either giving it or getting it—it's used in a very different way than I've come to think of it. You typically think of motivation (especially related to eating and fitness) as something someone does to you from the outside. If my job is to motivate you, then you think my job is to get you to do something—to pump you up, jack you up, glaze you over, and send you out with a "Rah rah rah!"

The problem is that there's no power in this concept of motivation. You are depending on someone else to give you the impetus to do something. It's short-lived, if it works at all. *You* need to find and generate the impetus, and this chapter will guide you in doing just that—in a new and positive way.

Informed choice replaces the traditional (and essentially bankrupt) concept of "motivation." From this point on, I won't even use the word. It's too much a part of the vocabulary of diet thinking, one of a number of words—such as "lifestyle"—that while not innately negative, have come to be associated with too many diet-oriented concepts. "Motivation" is a false, temporary push that you think you need to get started and "stay on" some rigid program. None of that applies to fueling.

SOMETHING NEW: IT'S YOUR CHOICE

"Personal responsibility" has become a buzzword that has nearly lost its meaning. Too often it's folded into the same old, tired "nag approach," as in "You really should be responsible for your body."

That's not my idea of personal responsibility. My definition doesn't say you "should" be responsible, but rather acknowledges that you *are* responsible— whether or not you accept that and use the freedom that accompanies it. Whether you're willing to exercise your choice or not, you do have a choice. Once informed about how your body works and what works best with it, what you do with that information will be up to you.

Fueling is not about what you can or can't have, it's about what you want. When you move beyond "have to" ("I have to eat better, I ought to change my habits, I have to get fit, I should be healthier") the only question that remains is, "If you don't have to, then why would you? Why might you *choose* fueling?" If "I should" was your reason, and we remove that reason, what reason do you have?

Just allowing that you truly do have a choice either way may prove more of a challenge than you think. "Of course I have to eat better!" you may say. "My doctor said I'll get sick if I don't! My wife will leave me! I'll never be successful if I'm fat! It's wrong to eat poorly!" Is it really? Just answer this: Where has it gotten you so far to *have* to?

There's a subtle but very powerful difference between "I have to do this" and "This is what it will take to get the results I want." Only the latter tells the whole truth. You don't really have to. You only have to if you want particular results.

"Oh, that's the same thing," you may cry. "That's no choice—obviously I want those results." Ah, but it *is* a choice. It's *not* necessarily obvious. One possible answer is, "I don't care, and I'm willing to pay the price." Getting sick *is* an alternative. People make that choice all the time. They just don't always admit it.

To insist that you have to is to insist you have no power, to remain subject to the will of someone and something else, to disclaim responsibility for your own body and the actions that affect it. Informed choice is supremely powerful, but it requires that you be responsible.

I could hold a gun to your head and say, "Eat this way" and you probably would, but what would that accomplish? That might change your eating, but not in the way I'm talking about. If I did that, *I'd* be responsible for changing your eating. What works is for *you* to be. Rather than "modify your behavior," I'd rather see you tap your ability to be the source of your behavior.

Therefore, I will not try to make you, get you to, shame, threaten, order, cajole, obligate you, or otherwise bulldoze you into fueling. What you do is up to you! Maybe you can tell kids to do something "because I said so!" but for adults it doesn't work. You need to have your own personal—and powerful—reasons to use the information here. Only you and your own plans will inspire you to care for yourself.

Once you've established that you do have a choice, it's most effective simply to explore what might sway your choices toward those that will best serve you. Thus, food choices become "I don't *want* what doesn't fuel my body" instead of "I can't have that."

Hear the difference? In "I can't have it," someone else made a determination and you followed—probably unwillingly. The fact is, you *could* have it. But you chose that you didn't *want* it, because something else is more important to you.

Cindy, a workshop participant who described herself as having "enough books about diet and weight to start a bookstore," saw this after BodyFueling: "Now, if I want a cream puff I can have it. But now I also know what I'm doing to myself when I do. I'm always aware that everything I put in my body is an investment—for better or for worse. It really works to look at it that way. I'm much more aware of what I'm building. I honestly don't *want* to drug myself with fat and sugar anymore—I see too much to live for and have energy for."

THINK FIRST, DO LATER

That we're looking at inspiration and your thinking *before* looking at the body and food is no accident. Like everything else in *BodyFueling*, it's totally by design. It's important that we go through this exercise; it's also significant and purposeful that it happens before anything else. Before I tell you what to do, how to do, how it works, and why it works that way, I want you to have a perspective in which to view the information, so it's a positive experience of choice—not a new bunch of rules to follow or just another high-carbohydrate diet. I refuse to simply throw information at you; there's already plenty of that going on.

Therefore, I don't present you with anything to do until we've addressed these issues: that you do have a choice, that you are responsible, and that there are things in your life—plans and purposes—that will influence and inspire your choices.

I agree that knowing how or what to do is definitely important. (That's why there is plenty of that later in this book.) But the key is to cross the gap between knowing and doing. Ask yourself how often you've known what to do—and not done it.

If you just want to change your eating for a little while, you can rush in and manipulate the eating itself. To change your eating to *a way of living* requires you to first transform your whole way of thinking. We can't just rush out and dump a pile of building materials on a rotten foundation. First we must carefully lay a solid foundation.

SUSPENDING JUDGMENT

This is likely to be a departure from approaches to which you're accustomed, where you just get handed the diet rules, shoulds, and recommendations. Typically, that's all you're trained to look for. This is the nation that worships "Just do it." The only problem is, you don't. It's a nice tidy idea, but it doesn't work—Americans' headline-making lack of success with fitness is proof.

Not only does the BodyFueling approach not supply instant answers, but the questions we explore initially may be unsettling. For many, it's much easier to avoid this kind of inquiry, focus instead on technical data, and then blame it for failure.

As a result, it's not surprising that I've run into an extraordinary amount of resistance to starting with the subject of your future. As Americans, we're listening for the how-to, for the what-to-do. We want to know how to get it before we know *why* we want it. We worship content, when context is of equal or greater importance. We worry endlessly about doing it or not, or doing it right, but we never take a step back and first ask why.

"Just tell me what to do," people insist, as if that will ensure they'll do it. "Let's get on with it," they say. Well, this *is* it—as big a part of it as any. "This isn't what I expected." You're right, it sure isn't. If it was what you expected, it would be the same old thing you've always known—which didn't work. It looks different because it is different. If you want "the same," buy a diet book.

If this issue makes you uncomfortable, know that you're not alone. Also know that it's not an accident. Be curious about why this makes you so antsy or angry or sleepy, rather than certain that your feelings of impatience are justified. If you're upset about "not getting down to the facts," that's a hallmark of the very thinking that keeps your efforts in the unsatisfying realm of "changes I have to make," "a diet I need to do." It immediately tips me off that you see your future and your life as unrelated to eating.

That flawed thinking helps perpetuate America's obsession with what we (unappealingly) call "sticking to it." Healing this rift between your eating and your future solves a lot of that problem (and getting informed about what really works, as you will see later, takes care of the rest). But trust that maybe what you think presents an even bigger hurdle than what you do.

BodyFueling is less something to do than it is something to know—something not to "follow," but to *live*. It's a profound change in perspective that will form the basis for your commitment. Don't rush headlong into doing it—or, as is more common, *trying* to do it. Suspend your thirst for content—at least temporarily. Trying to change your eating when you're wallowing in the midst of what I call "diet thinking" is like changing your clothes to a white outfit when you're still in the middle of a mud puddle. It just makes more of a mess.

IF YOU HAVE NO REASON TO GO, YOU DON'T NEED DIRECTIONS!

How come merely telling you what to do is so futile? Because it gives you no ownership in the data; content by itself doesn't demand your engagement. It's not personal; you don't connect with it. Information alone doesn't guarantee a response. The assumption that it ought to is a major and fatal premise of traditional diet-thinking education. I see lots of information thrown at you every day, and then I see the throwers whining, "They just don't do it!"

In fact, if being told what to do elicits any kind of response from a human being at all, it's defiance and opposition. Telling you what to do is probably a good way to ensure that you don't do it.

If knowing doesn't ensure doing, what does? Purpose. I'll demonstrate with a question: Are you going to Ohio tomorrow?

If you answered "No," then you probably have no reason to go there, do you?

If I gave you really great directions to Ohio, then would you go to Ohio tomorrow?

Highly doubtful—because you still have no purpose in being there. Directions by themselves don't get you on the road. If you have no interest in going, even the best directions won't get you there! If you're not going, you don't need directions at all.

On the other hand, if the fiery love of your life and a job of your dreams at a salary of $2 million a year was in Ohio, you might be interested in going. And if you were absolutely planning to go, then you'd need to know how to get there. Then you'd want the best directions you could find.

Some people think the entire eating problem is bad directions. I definitely agree (as you'll soon see) that's certainly part of it. But not having much of a purpose for using the directions is just as problematic. This book contains the best directions available for obtaining fitness, health, energy, and leanness. But if you have little or no interest in getting to where fueling will take you, you don't need those how-tos. Why dash for a road map if you aren't serious about the journey?

So begin asking yourself about this journey and why you're excited to use the "directions" you will get later. What interests you about what fueling has to offer? What could you use more vitality and more years for? What will you spend them on?

NOT JUST ANY REASONS

It's not enough to have just *any* plans or want *some* results. Chances are you already do. Chances are also that if they haven't inspired you to do much by now—if you have not made changes you think you "should"—those reasons are probably not very compelling.

Your reasons for wanting or using information typically influence whether you use that information, and how you use it—your perspective affects your actions. For example: I have the same information about car care now that I did when I owned a little econo-box hatchback. But the hatchback was a temporary car; I planned to keep it just for a year or two. And I didn't care for it well, even though I knew what to do. I never changed the oil, didn't tune it up once in 52,000 miles, and ran it out of gas three or four times.

When I replaced it with the convertible I'd been coveting, things changed. I still knew the same stuff about car care—but I started to use it. My appreciation of my new car, my plans for the future of the car, made the difference. I intend to drive it till I have a daughter to give it to. And I plan to enjoy it until then.

Of course you do all the right things to your car if it's very important to you to keep it for 20 years. If it's not important, you don't—or it's very hard to "motivate" yourself to. (Hear how that word becomes interchangeable with "make" yourself?) We can alter the way we look at our bodies in this very same way, making a shift from temporary to lifelong, from careless to caring, and from deprecating to appreciative.

What you think and say about something affects your experience and thus your actions. If you saw having a child as merely being pregnant—nothing more—you'd have a different experience of pregnancy than if you saw yourself as creating a product of love between you and a partner, a new friend to share life with, an expansion of family, a potential contribution to the earth. Hear the difference? You'd not only experience pregnancy differently; you'd probably also treat yourself and the pregnancy differently.

Here's another example. The person who is laying brick day after day for a wall, who is simply told that his job is to build a wall, will have a different experience than one who is told his job is to build the world's first center for educating physically handicapped children of exceptional intelligence. The latter will probably also build the wall differently, pay a different level of attention to it, than the former. One can see beyond the mere wall to what he is really building and what its purpose is. The other can only see a wall for the sake of a wall.

Compare this to the way you have looked at and spoken about your reasons for seeking an eating-related change. Has it sounded something like "I have to change my diet," "I need to lose weight," "I've got to stick to this program," "I must lower my cholesterol/blood pressure," or "I look awful; I can't wait to lose 10 pounds"? These are the kinds of "reasons" I hear constantly. "I've got to lose fat" is as about as inspiring and appealing as "I've got to clean the bathroom."

Compare those to "I eat to nurture my body so it is the natural representation of a person who is active in the community." Or "I eat to keep my body lean and strong so I can be the most outrageous mom of three . . . and grandmom . . . and great-grandmom . . . in this city/state/country (how adventurous are you?).'' Or "I eat to keep my body fueled for high performance on the job, since my work is about XYZ, and it's very important to me." "I eat to invest in the future of my real job—being a fun dad."

Does eating sound different now? What would *you* rather have your eating express? Which makes caring for yourself more compelling?

"SHOULD" IS A WORTHLESS WEAPON

One overused reason for pursuing fitness, which you may have been content with before, is: "Well, I should." But it's one that I assert won't get you to fuel your body (or do much of anything else). I don't see many people doing important things just because they feel obligated. If they do, they don't seem very happy, and it usually doesn't last.

When I ask people about their commitment to health and fitness, it frequently comes out as a thing they "should" be doing. "I am committed to working out three times a week." "I am committed to losing 15 pounds." Bring it back to *why? What for?* What is your body for, and *why* would you want it leaner, fitter, or more energetic or healthy? Don't cop out with "Well, I just do" or "Isn't it obvious?" or "Because I should."

WHAT ARE YOU FUELING?

If you're fueling a future, the most crucial question is: *What* future? Your answer makes the difference between *working on your eating* and *investing in your life*—two truly different experiences, only one of which I think you enjoy.

What do you want your body to be able to do? What beloved aspect of your life demands a fit, healthy, resilient body? What do you want to do and be that requires energy? Now . . . What if you ate for that? Fueled that?

Don't be modest. Something or someone out there benefits from you having optimum performance—and you benefit, too. It may be your work, your children, your hobbies, your community. Whatever they are, they are things that motivate you far more than "I should" or "I look terrible" ever will.

What are you for? Do you deliver babies? Father great children? Run triathlons? Teach our future generations? Write things that make a difference? Manage other human beings? Are you for your grandchildren? Your company? Your love? Your retirement travel plans? Eat for that.

Be specific. "I just want to be healthy and happy" isn't powerful enough to influence your choices on a lifelong basis.

Once you get started, it gets easier. One BodyFueling workshop participant envisioned herself like Kate Hepburn with a huge home and great gardens—which she'll have the energy to tend herself, well past her nineties. Tom wants to be "100, horny, and running triathlons." Peter wants to sail around the world and "not be a burden to my children, but rather a continuing contributor to their lives." Pam wants to be a 90-year-old racquetball competitor. Linda wants to teach her great-grandchildren to ski, just as she did her kids. Wayne wants to be an energetic manager—and when he gets home at night, an even more energetic dad to his one-year-old. Laura works in recycling and plans to have an impact on the way we treat the environment. Al wants to live in Portugal, where medical care is limited, demanding that he stay healthy. Carolyn, whose 30-year-old lover is 20 years her junior, wants to keep up with him—in every way. Betsy doesn't ever want to stop white-water rafting.

If there is a way to eat that will better their odds for achieving these things, they will eat that way—happily and enthusiastically. Eating becomes an opportunity for obtaining or achieving something great—not a means for "fixing" a "problem." They choose food that they know will fuel their dreams and ambitions.

BE WILLING TO EXPLORE

If you're like many people, you have been so busy railing against what you don't want that you haven't even bothered to consider what you do want. You haven't identified something that excites you, inspires you to feed your body, to treat yourself with honor rather than to inflict punishment on your body.

It can be hard to look that far ahead. People rarely come to this question prepared to discuss the next 75 years or their purpose on the earth. Not coincidentally, most people also don't have a way of eating that works, and don't see it as a natural, lifelong proposition. There is a connection between your vision of the future not extending very far, and your successful eating not lasting very long.

One highly successful stockbroker at a corporate workshop bravely admitted—among her peers—that she really had no idea what was in her future, what she wanted or pictured. She never thought past the current year. Not only was that disturbing in itself, but she had never connected that shortsightedness with her struggle against "weight." She was trying to make herself a "thin" person by chanting "I am a thin person," whenever faced with food. This is resistance to food, resistance to who she really thinks she is (why would she have to chant "I am thin" if she really believed she was?). The scariest part to me is that she *was* thin—for what little that word is worth—and on a commercial weight-loss plan.

Her whole focus was on thinness and how her body looked right now. Nothing about health, no sense of her body being a precious vehicle intended to carry her to her precious future. There was no precious future. She hadn't created one. So what else could she focus on?

"GOALS": THE A TO B MENTALITY

Yet another answer to what you're fueling that doesn't work too well is what I call the A to B phenomenon. Mostly, when you hear people talking about doing something for their fitness, it's limited to the confines of this context.

You start at point A, and there's a point B you want to get to. Rather than the whole rest of your life, point B is some event or arbitrary point weeks or months into the future. Sometimes it's a wedding—yours or someone else's. Sometimes it's a cruise, a class reunion, summer, a new love, a visit, a party, an athletic event.

This is how our culture has trained us to think. There hasn't been much encouragement to look farther than the tree in front of your nose (or in your mirror). You weren't taught to think of the forest. But there is a forest—a long, full life after point B that never gets addressed in this equation.

Approaching fitness as a short-term goal or a one-time fix has several flaws. Chief among them is that whatever changes are made in order to get to point B are dropped once point B is reached. Goals end—and your goal-related actions end with them. You make it, and you have no reason to keep going.

Americans are dieting en masse to lose "weight" so they can fit into their swimsuit or wear that dress to Aunt Mabel's wedding. Then summer's over, the wedding's over, the reunion is past. Whatever you did up till that day, that week, or that season you no longer have any reason to do.

This is related to another flawed assumption—the notion that fitness and health are somehow achievable by doing a certain thing for a short time and then having "gotten there." It holds out hope that there is someplace one gets to, some mecca, where one never has to think about one's actions again.

This is what diets have meant to people for as long as I can remember. When I was growing up, the idea—among kids, teens, and adults—was to go on a diet, lose the "weight," and that was that. We believed you could diet, then fall back into whatever groove you started from with no repercussions. If the diet didn't somehow leave you impervious to the effects of fried food indefinitely, something was wrong with it—or you.

The tendency to see fitness this way persists. I still encounter indignation at the idea that one cannot simply follow a plan, a set of rules—temporarily do things differently—and have the results last forever with no further attention. It would be as if one day we could put a certain type of gasoline in the tank that would leave the car never needing any gas again.

But that doesn't happen. So what does? The much-reported (but never adequately resolved) disaster is that you wind up back at point A. Almost everyone I've worked with has experienced this at some point in their lives. You get to point B—triumph!—and then six weeks or six months later, you're exactly where you started. Or worse.

(It's important to note that this is not entirely due to flaws in our culture's fitness *thinking*. What we're *doing* in the name of fitness doesn't work either. The methods most often used to get from point A to point B are flawed, creating *biological* reasons for the miserable recidivism rate associated with diets. Biologically, those methods make sustained fitness virtually impossible no matter what the state of mind. But that's a whole other story, begun in the next chapter.)

Focus on coming up with a context for your life rather than a "better" or longer-term goal. They are different. Sometimes people become annoyed with me when they say, "I know—I want to run a marathon in three years!" and I say, "Okay, but what about after *that*?" Athletes have a reason to fuel beyond how they look, and while they're competing they *appear* to represent the powerful pull of fueling something bigger than "thin thighs"—such as performance or victory. But even athletes, without a context beyond their sport, can easily turn their eating into a "should." As a result, they not only may struggle with eating disorders during their competitive years, but also often quickly become poor examples as soon as their athletic career has ended (about how many former athletes have you said, "Wow, look how out of shape he/she's gotten!"). They had nothing beyond their last event to keep them caring—that marathon victory wasn't a lifelong context; it was just a slightly longer short-term goal.

Plan for your life, instead of for tomorrow when you put on your jeans. Eating and exercising, when driven by a larger purpose, are a different experience than they are when you use them as a tool to "change right now."

GOALS WITHIN REASON

Short-term goals can be useful and fun. They become limiting only when they're *all* you've got. Without some impetus bigger than all of them—something that includes them but goes way beyond them—you're back to a dry, unappealing "have-to."

I love killer biceps, but if it were the daily focus of why I fuel—the sole reason—it would quickly become tiresome. What I plan for the next 100 years makes it very desirable to act for the preservation of my body. I want to. Every bite is an investment in a long future filled with books, screenplays, children, travel . . . Mmmmm!

If I eat to serve a lifelong commitment to educating other people, requiring a strong, resilient, energetic body—and yet I am working toward better biceps in the next six months—that's no big deal. I am not being ruled by the smaller goal. I have a way of eating that works, in which I am placidly and pleasantly engaged for life. Now I have this game to play for the next six months.

Investing in your life won't take you off the track of more immediate goals; it will naturally get you to the smaller goals along the way. (The leanness that makes you healthy, strong, and long-lasting also happens to look good, by our cultural standards.)

Goals and long-term vision work nicely together, actually. A goal gives you something in which to anchor the long-term vision day to day. Within a larger context, goals have a tremendously positive power—you own them, rather than their owning you.

WHAT IT'S FOR VERSUS WHAT IT'S NOT: FORGET WHAT YOU DON'T WANT!

A powerful purpose for fueling will be positive as well as open-ended. At first you may gravitate automatically to the negative–a *"not* something" rather than *"for* something." I've found people have an exceedingly difficult time getting past the "nots"—what they don't want, what they shouldn't eat, what their bodies are not.

If a baby is playing with something that's not too healthy for him to be playing with, it generally works better to introduce something new for him to focus on. It's far less effective if you simply try to drag him away from the current object of interest. This works for us, too. Instead of "Don't touch that. Don't be interested in that. Don't think about that," get interested in something else. Seek to turn up the volume of your passion for living—not squash your passion for particular foods. Instead of trying to stop something, start something.

Yet, when I ask workshop participants what their body is for that would make them want to fuel it, the first answers invariably come out like this: "I don't want to look like my mother." "I don't want to die young." "I don't want to look like this anymore." "I don't want to be fat." "I don't want to have such a hard time climbing stairs." "I don't like what I see in the mirror." "I don't want to hurt anymore."

That's eating *against* something. What DO you want? What DO you see? What could you eat for?

Culturally, we're trained to look for what's wrong: what's not possible; reasons we can't rather than reasons we really want to. People initially believe that what they don't want will jump-start them (even though it hasn't worked before). Are you really inspired after you've thoroughly whipped yourself? But you do it all the time; I see it in client after client. Self-deprecation, even self-hatred are the tools you reach for first—the only tools you may know.

Focusing on what your body is not takes you in an utterly different direction than what your body is for. "What you're not" takes you to failure—in fact, it is a response to failure. "What you're for" invites you to explore future possibilities. "For" is going forward; "not" is going backward or staying stuck in place, trying to avenge the past or fix the present. What you're not (or what you don't want) becomes a project of "fixing" what is (or isn't) instead of living toward and fulfilling something desirable.

WORKING ON YOUR EATING VERSUS WORKING ON YOUR LIFE

You may think you should be focusing on changing the way you eat, and if others are concerned about your "weight" (fat), they try to "get you to" change the way you eat as well. That's a mistake, and you've probably noticed yourself that it has limited (if any) success.

Inspiration comes from undertaking to create the life you want, not from working on your eating as if it were separate. Instead of an extreme close-up in which you zero in on your eating, pull back to a wide-angle view and get clear about how important your life is, and why. Toiling over your body, your weight or even your health is dull, dry, and limiting drudgery.

A man in his mid-forties saw lights go on in the middle of a recent workshop. "My God," he said, "I've been eating all my life to *fix* myself, instead of eating to have the energy to live my life!" Subtle? Maybe—but it changed his whole experience of eating. He called us three times in the three days afterward to excitedly talk about the physical energy he gained by feeding himself in a way that was scientific—and the mental energy he saved by abandoning the grind of trying to *fix* himself and *do it right*.

LIKE IT OR NOT, YOU ARE YOUR BODY

Americans seem to think about and treat the body as a *thing*, as if it's separate from us and somehow should run by itself. We take it for granted. We don't appreciate it. No mystery, then, that you don't even know how it works or what it needs, or make it your business to find out.

But to try to make your body beautiful, you're willing to do unthinkable things to it. You'll gladly run it out of gas all the time. After all, it's not really yours! From the neck down, it's something else. To mistreat the body the way some do, you'd have to be divorced from the body; you'd have to work up a disregard or disrespect for it. Otherwise, it would be too painful to live with yourself and the damage and abuse you inflict.

If you deny ownership of the body, you can also deny the facts about how it works—no matter how well you know them. I'll never forget the university biology department adviser with a master's degree in biochemistry to whom

I described my work as not new information but inspiring new education. She ruefully pulled a bag of corn chips from her desk drawer and admitted, "This is all I eat all day." Talk about knowledge not making the difference!

People who aren't happy with their bodies sometimes actively take the position that the body is only distantly related to their lives. "I'm not my body," they insist loftily. The mind and the spirit, they say, are far more important. I contend they take this position only because they're sure what they'll "have to" do to handle the body will be miserable, and/or because they've failed at handling it so often they've given up. That's understandable, since there's no way to succeed at that game.

But it's just not true that you're not your body. You can *say* it all you want, but when you're lying in the hospital after a heart attack, how can you continue the work or sport or whatever else you love, while your body stays behind and recuperates? There's no separating the two—in this life, at least. On this earth, your soul, mind, spirit (and anything else your beliefs say are part of you) all come in this package we call a body. That body is the machine that will support every activity you have planned for the rest of your life.

You decide how important those activities are to you. If you are to accomplish what you want to, your body is coming with you—in fact, it's propelling you there. Decide what kind of condition you want it to be in, given where you're going. Then learning exactly what affects its condition will have a solid purpose.

"IT'S ONLY ME"

Sometimes, the greatest roadblock to discovering an inspiring reason for eating well is the conviction that you aren't important enough to warrant excellent care.

In the April 1992 issue of *Bazaar*, there was a news clip that noted that Olympian women need to eat a loaf of bread a day (among other things), an amount that the magazine suggested "most American women couldn't imagine." But I may eat nearly that much bread in a day. It's not hard for me to imagine at all—and I'm no Olympic athlete. But I do think of myself as being as important as one—to myself, to my work, and to the people directly around me—and that's key. (I also know exactly what my body needs and what it does with bread, and that helps immensely, too.)

World-class athletes obviously need to take great care of themselves and "fuel" appropriately. In fact, athletes are the one group of people who do talk about food as fuel for their activities. Why not you? Most people think they are ordinary souls who don't need to bother as much with good fueling as athletes do. True, the costs of not doing so are less immediately obvious— you're not going to lose a gold medal or fall on your face during a sprint. But what about your world-class *life*? Life is an athletic endeavor. We are athletes in our lives and would do well to honor ourselves as such.

Think about your average day. You probably have a job or business, possibly a very demanding one. Maybe you have a lover or spouse, maybe kids, too. Social activities. Sports and exercise. Travel. Errands. Volunteer work. You think you don't need energy for those things? You think that those aren't Olympic trials? That getting through one of your action-packed days isn't an Olympic feat?

You are important enough! How many times do I hear "I don't have time to eat. I'm too busy taking care of . . ." Fill in the blank. My work. My office. My husband. My kids. My groups. My home. My car. My friends. My mother. More backward thinking (or nonthinking). How do you expect to take care of all those people and things if *you're* not taken care of? How well can you really accomplish what you're out to accomplish, when the machine you live in needs fuel and you're not providing it? When you maybe don't even know what that fuel is?

Every body needs fuel. Everyone who owns a body must fuel it the way it was meant to be fueled—if one's life demands high performance from it.

And whose doesn't?

INVESTING: PRECIOUS GEMS

Many people concern themselves with retirement planning and act to ensure financial security in later years. Yet in our culture it is not yet habitual to plan carefully for a "savings account" of health and fitness—to *eat* as if "investing" in one's future body.

People who are consistently, permanently inspired to care for themselves have the conviction that the body is precious and worth their investment. You don't treat precious things badly, only things you don't think are valuable. If you are deeply in touch with how precious you are, you won't want to mistreat the package you come in either. If you value yourself and the body you come in, fueling is then an obvious priority, an instinctive course of action.

As with financial investing, little can be done to suddenly turn a meager investment into instant fortune. Health and fitness—like savings accounts— are built consistently, not suddenly. And it's efficient eating, not money, that represents investment in your body. Money can't necessarily recover a deteriorated body. You can't buy health as easily as you can throw a greenback on your doctor's desk.

Even if you could, why spend money that way? Why abuse yourself in the hope that money will buy you out of the consequences later—when you can painlessly prevent costly ramifications and spend your money on something great instead?

JUDY: THE DIFFERENCE "WHAT YOU'RE FUELING" CAN MAKE

Judy, a morbidly obese 35-year-old woman who has been dieting since she was six, called us a week after our workshop to tell us this story. Her husband had bought a box of jumbo, greasy muffins, which she normally would have eaten four of immediately. She said that she looked at the muffins for a long time, then said to herself, "You know—there's no fuel in that for me." So she had a bagel instead—happily.

Judy was standing up for her body as she never has before—because she is now conscious of her body's value and necessity in a way she has never been. No longer is it this separate "thing" she must drag around. It's *her*. And it's the only one she's ever going to get. For the first time in 29 years, she's not trying to "fix what's wrong"—just fuel all the great things she sees as being possible from now on.

WHAT NOW?

I've introduced this inquiry. It's your job to keep it going. If you think you just want to skip to the how-tos without considering further . . . well, as I've emphasized, every choice is yours to make.

But I've been studying people and how they go about this for years. I've taken a close look at what's missing—why so few feel satisfied in the endless, universal quest for fitness and a way of life that supports it. I've learned from my own experience and that of thousands of others: *great directions are utterly useless without a journey planned.* In the case of eating, that journey must be a lifelong one, visualized in detail, for your experience to shift. If you don't develop and keep developing a perspective that goes far beyond next month or even next year, you'll probably never escape diet thinking.

The reward is a way of seeing your body, yourself, and your life—all connected—that lets you enjoy the possibilities, and relish how everything you do for yourself is contributing to those possibilities. Pair this with full knowledge of how your body ticks and how that applies to eating and exercise, and you've got power, choice, and freedom like never before.

I encourage you to use the worksheet on page 26 to continue the exploration.

FUELING YOUR FUTURE

Picture yourself during the following time periods.
Jot down 1 to 5 things you'd really like to be doing, or imagine yourself doing at that time. (e.g.: work, recreation, travel, hobbies, family, community.)

6 months from now I would like to _____

_____

2 years from now I would like to _____

_____

10 years from now I would like to _____

_____

30 years from now I would like to _____

_____

What role will your body and its condition play in the above activities?

_____

_____

I can envision myself active and healthy all the way to at *least* age _____

THREE things I would do if I had more energy are

1) _____
2) _____
3) _____

Other people in my life who rely on me to be healthy, alive, and strong are

_____

_____

I want to care for myself so that in turn I can take care of

_____

_____

Ultimately, the future I want to "fuel" is essentially about

_____

_____

2

WHAT'S WEIGHT
GOT TO DO WITH IT?

If I told people I've gained 15 pounds over the past two years, a likely response might be, "Oh, that's too bad," or "I'm so sorry." Sorry about what? That I now have 15 additional, active pounds of food-burning, fat-burning, metabolism-increasing muscle? That I can eat more food—*need* to eat more food—just to "feed" that muscle? That I look sculpted and toned? Please, hold your sympathy.

But that reaction is typical—and telling. *What is the reflex that makes people assume my added "weight" is "bad"?*

The use of weight to define, determine, and measure health and fitness is the pinnacle of diet thinking. "Dieting" has begun to lose favor as a means for weight loss, but "weight" has managed to remain at center stage. "Diets don't work" has become a familiar knee-jerk refrain, but it's not just that diets don't work—it's anything aimed at "weight" loss. *Weight doesn't work* as a unit of measurement.

Focusing on "weight" is the most basic and widespread mistake in attempts to become lean or healthy. To manipulate that number, you'll do things that change the "weight" but don't improve anything. You'll do things that are not only unhealthy but also counterproductive to what you really mean to accomplish. "Losing weight," as you probably currently pursue it, is not only *biologically predetermined to fail*, but also *compounds the original problems* and diverts attention from real solutions.

If what you weigh has nothing to do with how healthy, fit, or fat you are, why will I spend time on it? Because even though there is no sensible premise to support loss of "weight," more than half of all Americans are trying to do it. Because you *think* weight matters. And because understanding why it doesn't helps you to understand your body, and to fully distinguish diet thinking.

WHAT IS "WEIGHT"?

Let's start out by examining the word "weight" itself. It's such a common word, so massively overused, that it's probably something you never even think about, let alone question. "Lose weight"—everyone knows what that means!

But what are you really trying to say? What is "weight"? Think about that for a minute. "Weight" is a generic term, a measurement that could refer to anything. Virtually any object you can touch has a weight. Everything on your body has a weight. So does your car. Do you say, "Honey, I'll need the weight tomorrow?"

What do we mean?

In one workshop, I asked a client, Nancy, to show me where the weight was that she wanted to lose. "All over," she replied immediately. "Oh, okay," I said. "Your hair, too?" Everyone laughed. "No, no, not my hair."

"Oh, you said all over," I reminded her. "What about your teeth?" More laughter.

"No."

"Your bones?"

"Nope."

"Skin. Arms? Legs?"

"No!" she protested, laughing. "I want to lose *fat*."

Ah, fat.

But that's not what you say. Virtually everyone starts out talking *weight*. Of course, they don't mean "just anything." Almost everyone I have ever talked to about this wants to lose fat and fat alone; almost no one wants to lose anything else.

Still, it doesn't matter what you meant. Sometimes in life you get exactly what you ask for. And that is exactly the case with weight loss. Unfortunately, not saying what you really mean can get you into real trouble—and it does here. Really, how can you expect to lose something efficiently when you can't (or won't) even say what it is?

So you want to lose fat, but you say weight. Now let's examine something else: The Formula.

What do you do to lose that "weight" (though you mean fat)? What is the timeworn, generic, everybody-knows formula that losing "weight" always comes down to?

Eat _____, Exercise _____. Fill in the blanks.

In every group I've ever led, this phrase is sadly easy to complete. I just say, "What does everyone know is the formula to 'lose weight'? Eat . . ." (And I pause.)

"Eat less and exercise more."

No matter who they are—homemakers or executives, teenagers or senior citizens, white-collar professionals or welfare mothers, athletes or accountants, physicians or plumbers—people obligingly regurgitate this formula like robots. It rolls off their tongues.

DRIVE MORE, USE LESS GAS?

Remarkably, this formula has gone unquestioned—until now. Let's look at "eating less and exercising more" in the context of food as fuel. If food fuels the body, can you see how "eating less and exercising more" presents a problem? Decreasing the fuel supply while increasing the demand creates a deficit. You put in less fuel, and drive the machine harder than ever. That's like running your car twice as fast, twice as hard—and expecting to put in less gasoline. It doesn't make much sense, does it?

Except that the formula purposely creates the shortage. What Americans have always assumed is that fat will conveniently and completely fill in that gap. You deprive your body of fuel with the thought that if you create a void, the body will automatically choose fat to fill it. Then, according to this reasoning, you'll lose "pounds" (of fat, though you don't specify).

There's just one problem with that: *It's not what happens.* Fat can't pay back the deficit you create by "eating less and exercising more," because *the body doesn't run on fat alone. Carbohydrate is the human body's primary source of fuel—the immediate source of energy we use constantly to fuel our activity and most of the work of our cells.* The body must always have glucose—the carbohydrate found in your bloodstream at all times—and *virtually no fat can be made into glucose.*

Ideally, your body makes glucose out of food—carbohydrate food. But it's common to cut out food, thinking that's the key to "thin." Perhaps you're on a weight-loss diet that specifically restricts carbohydrate (as most do). Or else you're too busy. You don't have time for food; you forget.

So where does your body get glucose if you're not providing it? If you don't eat enough carbohydrate—whether purposely or thoughtlessly—your body manufactures carbohydrate fuel using existing materials. *But not the materials you may have always assumed.* While your body cannot turn any significant amount of fat into glucose if you come up short, the system can make glucose by grabbing protein from your lean muscle tissue and converting it to carbohydrate. *Your own muscle tissue is destroyed in order to replenish the too-low glucose supply.*

This is a survival mechanism; as you'll continue to see, your body is efficiently geared with numerous safety features to ensure that you stay alive. And since we're designed to use glucose at all times, this is your body's way of making glucose when you don't keep it well supplied with the food to do it.

So the assumption that your body will manage somehow on its own if you expend more energy while consuming less is half right—it just doesn't do it the way you may have hoped. Fat is not the crutch your body leans on in a glucose deficit. Fat has other functions, which you'll learn later.

But at least if your muscle can be used to make fuel, your body's needs are handled, right? Well, in a way. Your survival is ensured, and you even lose "weight"—because the lost muscle weighs something. The problem is that losing pounds of muscle is nothing to celebrate. In fact, it's dangerous and counterproductive. This kind of "weight loss" worsens the immediate bodyfat situation *and* the long-term outlook for leanness. Here's how.

DANGEROUS

Destroying your own muscle for the purpose of creating glucose during a shortage is dangerous for several reasons. One, your muscle obviously has a purpose. Your muscle mass is your strength; it supports your skeletal structure and protects your bones. As physiologists William Evans, Ph.D., and

Irwin H. Rosenberg, M.D., of the U.S. Department of Agriculture Human Nutrition Research Center on Aging at Tufts University, declare in their book *Biomarkers*, "Muscle, to a far greater extent than most people realize, is responsible for the vitality of your whole physiological apparatus."

Two, burning muscle for fuel is inefficient and wasteful. It's "environmentally unsound" to your insides. It uses a process that leaves toxic biochemical by-products in its wake. Because protein is nitrogen-based, nitrogen is given off when muscle protein "burns," leaving your body an unpleasant mess to deal with. Organs such as the kidneys and liver are unduly stressed as they are saddled with the task of safely processing and excreting these by-products.

Three, the heart is a muscle. You might hope your body has the good sense to save that muscle for last—and in fact it does, attacking the muscle tissue of the larger extremities first. But how far do you want to push it? People can and do damage heart-muscle tissue through constant dieting.

Four, along with loss of muscle protein comes the loss of other important body proteins. The antibodies that defend you against illness are proteins. Muscle contains enzymes designed to metabolize fats, which are lost when muscle is lost. And when your body is struggling to process muscle protein into carbohydrate fuel, the liver produces more low-density cholesterol, and fat-storage-assisting enzymes build up.

Five, it is impossible to completely break down fat without carbohydrate—which diets usually restrict. Fat that breaks down without carbohydrate's help does so incompletely, leaving more harmful by-products behind to join the poisonous "leftovers" of muscle/protein breakdown. More processing nightmares for your organs.

And six, if more than about one-fourth of weight lost is muscle, and/or if the loss is very rapid, serious protein deficiency and electrolyte imbalances can cause heart irregularities that could result in death.

Enough? And to think you could have just eaten a roll and avoided all that!

(You'll gain further insight into this entire process in Chapter 3, "Fueling the Human Body: Your Owner's Manual.")

TOTALLY COUNTERPRODUCTIVE: THE BIG IRONY

The counterproductive aspect of "weight" loss by fuel deprivation is almost more compelling than the idea that it's dangerous—and it's certainly more ironic.

Converting muscle for use as fuel leaves you less lean in the short term, since you're losing lean tissue and thus your overall percentage of lean mass goes down. Even more significant, though, using your own muscle for fuel in an effort to lose fat is counterproductive because *it sets you up to gain more fat, and have a harder time losing it later.*

That's because muscle is what scientists call metabolically active tissue. It's the part of your body that demands fuel be burned—including fat. Muscle demands 98 percent of the fuel you consume. Only about 2 percent of the energy in the food you eat is required by the fat on your body. When your body converts muscle to fuel, it is destroying a gas-guzzling engine because you let the tank go dry.

And since a smaller engine burns less fuel, your rate of fuel consumption decreases. Losing muscle "weight" is like going from an 8-cylinder to a 6-cylinder engine—or less. A big engine (even in a compact car) will demand and use more fuel more quickly. A small engine "conserves."

When you lose muscle, you lose the very thing that burns what you *really* wanted to lose. Isn't that crazy?

The more muscle you've got, the more fuel you burn, and the more food you can eat—in fact, the more you need to eat to support that muscle. The less muscle you've got, the slower and less efficiently you burn fuel. Muscle is the most influential factor in your metabolic rate. Clearly, it's something you want to have as much of as possible. The loss of even one pound of muscle is devastating.

The loss "dieters" experience when they lose pounds rapidly is excruciating. If muscle is a huge factor in your overall metabolism, imagine what losing 40 pounds of it does to your ability to burn the food you eat. Yet that's often what people who lose 75 or 100 pounds or more do lose. We all know that liquid diets on which people lose hundreds of pounds are doomed—but very few know this is a key reason why.

YOU'VE LOST WEIGHT—BUT WHAT HAVE YOU GAINED?

When you lose "weight" by eating less and exercising more, you get exactly what you asked for. You lose "weight." But it turns out to be a booby prize. You can lose "pounds" this way. The question is, pounds of what?

"Weight" could be anything—your hair, your hat, or your shoes. *You haven't necessarily lost fat.* Muscle weighs! If you tell me you "lost weight," I don't know what that means. You might have lost fat, but you might have lost muscle, too. You might have lost an arm or a leg.

"Weight" isn't innately bad, and before we judge pounds—lost or gained—we ought to distinguish what they are. "Weight" isn't necessarily fat. *It's not inherently healthier to weigh less—it's healthier to have less fat.* The weight-loss movement of the last 40 years has never clearly distinguished this—and still doesn't.

Historically, the dieting world has been happy to part with "pounds" without a care for what they're composed of. People who proudly chirp about having lost massive pounds are bragging that they have just destroyed tissue that would have burned fat for the rest of their lives. I think of this when I overhear someone excitedly boasting to a friend or store clerk: "This cappuccino is the first thing I've eaten all day, but it's worth it—I've lost 13 pounds already." I have to fight the urge to walk up to them and say, "Why didn't you just amputate your legs? It would have been faster, more permanent, probably less painful in the long run, and not a whole lot worse for your body."

What do you think is going to happen when they start eating something besides cappuccino again? Far from having successfully handled their fat problem, as diet thinking believes, they've *destroyed fat-burning machinery and switched on fat-making machinery.* (Not to mention what's been lost as the body tries to function without the variety of nutrients it needs.) They will be having this conversation again with a different person, maybe in two months, maybe in six months, maybe in a year.

WEIGHT CAN BE GREAT

My own experience is a positive example of how meaningless "weight" is as a measurement. After two years of consistent, purposeful "fueling," I had my body composition tested. In those two years, my bodyfat went from 27 percent to 17 percent. It showed: My dress size had gone from 6 or 8 down to 2 or 4.

Even more noteworthy, given the way the world measures body progress, is that I weighed exactly what I had two years prior. I lost no "weight." And I still haven't.

No weight loss? Didn't "fueling" work? Yes—beautifully. When I started, 27 percent of my 130 pounds were fat pounds. That's about 35 pounds of fat I was carrying on my 5'6" frame. Two years later, only 17 percent of my 130 pounds were fat pounds. That's 20 pounds of fat. From 35 to 20 pounds fat; net loss—15 pounds of fat.

So why wasn't I 15 pounds lighter? Because even better than the 15 pounds of fat I lost were the 15 pounds of muscle I gained. With moderate exercise plus good fueling, I added 15 pounds of lean, metabolically active, fat-burning tissue.

In traditional "weight loss" terms, those two years would be considered a failure because I lost no "weight." But I replaced 15 pounds of unneeded feathers with 15 pounds of valuable gold. The net weight is the same, but 15 pounds of gold takes up a lot less space than the same weight in feathers, so I'm smaller. I'm also stronger, healthier, less at risk of disease, and, yes, most people would agree I look better. Muscle is *good* weight.

IT'S NOT "HEALTHY EATING"!

"Eat less/exercise more" not only isn't about fat loss, it does nothing to address health, nutrition, and energy—which are also concerns for most people. In fact, "eat less/exercise more" runs entirely counter to "healthy eating." It bears no connection and no resemblance to what's healthy and makes you feel good, because the effort on which it focuses—weight loss—has nothing to do with either fitness or health. Fat loss may, but fat loss is something else entirely.

In late 1992 and 1993, many commercial diet companies began desperately trying to repackage their products to associate "weight loss" and "diet" with "healthy." Ultra Slim-Fast briefly switched from "Give us a week—we'll take off the weight" to "The healthy way to lose weight." NutriSystem and Jenny Craig suddenly began talking about "learning to eat right."

The problem is that just mouthing the words doesn't change the content or intent. Simply saying so doesn't make drinking glorified milk shakes "healthy living." Besides, eating "right" (as opposed to "wrong") is just more diet thinking. Most of all, the programs were still the same higher protein, too-low-carbohydrate, "diet-like" . . . well, diets—and they still focused on weight loss. The companies just painted over the outside to appeal to a growing public concern.

Despite the "education" claims, a size-6, already-lean young woman I know was eagerly accepted into one of these commercial programs, lost 15 pounds (mostly muscle, since the leaner you are when you lose "weight" via carbohydrate deprivation, the more muscle you lose), and rapidly gained 15 pounds back (all fat) when it was over. Now she struggles with food and fat even more than she did before, having shrunk her engine and thus reduced her total requirement for energy from food. And, after all that, she didn't understand what had happened and *still* didn't know how to eat for leanness.

Weight loss is designed only to make your weight smaller. It's ironic enough that it doesn't necessarily make your body smaller. It's even more ironic that people try to lose "weight" for their health—when the typical "weight"-loss method is 100 percent removed from being healthy. It is, in fact, *damaging* to energy and health.

IT DOESN'T TAKE MUCH

Losing fat affects the scale differently than losing "weight" which includes muscle. Of course, you'll lose some pounds if you lose fat. The important part is it won't take as many pounds of fat as you might assume to look and feel the way you want.

People often say, "I know why! Muscle weighs more than fat!" That's more unexamined nonthinking. Does turkey weigh more than ham? A pound of fat weighs the same as a pound of muscle—they both weigh a pound.

More accurately, a pound of fat takes up more space than a pound of muscle (fat is lighter by volume), so when you lose a pound of fat it really shows. You can lose a great deal of muscle, however, and not improve the size, shape, or tone of your body (in fact, it will ruin the tone). That pound of muscle wasn't taking up much space. It was sitting there looking good and demanding fuel.

This means you can forget whatever your preconceived notions are about how much "weight" you "need" to lose to achieve the leanness you want. You really have no idea. The number of fat pounds it will take is far less than the number of generic "pounds." Remember, those undistinguished "pounds" include the muscle donated for fuel when you diet yourself short of glucose.

Women have informed me that 10 to 15 "pounds" is "what you have to lose" to drop a dress size. I dropped a dress size after losing 3 pounds—of fat. How's that? Women who lose 10 to 15 pounds the usual way lose the same thing—2 to 4 pounds of fat. You can guess what the rest is. That's the "rest" I *didn't* lose.

By the same token, a fat gain that scarcely shows upon the scale shows quickly on your body. You may not notice a half-pound on the scale, but because even a half-pound of fat (think feathers again) takes up significant space, your belt notch may change. On the other hand, my 15-pound muscle gain only improved the lean look (though my broad shoulders require my tops to be a size larger than my bottoms!)

NO FAST FAT LOSS

There is no such things as fast fat loss—it's physically impossible to lose significant amounts of fat "overnight." You didn't gain it all overnight, either, no matter what you think. There is only fast "weight" loss—and fast weight loss means muscle loss.

Ask marketing representatives of a certain commercial diet claiming 30,000 users if you lose only fat on their program, and they say, "Yes, only fat." It's a lie. They also promise weight loss as fast as 10 pounds a week. It is virtually impossible, physiologically and biologically, to lose 10 pounds of fat a week. Ten pounds, yes—muscle, water, fat, glycogen, other waste products—but pure fat, no. Ask them to prove it's only fat, and they avoid the question, talking instead in generalities about how much research backs them. Ask them to provide the research and they get very nervous.

Weight loss is about speed. It's not about transforming the way of thinking, eating, and living that spawned the fat, or learning how it happened. It's about getting pounds off, fast. You worry about the ramifications later.

THE MAGIC NUMBER—WHO CARES? YOU DO.

You can see now that weight is not relevant to how you look or feel or how long you live. There is no such thing as a "weight problem," "overweight," or "ideal weight." That number upon which America is fixated—and spends tens of billions annually to manipulate—is utterly inconsequential to fitness or health.

You could argue that if I was 5'1" and weighed 750 pounds, that would be a problem. And it certainly would. But it would still be a fat problem, not a weight problem. And we'd probably notice it even if I never weighed myself.

Who cares what you weigh, if you look and feel great? More people are saying, "I don't care—I just want to be fit and healthy," but there's still a frighteningly large group who believe that the number tells all. They don't care what the mirror says; the number rules. In my classes I have spent hours outlining the concepts in this book, providing graphic demonstrations, distributing textbook page copies—and had people ask at the end, "So how fast will I lose weight?" It's both fascinating and horrifying.

Despite the facts, most everyone I have worked with has had some number in mind. There's a weight they want to weigh, used to weigh, have never weighed, or have been told by their doctor they should weigh. (One client's doctor told her to lose 20 pounds and come back in a month.) Many people have an entire chronicle of their lives based on what they've weighed at various times. They'll tell a story something akin to "weights I have known." Clients have recited narratives that go something like: ". . . and then, in 1984, I got down to 127, but that only lasted for two months. After that I went up to 143 and stayed there until the spring of '87, when I went on the XYZ diet. I was a size 10, but lost 6 pounds by . . ."

A woman in a recent workshop admitted that even if she were a perfect size 6 and had enough energy to make people envious, she wasn't sure it would be okay with her to weigh in at her current number of pounds. Another client, Dawn, tells the story of her boss down-dialing the scale in the ladies room because he got tired of hearing them chatter about losing weight. She walked into the ladies room one day, weighed herself, and was

10 pounds lighter. She thought to herself, "Well, I guess I don't need to lose 'weight' after all,"—even though she felt terrible and didn't like how she looked.

At a health club, I overheard two women in the locker room wondering whether the club scale or the Weight Watchers' scale was right. They were talking about a difference of 2 pounds. "Well, it was 138 at home, but 140 there, but of course I had clothes on then, but . . ." If I had had more guts, I would have shouted, "Who cares whether you weigh 138 or 140! There's a mirror right in front of you! Do you like how you look or not? Did you lose fat or not?"

"Greg," a Fortune 10 vice president, reported three months after we worked with him: "I've missed only one snack since the workshop, and I rarely eat junk anymore. I grab apples, bananas, bagels—it's just something I do now. It feels right. This was the first Thanksgiving I didn't feel bloated and lethargic after dinner. I don't *like* fat or grease anymore. I love eating this way. I feel very different, look very different. I don't feel tired in the morning anymore, and I don't feel fatigued at the end of the day. And I've been steadier than ever with my exercise program." His waist had shrunk several inches as well.

But. "I'm still concerned," he said. "I haven't lost any *weight.*" Aargghh! One of the sharpest, most on-the-ball managers I have ever encountered, Greg leads one of the most progressive international companies in the world. He looks and feels better than he ever has, by eating in a way he never dreamed he could—yet he was still concerned because the scale didn't say what he thinks it should. That's how totally crippled this culture is when it comes to weight. It defies all logic.

How many times have I seen this question (or some variation) in womens' magazines over the last 10 or 15 years—right up until today—"A friend told me I shouldn't do weight training because I'll gain weight." Yes, you will! That's great. Gain, gain, gain! Just be sure of *what* you're gaining!

Or how about this one: "If I wear navy, will I lose more 'weight' during my workout?" Thinking more *sweat* loss, being "weight" loss, counts for something.

I gain 3 pounds after I eat my breakfast in the morning: two slices of toast, 2 ounces of turkey or chicken, a giant bowl of oatmeal with raisins, a cup of coffee, and four or five glasses of water. So *what?* Pounds of *what?* I gain 5 pounds when I put my winter coat on. As an experiment, I weighed myself before a run (132) and then after (128). Then I drank four or five glasses of water (131).

While the number may be impotent and its fluctuations meaningless, such fluctuations have the potential to dominate your life—*if you validate them*. I've seen many people truly overwrought based purely on what the scale says—and taking dangerous, *needless* action as a result.

One of our first clients, Sue was an intelligent and wealthy businesswoman who also happened to be a golf champion. She had everything going for her—and was ravaged by concern about her "weight." She had stopped eating dinner by the time we worked with her because, she said, she was several pounds "fatter" every time she got on the scale after dinner.

Bright and successful as she is, she somehow didn't connect that swallowing a bunch of food might affect her total body weight, in the same way that putting a bunch of rocks in her pocket might. She really believed that the food she ate could instantly become several excess pounds of fat.

By the time we got to her, she *was* beginning to put on actual fat—because she was starving herself. Skipping dinner—and sometimes lunch, too—while following a rigorous athletic training schedule, she was "eating" precious muscle tissue and slowing her metabolism down. She was terrified to begin eating the quite moderate amounts of food we recommended—they seemed massive to her. Three meals plus snacks? Believing her meager food "allowances" had actually been staving off further disaster (not realizing that these scale-inspired cutbacks were causing, not treating, the problem), it seemed that such steady eating would really do her in.

But just the opposite occurred. While it can take more time to retrain bodies that have grown accustomed to years of starvation, Sue had been athletic all her life and hadn't been "living off her lean" for very long. She found her too-tight clothes to be comfortable again within a month of fueling.

The exciting part was that the results came from eliminating the suffering of starving. She got to eat. As she said: "It's wonderful to eat without a constant emotional battle. The charge is off; it's relieved a huge frustration. I think, 'I can do this [fuel] or not' and usually I choose to. I have desserts, but now that I know I can have them, I don't *want* to eat them all the time."

WHAT TELLS THE STORY THAT WEIGHT DOESN'T?

Diet thinking keeps people looking at the scale, even though it tells you no more than your wall clock. When you jump on a scale immediately after eating something, added pounds don't reflect fat that instantly got stored from the food you just swallowed. When you jump onto the scale after a workout, lost "weight" isn't pounds of fat that have just been "burned off" your body. When you learn the actual "specs" of the body's design and operation, you'll realize it just doesn't work that way.

The scale doesn't define which pounds are fat and which are muscle—any more than the meat scale in the deli department tells you how much of a pound of meat is ham and how much is turkey. You have to look at what's on the scale!

There are a number of different ways to get your body composition tested. These tests will tell you approximately how many pounds of muscle and how many pounds of fat comprise your total body weight. If you're seriously interested in testing your body fat, I suggest you consult a health clinic or exercise physiologist in your area. The tests range in cost from about $25 into the hundreds of dollars, depending on where you live.

▶ *Dual-photon absorptiometry* (now considered the most accurate test). NASA uses this. You probably won't.
▶ *Skin-fold calipers* (the "pinch"—considered the least accurate test). The Accu-Measure is an at-home test of this kind. Athletic clubs frequently use this method.
▶ *Bioelectrical impedance analysis* (measures the degree to which fat impedes the travel of a mild electrical current)
▶ *Total-body electrical conductivity*
▶ *Hydrostatic* (underwater weighing—long considered the most precise). You sit in a scale above a tank of water and exhale as much as you can. You're then lowered into the tank, and your rate of descent is measured and factored into a formula. You usually need to do this three or four times to obtain an accurate average. Your lung capacity may also be measured using a spirometer.
▶ *Futrex.* An electrode is attached to your ankle, some basic body dimensions and activity information are computed into the machine, and a laser beam uses refracted light to measure the density of fat in relationship to muscle.

Recommended ranges for bodyfat from the health and medical communities vary, from 16 to 25 percent for women, and 10 to 20 percent for men. Both male and female athletes can get into the single digits; this is not recommended for the nonprofessional athlete, nor is it necessary.

If you feel you must measure yourself with some kind of machine and don't want to spend money on bodyfat testing, there is one advanced way to use the scale with a moderate degree of accuracy—but it works only if you're fueling consistently. If you've truly been giving your body exactly what it needs, it will not make glucose out of your muscle protein. So if the scale consistently shows a loss of "pounds," you can count on them being fat. And if you've truly been giving your body exactly what it needs and not much fat, a consistent increase in weight is likely to be muscle. This should be measured over a period of weeks or, better yet, months—daily weighing won't work.

YOUR EYES ARE THE BEST MEASUREMENT TOOL

Still, the first way I knew exactly what I had lost and gained was by *looking* at my body, *feeling* my strength, and *seeing* the way my clothes fit. The scale said nothing; my first 6 pounds of fat loss happened to occur simultaneously with a gain of that many pounds of muscle. I was two sizes smaller, I was "harder," and I could do chin-ups for the first time in my life. What more evidence could I want?

It is almost as unnecessary to measure your bodyfat as your weight, in my opinion. Given the numbers-crazy measure-mania to which we're prone, I *don't* recommend it. I didn't test my body composition for more than two years after I began "fueling." When I did, I was able to guess the figure, right on the nose, before I found out what it was. It's not that hard to tell— once you start looking beyond weight and even "thin." I've been quite accurate guessing my clients' bodyfat as well—as close as Santiago Burastero, a physician conducting a study on bodyfat at St. Luke's-Roosevelt Hospital in New York. "In the last three years, he has observed almost 2,000 volunteers, measured them with every state-of-the-art technique he knows, and discovered that his eyeball estimates usually come to within two percent of what sophisticated body-fat tests come up with" ("Fat Gauge," *Allure*, January 1993).

Sometimes, in our eagerness to measure everything we forget to look and listen to *us*. Like Dawn, who believed the tampered-with scale even though her experience told her nothing had changed, we trust machines and numbers more than our own eyes and sensations and experience. This can be dangerous as well as discouraging. If your reddened, screaming baby felt like an oven, but the thermometer indicated a mild 99°, would you say, "Oh well, she doesn't have a temperature!" Of course not. But that's what we do with the scale.

In this culture we count everything. When it comes to fitness and exercise, we not only count calories consumed, calories burned, and pounds gained or lost; we rigidly monitor every morsel we eat; we chart how much weight we lifted today and compare to last time and next time and the national average; we count the number of times and hours we exercise and how many miles we went and compare that to others; we measure our heart rates and our bodyfat and our inches.

The "right" numbers—body composition—can become as oppressive as the wrong ones if you fully substitute them for your own instincts and sensibilities. I gave a series of workshops at one very exclusive athletic club whose manager and assistant manager (both highly educated in the physiology discussed in this book) confessed to testing each other weekly and, in the words of one, "freaking out" about their bodyfat. Both are beautiful, extremely fit athletes with substantial, sculpted muscles. I certainly didn't need data to tell that they were each 13 to 14 percent fat. Why did they?

There is a theme here: Misplaced concern. Just as we worry about the pesticide on the food we eat without worrying about the fat content—or don't put fuel in the "tank" because we're too busy grooming some small, insignificant piece of the vehicle's exterior—we become fascinated with high-tech diversions that only distract us from the more important matters at hand.

Now that you're learning to think and act, rather than simply believe and react, start learning to see and hear your body, too.

THE "OLDER EQUALS FATTER" MYTH

"All of a sudden some metabolic switch deep inside me flicked to a slower setting."
—PENNY WARD MOSER,
    "Anti-Aging Fitness Program: The New Fountain of Youth,"
    Self, September 1992

Muscle loss makes sense of the A to B goal phenomenon I presented in Chapter 1, "Fueling Your Future." Your ascent back to point A, while hastened by lack of impetus to move beyond point B, is further hastened by the metabolic damage resulting from a faulty method of "travel."

But the irony goes beyond the fact that a "weight"-loss diet damages your body's largest contributor to fat burning. That fact triggers a vicious cycle: After your weight-loss diet has caused deterioration of fuel-burning muscle, you find yourself gaining fat more easily. But since you mistakenly gauge that fat gain by your "weight," you turn in panic to another "weight"-loss diet, and that digs a deeper hole in your fuel burning, to which you still see only one alternative—and on it goes.

As a result, the average American loses a full 25 percent of the lean body mass he/she had at age 20 by the age of 70. That's one-fourth of your fat-burning, metabolically active tissue—a quarter of your engine over 50 years, or about 5 percent per decade.

You can see that even if food intake remained identical day to day—bite for bite—at some point the shrinking muscle mass would demand less fuel than what the fixed intake kept providing. You'd be eating the same, but needing less. That gap between what you eat and what you need grows as the muscle mass decreases further and metabolism slows. Thus more and more of the resulting excess is stored as fat.

No wonder people say, "You get fatter as you get older." You will gain fat more easily *if* you lose muscle as you age. And you will lose muscle as you age *if* you continue to sustain your energy by using muscle for fuel. What's never pointed out is the "if"; people don't question why that muscle loss happens and don't learn that it doesn't have to. The way muscle loss is reported makes you think it's "just the way it is"—a prediction of *everybody's* future, rather than a mere observation of the past.

But muscle loss is not an inevitable process we're helpless to control! These reports don't cite the simple biological data that clarify how dieting, skipping meals, and "cutting back" on carbs or food in general facilitate your reliance on muscle as a fuel crutch. If fuel deprivation causes muscle loss, and if half of all Americans are dieting—can you see what is happening?

And don't think that the nondieting half aren't depriving themselves, too. The American way of eating in general tends toward the erratic. You may not be doing it purposely, but even those who aren't trying to go hungry often do so unwittingly. You don't remember to eat, don't have time—but you don't know what it is costing you.

STOPPING THE DOWNWARD SPIRAL

Muscle loss isn't a "natural" genetic legacy. The downward spiral—losing "weight," gaining fat as a result of the damage, and thus trying to lose more "weight"—can be stopped or reversed by *fueling*. Give the body quality food with consistency and regularity, and your body need never "withdraw" muscle for fuel. Best of all, with consistent and widespread education that starts early, the downward spiral need never begin. Kids start life by eating in a way that instinctively provides them with what they need. They may learn to like junk, but at least they don't starve themselves. It was probably sometime between puberty and your twenties that you had your initial first-hand experience with a diet. Something happened: You heard, saw, or read something; your mother, dance teacher, boyfriend, or girlfriend made a remark. Maybe it was a picture, or someone else's body.

Something had you convinced that you should lose "weight." So you began—using the only tactic you knew, the one already branded in your consciousness. It's the same thing our culture is still offering up, blindly and unthinkingly: Eat less and exercise more. The more you did it, the more "weight" you lost. The more weight you lost, the more muscle you lost. And the more muscle you lost, the easier it got to gain fat. And the more fat you gained, the less you ate and the more you exercised.

This is the core of yo-yo-ing. The fatter we get, the more society tells us we must starve to "fix" it. The more we starve, the fatter we get. Until recently, society has never questioned the worth and effectiveness of this starving business; it has instead questioned those who fail at starving. Now that it's begun to question starving, it's still confounded about why it fails.

If we truly and deeply believed that shooting your foot off helped you walk better, and no one ever questioned it (even though, in practice, it never quite seemed to work), there would be a lot of very frustrated and pained people limping around. Maybe worse, they'd feel inadequate because this "tried and true" method didn't work for them. Isn't that how it is with "weight loss"? People are ashamed because what everyone "knows" should work doesn't work for them.

MAINTENANCE

Weight "maintenance" is now considered to be the true challenge of weight loss. The battle may be over, but a new war has been declared. Just the idea that you need another program to "maintain" the first says it's going to be rough—expect defeat. Poignantly, one client (and weight-loss program veteran) concurred: "You hope you won't gain the weight back. Actually, you don't hope. You know you're going to gain it back. Everyone knows. We pretend to hope." That's because "weight" loss is by nature physically and psychologically unmaintainable.

BIOLOGICALLY UNMAINTAINABLE. A series of congressional hearings chaired in early 1992 by Rep. Ron Wyden of Oregon revealed that 90 to 95 percent of those who use the programs gain back all their "weight"—if not more. (Of course, they're not just gaining "weight," but pure fat.)

That's not a mystery, though researchers and health professionals continue to call it that. You can see that given the biology of weight loss via "eat less/exercise more," what is called "maintenance" in the diet industry is a lost cause. Physiologically speaking, you haven't got a hope in hell of "keeping it off."

New research or not, weight is still what the researchers talk about. What's "new" is they warn that weight loss must be "permanent" or it's unhealthy. What's nuts is they never say that "permanent" *muscle* weight loss makes permanent *fat* loss unachievable. They promote generic weight loss, achieved by the same classic one-size-fits-all deprivation formula. A permanent struggle is all you can count on.

PSYCHOLOGICALLY UNMAINTAINABLE. Even if weight loss/maintenance worked physically, the old, tired thinking doesn't. It's never about a life of fueling yourself to live fabulously. It's about "losing 20 pounds." It's never about what bigger, greater possibilities you are moving toward—just the drudgery of "keeping it off." Weight maintenance isn't about living—it's about your weight.

You're still "on" a program, but now it's a maintenance program that simply extends the grim, hopeless cycle—shifting attention from lowering a meaningless number to keeping it there. You replace your short-term diet with something almost worse: a diet you're supposed to stay on for the rest of your life.

At one recent workshop, a woman struggled for words as she tried to describe what it was she really wanted. "I think," she said haltingly, "what I want is a weight-loss program that will work, and then to integrate my weight-loss program so it's a part of my life." Of course, she quickly learned that BodyFueling is not about weight loss, that it's not a program, and that her weight was irrelevant. What struck me was the unlikely idea of shoehorning something as unnatural as a "weight-loss program" into your life.

I knew what she meant, though: She wanted it to blend in and just become *eating*. But she had no language to articulate it, because "program" is all the vocabulary she had. Where is this language reinforced? In articles like "The Finish Line" in the August 1992 issue of *Self*. " 'What is needed is a phased, long-term eating plan that incorporates both a weight-loss phase and a longer weight-maintenance phase that builds on it,' said Johanna Dwyer, D.Sc., R.D., director of the Frances Stern Nutrition Center and a professor at Tufts University Medical School." What a mouthful! I'd simply say what is needed is eating and living.

When the now-famous "yo-yo study" (which linked the repeated losing and gaining that marks chronic dieting with coronary artery disease and premature death; profiled further in Chapter 5, "Diet Thinking") hit the streets and the anti-diet movement began to swell, companies scrambled to repackage their programs to capitalize on the negative publicity, rather than perish by it.

Having weight-loss companies go into a huddle and come out grinning with "weight management" is like finding kids with chocolate all over their faces, swearing they just ate green beans. They didn't go back to ground zero or update the old thinking. *Weight maintenance* and *management* are built squarely on the paradigm of diet thinking—it's just "weight loss diets" with a new name.

CONTROL: THE BOOBY PRIZE OF MAINTENANCE

Especially where maintenance is concerned, much is made of *controlling* your weight (or food or your body). But in this context, control is the furthest thing from real power. Power is relaxed and implies choice: "I know what I want, need, and will have." You hold all the cards and do with them what you wish.

By contrast, control implies that someone or something else holds the cards. You can't own it, only manage it. You've barely got a handle on it; if you get the upper hand, you must be forever on your guard.

Control also means denial and resistance: "I'm not having ice cream . . . I'm not . . . I'm *not* . . ." People think if they can gain "control" of something—weight, fat—it won't run them. But to resist something is to validate its existence. "I will not get fat; I will stay thin" dominates your life just as "I'm fat" does.

Maintenance promises a life that is centered around reigning in or holding back one of the most natural human instincts—to eat—and that is so oriented around reduction (of pounds, portions, calories, sizes, body parts) that it reduces life itself. It is managing your own starvation by seeking to control an irrelevant number.

Think of Weight Watchers. The name tells all. "Watching your weight." What a concept! What a life! Imagine: Your eyes are glued to the dial on the scale. I'd rather watch the most boring TV in the world than my "weight"—as if it had anything to say about me anyway!

Ironically, those who manage to stay the same weight their whole life— thus supposedly winning the maintenance game—usually still gain fat over that period. As you've seen, body composition can change dramatically— for better or worse—without weight changing at all.

"WEIGHT" REGAIN IS ALL FAT

Failure to "maintain weight" is actually much more of a disaster than most people realize. You may think the worst part of "regaining the weight" is being back where you started—but you're not.

If you lose, say, 50 pounds—and 25 are muscle—you can easily gain 50 pounds back. After all, 25 pounds of muscle is a *lot* of engine. (Plus, fuel deprivation causes additional metabolic changes that further hasten fat gain, as you'll soon see.)

Then you say "I gained all the weight back." But that's not all. When you lose weight that way, you don't gain back the exact weight you lost. Those 50 regained pounds are not 25 muscle and 25 fat. *They are all fat.*

You don't just pile on 25 pounds of muscle in a few weeks and with no effort (though it is possible to lose them nearly that fast, if you're really starving). It takes months or years to build muscle—and not only good fueling but also exercise is required. It's a lot easier to lose muscle than to gain it. (More on this in Chapter 4, "Exercise.")

So you lose 25 pounds of fat and gain 50 back! And you have 25 pounds less lean muscle than when you started. Your total bodyfat percentage has increased.

LOSE NOW, PAY LATER

Weight loss creates a repeat customer. Each time you lose "weight," you're more likely to be fat again in the future.

Why? Every time a "weight-loss diet" has you lose a bunch of pounds that are mainly muscle—by creating a fuel deficit your body can fill only by "dipping" into the muscle protein tank—you lose pounds of metabolically active tissue that was once "on your side." You're locked in a cycle in which the regain of fat is imminent. So your need for "weight loss"—if you remain uneducated about what is really going on—stays firmly in place.

"If doctors know all that, why do they get on TV and swear up and down that they're doctors and it [the diet] works?" Dawn, our participant with the scale-tampering boss, asks plaintively, echoing the obvious question that at least one participant in every workshop arrives at eventually.

I offer these possible answers:

1. I don't know. I ask exactly the same question every day.
2. Money.
3. America wants speed, and weight loss does do *something* fast (it's just that what it does isn't what you really want).
4. It does work, in a sick sense, in that you do lose what it promises—you do lose pounds! But these diets and their advertising play on your vagueness, your not having distinguished that you want to lose fat. And they will continue to do so until Americans demand complete education, not a temporary quick fix that makes some arbitrary number smaller for a brief time.
5. They don't know.

The average medical doctor has had about as much nutrition training as the average anybody else. Our culture has elevated medicine to a level where we expect doctors to know everything and do everything—in fact, to be more responsible for our health than we are. But Western medicine hasn't focused its training on keeping healthy people healthy; currently, it emphasizes fixing sick people.

On one talk show, I heard Covert Bailey, the highly respected MIT microbiologist and fitness educator, poke fun at "medically supervised" diets. "What does that mean? Why would I want medical supervision for a diet? I'd want medical supervision if I was gonna have surgery, but for a diet?"

A friend in medical school, who took a "sub-elective" course in nutrition her first year, told me: "The instructor said, 'Enjoy this. It's the last chance you'll have for the next four years.' " And our clients notice. I long ago stopped counting how many have said, "Well, everyone knows doctors don't know anything about nutrition anyway." Many clients first came to BodyFueling because their doctors absently mumbled, "Lose XX pounds and call me in a month." Some have confided they wouldn't listen to their doctors' guidance anyway—because their doctors are fat.

Dr. Anthony Sattilaro, who eventually cured his cancer by eating a more particular version of the diet now recommended for its prevention, is candid about this in his book *Recalled by Life*: "As with most physicians, my medical training did not include the study of nutrition. I understood the need for certain nutrients and the problems associated with nutrient deficiencies, but I had little understanding of how the overall diet promoted health or illness . . . Since doctors don't receive much training in preventive medicine, or nutrition, they don't place much emphasis on it."

This fact is underscored by a report in the April 1993 issue of *Nutrition Action Newsletter* noting that when New York Hospital Cornell Medical Center sent a survey on diet and disease to 30,000 practicing family, general or internal physicians listed with the American Medical Association (AMA), only 11 percent responded. And of those who did respond, only 23 percent asked patients about food and fluid intake; only 34 percent used nutrition research to improve patient care; and little more than half recommended dietary solutions to blood pressure or cholesterol problems.

One client revealed that she was shocked when she first learned that her doctor was on a popular commercial diet program. "I thought, shouldn't he know how to do this? But I realized he didn't, not any more than I did." Another client challenged her doctor after BodyFueling: "What kind of weight did you want me to lose—fat or muscle?" She said he replied, "I don't care which. You've just got to lose 60 pounds."

A SOBERING EXAMPLE OF WEIGHT TREACHERY

Arbitrary "weight" standards keep fit, muscular people out of weight divisions in sports, and even jobs. The story of Tenita Deal, an American Airlines flight attendant, makes this excruciatingly clear. As reported in *Health* magazine in February 1992, this beauty-contest swimsuit competition winner was first hired by American Airlines in 1961. She weighed 118 pounds. The airline insisted even then that she lose 5 pounds. To do so—and to stay that way—she consumed "a protein diet of meat and eggs" for 15 years. (The human machine requires the food/fuel we consume to be only 10 to 20 percent protein.) Diagnosed with cancer at 34, Deal's doctor suggested her diet "may" have been a factor, so she integrated more fiber into her diet.

After having a son at age 37, Deal gained 15 pounds. The airline had loosened its weight restrictions a bit by then but still required Deal to lose 5 pounds. As she reported in *Health*: "I would fast on juices for almost a month. Before getting my weight checked, I'd take diuretics and laxatives and almost faint on the scale. It got harder and harder to lose. When I couldn't get my weight down, I'd move up my vacation and literally stop eating. At one point I ended up in the hospital thinking I'd had a heart attack. The doctors said my potassium was low and my electrolytes had been thrown off from starving myself."

Deal also tried a liquid fasting program: "I spent all that money, did what they said, hard-walking for an hour every day. I weighed one hundred forty-six pounds and it just wouldn't go lower. My counselor said 'Why not settle for the higher weight? You look great!' I told her I'd be happy to—I mean, I'm fifty years old!—but I'd get fired."

Deal finally did decide to put an end to the "not eating for three or four days, exercising till I was in pain, and being totally focused on my weight." In September 1991, American Airlines settled weight discrimination lawsuits filed by the flight attendants' union and the Equal Opportunity Employment Commission.

The stark horror of what this woman sacrificed in the name of weight is a monument to diet thinking: *three decades* of serious, near-fatal destruction of her own health, marked by cancer, electrolyte imbalances, and long stretches of starvation. Desperately damaging a normal, healthy body so as not to get fired—this is "weight" mania gone awry.

It's also what's dangerous about not understanding the body. Because someone didn't understand the difference between weight and fat—between muscle and fat—or the precise costs of manipulating "weight," someone decided that a stupid number meant more than Tenita Deal's looks, overall health, or vitality as an employee and a human being.

And it is education that's missing, not a "fuller-figured standard" (as some fashion-model-bashers claim). Note that the problem here was not the standard of looking "slim." If that alone had been the issue, Tenita Deal— at size 10, described as muscular and compact, certainly not fat—would have been fine. No, it was the weight, the number. (Note: In May 1993, the same story was front-page headlines all over again—only the names had changed. The airline was United, the woman was 44-year-old Catherine Brewer [5' 4" and 150 pounds], and she was to be suspended without pay unless she lost 18 pounds. Like Tenita Deal, she and other men and women resorted to crash diets and appetite suppressants to meet the airline's weight restrictions. In this case, too, a lawsuit was filed.)

OFF THE CHARTS!

The *Health* article admits that a weight chart is not a precise measure of fatness, yet the whole piece pushes new, more "forgiving" weight charts.

Dr. George Bray, Director of the Pennington Biomedical Research Center at Louisiana State University, "believes that women can safely add some pounds as the decades pass, but not more than 11 over the life span." Oops! Sorry, Dr. Bray, I put on 15 already. Want to tell me those pounds—of lean muscle—were unhealthy?

You think these semantics don't matter? Sit in on one of my workshops sometime and listen to people's stories. See their confusion, their obsession with the number. See how many "normal"-weight people feel awful, and don't look so great, either. See how many overfat people think they're safe because they fit neatly onto the range of a height-weight chart.

It's impossible for any chart to identify a weight that is healthy. No matter how low your weight, bodyfat can be high. No matter how high your weight, bodyfat can be low. A person could weigh in the "ideal" range with 40 percent bodyfat (not healthy) and a very low lean-body mass. Arnold Schwarzenegger does not conform to "ideal weight" charts—yet he is clearly not "fat." Think about it.

But the media and medical professionals still are saying weight. Here, from my ever-growing file, are some choice items I believe keep this nonissue alive. The italics are mine for emphasis:

▶ "I think women should be even *lighter* than the 1959 tables," says Robert J. Garrison, a National Heart, Lung and Blood Institute statistician.

▶ "If that person has high blood pressure, angina, congestive heart failure, or arthritis of the knees, I can get quite excited because he'll improve by losing *weight*," says Theodore VanItallie, a Columbia University obesity researcher.

▶ William Castelli, director of the well-known Framingham Heart Study (on which the "yo-yo study" research was also based): "Look at all the bad things that follow *weight* gain . . ." (But nothing bad follows *muscle* gain!) "The real question is, is *skinny* better?" (No, but leanness is. Skinny and 40 percent bodyfat is terrible.)

In the next sentence, the article's author refers to Castelli as a "leanness advocate." But he isn't—he's a "skinniness" advocate. Do they think it's obvious what they mean? Do they think it's all the same? I talk to people about this every day, and it's not. *They don't know!* They don't differentiate, and it's dangerous.

▶ C. Wayne Callaway does acknowledge, "I also see men who meet the weight guidelines and who have no buns and are all belly and are already having their first heart attack at age forty-six." Yet the rest of the article supports weight as *the* marker of future disease.

Most of the researchers concur that fat is unhealthy, and they provide ample evidence to show it. This we agree on. The trouble comes when they use the word "overweight" interchangeably with "fat," so that people associate the two, look at their weight, and begin to manipulate it in ways that just make their bodies fatter. Dr. Bernadine Healy, National Institutes of Health Director, has said "There is no more important issue in nutrition at large than weight loss and weight control" (*USA Today*). I think there is no more important issue than having professionals and health leaders stop calling it "weight" and start calling it what it really is.

DE-EMPHASIZING SIZE

To a lesser extent, I would encourage de-emphasizing size as well as weight, because even it becomes irrelevant when health and leanness are the real concern. It can be misleading when I say I am a size 2 or 4 if you think I mean that's an ideal size, or that the size alone means I'm healthy and fit. It doesn't.

What's significant is the *change in size*, because when you lose fat, you do get smaller. It's more telling that I dropped sizes by fueling and losing fat than it is to say what size I am now.

To a point, size is also useful to demonstrate why weight is irrelevant, since people who weigh the same weight may differ in size due to vast differences in what constitutes the "weight"—muscle or fat. So it's also telling that others who weigh what I do may be much larger, and therefore probably fatter.

But people of my size can be much fatter as well. One can be a size 4 and be quite fat. You could call such a person "skinny," but not lean, which is why skinny and thin are pretty meaningless. You could also be a size 12 and lean as a rock.

I'd rather be the rock than the mush, regardless of size. I just happen to be the size I am because of my body shape and type, which you can't do much about—not that I can see any reason to want to change that part. There's plenty you can impact. You can't control how far apart your hipbones are spaced; you can affect how much fat is piled on top of them.

I used to care a lot about being "thin." But when I began to think differently—when I began to consider my health and future and strength and stamina, and learned exactly what would give me all of that—well, let's just say being "thin," sickly, flabby, and hungry became decidedly less appealing than being lean, fit, glowingly healthy, and full of food all the time.

3

FUELING THE HUMAN BODY:
Your Owner's Manual

I hope it's clear to you now that directions all by themselves won't inspire you to go somewhere. Once you have a journey in mind, however, good directions are of utmost importance. And now that you've thought a little about where *you're* going, you need to know how to get there!

If you wanted to get to Boston from Los Angeles, and you had a vehicle, fuel is the one thing—the first thing—you would be sure to have in that car. Without it you simply could not budge. What fuels make your body, the vehicle, run—and what makes it run best?

UNDERSTANDING YOUR FUEL SYSTEM

There is unquestionably a system design to the human body that has fundamental requirements. The problem is that we're given this very sophisticated and important machine without basic instructions. If you don't know precisely what you need, feeding yourself is hit or miss. When you miss, you start breaking down and losing efficiency.

What follows is the education we should all have had as a natural part of growing up—and which I hope future generations will have. It will provide an essential understanding of why I (and virtually every expert on the subject today) recommend you eat the way I call "fueling."

Fueling means learning to work with the way the body works, not the way you think it works, hope it works, or wish it would work. Learning how your body really works is worlds ahead of merely learning "how to eat." If you can predict accurately how your body acts and reacts, you can fuel yourself accordingly, and that understanding is crucial to the sense of ownership that makes fueling something you *want* to, not *have* to, do. Basic science will show you what you need to do to get what you want. It will be obvious what works, what doesn't, and what's optimal.

The following material is based purely on textbook biology and physiology. It's not my theory or viewpoint, nor is it a "philosophy." I've synthesized science and put it in language you can understand. I believe you have a right to this information, even a responsibility to know it. It's the informed part of being able to make informed choices.

THREE DIFFERENT "BRANDS" OF FUEL

Nutrition science defines the six nutrients as protein, carbohydrate, fat, vitamins, minerals, and water. Vitamins and minerals are *micronutrients* while protein, carbohydrate, and fat are *macronutrients*. That's because protein, carbohydrate, and fat are the three primary nutrients your body can burn as fuel, convert to fuel, or store as fuel. Your body runs on them. Without them, your body would be like a computer without an operating system.

What follows is the complete "manual" on each of these fuels and how they operate, so that you know how the body uses each and what happens when they're missing or imbalanced.

PROTEIN (UNLEADED)

Protein is the simplest fuel of the three to explain. The reason it's the simplest is that it's not actually intended to be fuel at all. It can become fuel—that is, the body has the ability to convert it to useable fuel. But protein *as protein* is not utilized by the body to provide energy—to "fuel" or run the body.

So what is protein for? You may remember from high school or college biology that protein was referred to as "the building blocks of the body." And that's exactly what protein is. The body uses protein to repair, maintain, and build tissue. Your body is constantly regenerating and repairing cells and tissue. Protein is critical to this renewal process.

When you exercise muscles regularly, creating a continuing demand on those muscles, the body responds to the need for strength at those locations by reinforcing them. Your muscles "build," or grow bigger and stronger. Protein is needed to do that "building." The antibodies that protect you from disease and heal you are proteins as well.

Protein itself has building blocks of its own: All proteins are made up of chains of substances known as amino acids. There are 22 known amino acids, and the body can manufacture most of them all by itself. But there are eight amino acids that the human body cannot produce on its own, yet that our bodies need in order for protein to perform its necessary functions. These amino acids are called "essential amino acids" because we cannot do without them.

That's why it's important that we eat protein, even though it does not directly fuel the body. If our bodies could manufacture all 22 amino acids, ingestion of protein might be optional. But that's not the case.

Where can we obtain these essential amino acids? By eating protein. What kind of protein? When choosing protein to eat, we have two general types from which we can select: animal protein or vegetable/plant protein. There can be advantages and disadvantages in both groups, but we can choose wisely from either or both and do very well.

From a health standpoint, there are two main considerations when selecting proteins: whether it is a complete protein and whether it is a low-fat (or lean) protein source.

Complete protein is that which contains all eight of the essential amino acids your body needs to run properly and that it cannot produce on its own. All animal proteins are complete proteins; this is an advantage of eating animal protein.

One of the disadvantages of animal protein is that it can be very high in fat. Many meat and dairy products contain well over the 30-percent-of-calories-from-fat-or-less recommended in the new government guidelines, and way beyond the increasingly common suggestion by health and nutrition professionals that we limit our intake of fat to 20 percent of calories or less. However, this doesn't have to be the case. There are plenty of animal protein sources that meet these standards: Lean white-meat poultry, fish, shellfish, very lean cuts of pork (such as tenderloin), low-fat or nonfat cheeses, and other skim dairy products such as yogurt and milk. Even eggs actually contain only 6 grams of fat each. While an egg also contains 275 milligrams of cholesterol, people whose blood cholesterol is below 200 and whose intake of saturated fat is low (less than 10 percent of calories) should not have a problem with eggs a few times a week. It is possible to find special cuts of red meat with fewer than 30 percent of calories from fat, and an occasional (once or even twice a week) serving of beef should not be a problem, especially if you are otherwise fueling yourself consistently.

In my work, I take no personal position about eating animals; that is for other authors to explore. My concern is for humans to be able to eat a 10 to 25 percent fat diet that is delicious and satisfying and that provides all necessary nutrients. So I have no "beef" (okay, pun intended) with any animal protein *that is lean.*

By the same token, I have no disagreement with people who choose to eat only plant food. I applaud that decision, whether it's based on human or planetary health, or both. Again, my one concern about vegetarian protein is that it be low in fat. It's a common fallacy that a vegetarian diet is automatically a healthy one. I've met numerous vegetarians who prided themselves on their natural, organic, earth-friendly diets, but who fueled so poorly (so little food, so infrequently, and/or so much fat) that I doubt the lack of additives made much of a health impact.

A vegetarian diet is not inherently low in fat. Vegetarians may load up on cheeses, nuts, and nut butters, eggs, beans, and bean curds made with lots of oils, and other greasy fare. A vegetarian may consume more fat than someone who eats burgers regularly!

It's certainly just as possible to eat low-fat vegetarian protein as animal protein. This is done by choosing low-fat and nonfat cheeses and other dairy products, eating nuts and seeds and eggs sparingly, and making beans and legumes the greatest share of protein intake.

The bottom line: Both a vegetarian diet and one that includes animal product can provide adequate protein and remain low in fat.

When choosing plant protein—beans, legumes, grains, nuts, or seeds— you need to combine several foods in order to get a *complete protein,* which provides all of the amino acids you need. While any animal protein contains all eight essential amino acids, plant proteins do not. Each contains different combinations of some of the eight. Some plant foods contain amino acids that others do not. Therefore, you can obtain all eight by eating plant foods that, when combined, provide complete protein. Beans and rice is an example of one such combination, reflecting the instinctive wisdom of many ethnic cultures and their cuisine.

By combining the two foods, you get as complete a protein as if you'd eaten animal food. On the next page is an easy-to-use chart that will guide you in combining some commonly eaten foods in order to get complete protein.

Also be aware that a 1987 study at Loma Linda University in California showed that animals fed rice and beans separately grew as quickly as those fed these foods at the same meal, so the idea that you must combine your proteins at exactly the same time may be outdated. If you eat a wide variety of foods throughout the day, it appears you'll absorb the full complement of amino acids.

One more important thing about protein: The body cannot store protein as protein. There are no caches of protein socked away for "rainy days," on call to fill in if we don't happen to eat protein for a while. Therefore, since the body is always using protein but lacks the ability to store it, we need to eat protein on a consistent basis.

That doesn't mean we need to eat a lot of it. Be sure you don't confuse consistency with volume, because it's a common mishap. The typical American, having been taught that protein is the "ideal" food, harbors related misconceptions (such as that eating a lot of protein builds muscle even if you don't exercise). While protein is necessary, we don't need heaps of it—and we certainly don't need it loaded with fat.

The U.S. Recommended Dietary Allowance for protein is 58 to 63 grams for men and 46 to 50 grams for women (60 to 65 grams for pregnant and breastfeeding women). Some nutritionists consider even that to be too much. But let's say that's the place to start—certainly it is a maximum. Think of it this way: Even breast milk is only about 5 percent protein—and it's designed for an infant's body, which is doubling in size during the first year of life. If a baby can grow on a 5 percent protein diet, then we ought not need much more than that.

Let's put these recommendations in better perspective: A 6-ounce sirloin steak has 45 grams of protein. A cup of nonfat milk offers 9 grams. A cup of cooked pinto beans provides 17 grams. A 2-ounce serving of tuna has 12 grams of protein. An eight-ounce yogurt plus an ounce of nonfat cheddar cheese would equal 24 grams.

Most people I've worked with either consume way too much protein or little to none. Some people alternate the two, eating none for a while and then gorging themselves on, say, a huge serving of beef. This is especially inefficient. Remember, your body cannot store protein as protein. The result of such erratic protein intake is a body that is without the necessary repair

COMBINING FOODS TO MAKE COMPLETE PROTEIN

GRAINS

Rice, wheat,
rye, oats, corn,
millet, buckwheat,
barley, bulgur,
corn, quinoia

NUTS/SEEDS

Almonds, walnuts,
cashews, pecans, Brazil
nuts, pistachios;
sesame, sunflower,
pumpkin seeds

BEANS/ LEGUMES

Dried peas;
lentils; kidney,
pinto, lima, navy,
and black beans;
soybeans;
chickpeas

*Combine beans/legumes with either grains or nuts/seeds for complete protein if
you eat no animal proteins (meats, eggs, dairy). Recent studies show that you need not
combine them at the same meal in order to absorb all the essential amino acids.
Simply eat the complementary proteins sometime during the same day.*

and maintenance tools much of the time, yet is occasionally overloaded with more than it can use.

If the body can't store protein as protein, what can it store protein as? Well, you've already seen that the body can turn protein (either dietary or from your lean-muscle tissue) into carbohydrate fuel if you run low on carbohydrate (glucose). Protein can convert itself in another way, too. When you've consumed more protein than the body can use in the next several hours, your body will break down the excess protein and convert it to fat. Protein can be stored as fat. (That's in addition to the fat that was already present in the food.)

Few people need the extra fat converted from excess protein "runoff," but there are other good reasons not to leave your body consistently converting protein to fat. Your body is no happier when you are de-aminating (breaking down the amino acids) for conversion to fat than when you are de-aminating to make glucose. Since protein is nitrogen-based, nitrogen is one of the waste products given off by this breakdown, and that toxin must be treated and excreted. You place undue stress on organs that wouldn't be called on otherwise. It's a lot of work to take amino acids apart and clean up the "ash" they leave behind.

Also, too much protein in the body has been shown to "leach" calcium from the system, and American women tend to have difficulty maintaining adequate levels of calcium in the diet and in the body to begin with.

Water loss is another result of protein breakdown, because the body uses as much water as possible to flush the poisonous ash of protein-burning out of the body. (This water loss caused by carb-deprivation protein breakdown is misinterpreted as a happy circumstance by people who confuse "weight" loss with fat loss.)

So if protein isn't supposed to fuel the body, what is? Both carbohydrate and fat do—and here's how each of them, in their own way, provide fuel for the human body to run.

CARBOHYDRATE (SUPREME)

I've already gone into carbohydrate in some detail because an understanding of its functions is so critical to eliminating "weight" as an issue. We've also discussed why carbohydrate deprivation has terrible consequences for your body. But how exactly do we fuel the body to circumvent muscle breakdown?

Carbohydrate is the human body's primary source of *immediate fuel*. Most of the time, our bodies use more of it than anything else. Even at times when the body may use more fat than carbohydrate, the body is still using some carbohydrate—it cannot run without it. The brain and central nervous system run purely on carbohydrate, and would cease to function if none was available.

Since the human body is brilliantly designed for survival, a built-in mechanism kicks in another fuel source when carbohydrate runs low. Your body's ability to take protein (from the diet or your muscle) and convert it to carbohydrate fuel is one of the key mechanisms your body has to guard against carbohydrate shortages.

You've already seen how the loss of muscle adds up to loss of "pounds"— loss of metabolism-raising, fuel-burning tissue. If dietary protein is diverted for use as fuel, it is not available for its primary functions of cell and tissue repair and maintenance. Any muscle tissue broken down by exercise and daily use does not get replaced, because dietary protein is being "stolen."

Under ideal circumstances, your body need not turn to this emergency action. To prevent the unnecessary diversion of muscle or dietary protein for conversion to carbohydrate fuel, you can do something very simple: *eat*. Delivering carbohydrate fuel to your body means eating carbohydrate food. Clearly, this makes eating not only normal and healthy, but necessary.

Complex carbohydrates make the best fuel—whole-grain breads, cereal, rice, pasta, potatoes, fruit, beans. (Beans also provide protein—in fact, most foods provide some of all three fuels we discuss here, but in varying proportions.)

In the process of digestion, carbohydrate is eventually broken down to a simple, useable form called glucose. Glucose is the form of carbohydrate the body consistently draws on as its energy source. Glucose operates from the bloodstream; that's the "rendezvous point" for delivering fuel to the muscles.

There is a blood level of glucose that is appropriate for each of our bodies. Too much—high blood sugar—is a manifestation of diabetes, in which insufficient levels of insulin inhibit glucose's ability to enter and fuel the muscle cells. Too little glucose in the bloodstream to adequately fuel you— "low blood sugar"—is also an undesirable condition. As a chronic condition it can be the result of a disease called hypoglycemia (although true hypoglycemia is rare).

Many people diagnose themselves as having hypoglycemia, when in fact their blood sugar is low simply because they haven't replenished it by eating enough carbohydrate food, or eating it often enough. People starve themselves, either unwittingly or consciously, and then declare themselves hypoglycemic. That's not being hypoglycemic. That's being human. "Low blood sugar" is descriptive; it is a symptom, not in itself a disease.

Since your nervous system runs on glucose exclusively, you can bet you'll feel dizzy, headachey, and unable to concentrate if your brain's precious glucose supply is dropping. But that it drops is a normal, predictable occurrence. If you have a tank full of something you use all the time, what will happen to what's in the tank? Your car's gas tank can be filled only to a point; if you drive constantly, the level falls until at some point you must refill it.

Most people regularly experience low blood sugar, yet don't connect the symptoms to how long ago they last ate. If they do make the connection and recognize their need to eat frequently to avoid these symptoms, they think they are "special." This is analogous to believing your car is broken—or special—because after a full day of driving, you actually had to fill the gas tank again.

Now you know that you use carbohydrate constantly, and that blood glucose is the primary end product of the carbohydrate you eat and the form that the body employs as fuel. Given that, the key to keeping your energy level high is to keep carbohydrate intake consistent so that the glucose level remains steady. Your blood glucose level is practically synonymous with your energy level. If your energy is low, how much carbohydrate you're eating and how often is a good place to look first. It's the bottom line.

GLUCOSE ISN'T STORED. Glucose in your bloodstream does share some characteristics with fuel in a tank. But your bloodstream is not a storage tank for glucose; it is better thought of as a "rendezvous point." Your blood is where it hovers or "hangs out"—kind of a stopover—prior to its delivery to muscle cells, where it is burned for energy.

There's only so much glucose that your body will allow to "wait" in the bloodstream at any one time (as you can probably imagine, there are many other things going on in your blood—and in your whole body—besides the ones we're examining). That means there's not only a minimum level of blood glucose you want to maintain, but also a maximum that your bloodstream can bear. You cannot jam endless amounts of carbohydrate into your body and keep it all as glucose for later.

The amount of glucose your bloodstream can "hold" will last from about three to five hours. This amount varies depending on the individual, and is a factor of how quickly you burn fuel in general (primarily determined by how active you are, how much lean mass you have, and how effectively you utilize fat as a "supporting fuel").

This means that *a crucial part of fueling is eating carbohydrate every three to four hours*. While you may be able to go a little longer than that without feeling it or triggering a deprivation response, this time frame will cover just about everyone. In fact, in my experience, most people feel better if their carbs come less than four hours apart. It certainly won't hurt you to "re-fuel" sooner than later. Doing this keeps blood glucose steady and energy up, and ensures that you never need to steal muscle to make the precious glucose that fat cannot adequately replace.

Obviously, regularity and consistency is significant to carbohydrate fueling. Given the system's design, the same amount of carbohydrate eaten all at once (instead of in many snacks and meals) will not be efficient. You cannot make carbohydrate last twice as long—say, six to 8 hours rather than three to four—by eating twice as much at once. That's like trying to put 20 gallons of gas in your car's 10-gallon tank, hoping that you can drive twice as far without a re-fuel. You'll get only 10 gallons in the tank, the rest will slop over the side, and you'll still have to re-fuel after the 10 gallons are gone.

What if you do eat "20 gallons" of carbohydrate when "10 gallons" would do? What if you consume more carbohydrate than your body can use as glucose over the next several hours? You still won't be able to go twice as far without re-fueling—because you can't "stock up" on glucose, and so the excess is not stored as such. But fortunately, if it's complex carbohydrate, neither will it make much of a mess (the way the extra 10 gallon of gas does as it drools over the side). To understand why, first you must see why quality fuel is *complex* carbohydrate.

COMPLEX VS. SIMPLE. Your choice of carbohydrate fuel is as important as its timing. The complexity or simplicity of a carbohydrate determines how rapidly it reaches the bloodstream as glucose. The complex carb, as its name implies, is complicated; it has many parts and pieces to it. Therefore, it will take more time to disassemble and will reach the bloodstream more slowly.

The simple carb, as its name indicates, isn't at all complicated and takes very little effort to break down. In fact, a simple carb (such as refined flour and sugar) is already nearly broken down. It arrives in the bloodstream almost instantly. This makes it an inferior choice for energy, health, and fat loss.

Why would a simple carb's speedy arrival represent a problem? You want to get your blood sugar up as fast as you can, don't you? No. The longer amount of time complex carbohydrate takes to break down and reach the bloodstream is healthier. And it won't feel like too long unless you've already dipped into the hysterical zone and are hungry enough to eat cardboard.

(Ideally, you don't let it get to the deficit point; that's part of what "fueling" is about.)

The "rush" of glucose you get from simple sugar is counterproductive, and here's why. As glucose arrives in the bloodstream, your pancreas, a gland, is signaled to produce a hormone called insulin. Among other things, insulin manages the metabolism and delivery of fuel—including carbohydrate fuel to cells that can burn it for energy. Sufficient levels of insulin ensure that blood glucose is metabolized and escorted to the cells that need fuel.

When blood glucose levels rise moderately—via the slower, steady breakdown of a complex carb—the pancreas has sufficient time to gauge precisely how much insulin is needed to manage that amount of blood glucose. But when blood glucose levels suddenly soar, the pancreas does not have time to accurately match insulin to the new glucose level. It has to act rapidly on limited information.

Yet it must get some insulin into the bloodstream immediately. That's a safety mechanism to keep blood sugar from remaining unnaturally elevated, which is what happens when the pancreas does not produce enough insulin, or any insulin at all. (That's diabetes. Unless insulin is artificially provided, blood sugar is "stuck" at the rendezvous point—the bloodstream—unable to gain access to the muscle cells that desperately need it. Untreated, in extreme cases, this can result in coma and/or death.)

A non-diabetic body will not allow this to happen. Since it hasn't been given sufficient time to act accurately, our clever survival machine selects the lesser of two evils—too much insulin rather than too little. It reacts to an instant surge of blood sugar by overshooting its mark. This ensures that at least the burst of sugar will be safely cleared out of the bloodstream, rather than stranded in the blood without proper management.

The problem is that oversecretion of insulin produced by your panicked pancreas overclears the blood of glucose. Insulin stimulates the liver and muscle and fat cells to remove glucose from the blood and use or store it. You're left with a blood sugar level lower than when you started—and you're hungrier and more desperate for fuel than ever. You experience what you may have called the "sugar blues," "sugar blahs," or even "hypoglycemia." But it's not a sickness—just your body's way of handling an inefficient fuel source.

A very large meal (the kind after which you are stuffed to the gills), incidentally, has about the same effect on the pancreas as simple sugar overload. The pancreas is overwhelmed and again produces too much insulin in its effort to manage the onslaught of fuel.

Now you're back at square one, low on glucose and needing more carbohy-drate. At this point, if you don't understand what is happening in your body, you might eat more sugar—seeking the quick burst you got the time before, hoping this time it's not so short-lived (but it will be). You might soar and crash many times over before you figure out it never will work. I remember riding that roller coaster, and I know it's frustrating.

Or, at this point you might say, "Forget it! I ate something and it just made me feel worse, so I won't even bother." You let your body handle the glucose deficit in a makeshift way. And it does: Desperate for glucose and unable to get a meaningful amount from anywhere else, it turns to your muscle, and/or any protein you've eaten.

In addition to being a poor strategy for maintenance of steady high energy, flooding the system with simple carbohydrate also encourages fat storage. The attendant oversurge of insulin not only ushers away too much glucose too quickly but also creates an easy pathway for fat to enter fat cells. That's because insulin acts somewhat like a key unlocking cells. It's a master key: It unlocks muscle cells to let the glucose in, but it also unlocks fat cells. When an excess of insulin is circulating in the system, it will routinely unlock fat cells for the entrance of any dietary fat also present in the blood (triglyceride). (And triglyceride levels are likely to be elevated since sugar and fat often come in the same package.)

If you value high energy, you need fuel that gives good mileage. That means carbohydrate whose complexity allows the pancreas time to process and respond with precision, providing insulin appropriately to manage a stable blood glucose level.

COMPLEXITY DEMANDS ENERGY. A carbohydrate's complexity pro-vides a second important advantage. A complex carbohydrate will expend not only more time but also more energy in processing—and that makes it less likely to wind up as fat. Technically, excess carbohydrate can be converted to fat and stored as such—just as excess protein can and will be. But it's downright difficult to eat "too much" of, or "get fat" on, complex carbohydrate.

For one thing, a high-carbohydrate diet gets your body burning. The energy required to process the "complicated" complex carbohydrate elevates your metabolism.

For another, excess carbohydrate has other potential destinations besides fat storage. There is a special "fuel tank" I haven't mentioned till now—a small stash of a carbohydrate called *glycogen*, which is stored both in the liver (for use by the whole body) and in the muscles (for use by the muscles themselves). The body cannot store glucose in the bloodstream, but glycogen is a way the body can store carbohydrate fuel.

The body can't store very much glycogen—that's why you can't run indefinitely on glycogen when glucose runs low. In fact, the body stores just enough glycogen to fit in the palm of your hand—1,200 to 1,400 calories worth. Glycogen is true emergency carbohydrate: While glycogen in the muscles will be called upon in a carbohydrate deficit situation (typically athletics), the liver usually hoards its cache until the situation is far more dire.

So the first stop for excess carbohydrate after blood glucose levels are maxed is to replenish glycogen stores. When those tanks are "topped off," any remaining excess can potentially be stored as fat. But wait! The body disdains storing carb as fat. It's a lot of work. Your body expends three calories to turn 100 calories of dietary fat into bodyfat—but to convert the same amount of carbohydrate calories into fat, it will expend 23 calories of energy.

In other words, it costs your body about one-fourth of any excess complex carb to turn the rest into fat. If you eat a bagel and the entire thing is more than your body needs anywhere else at the time, one-fourth of the bagel will be "donated" as energy for the processing of the rest.

Another plus: Complex carbs tend to be high-fiber foods. That means that if 65 percent of your fuel comes from complex carb food, you don't have to wonder if you're getting enough fiber or count fiber grams. And since high fiber, complex carb foods are filling, they'll probably keep you too full to eat enough junk to do damage if you make them your priority fuel.

REAL-LIFE PROOF. This is partly why I was slowly able to increase my fuel intake to 2,500 calories a day—even while cutting my exercise to half of my previous routine—and drop several dress sizes in the process. About 70 percent of those calories were complex carbs and only 10 percent were fat. My body expends a great deal of energy just to break down all that carbohydrate to simpler forms such as glucose or glycogen. Of the carbohydrate that remains, much is distributed to the bloodstream as glucose for energy, routed for conversion to glycogen stores, or delivered directly to cells for use as fuel.

If there's still excess carb after all that, my body will convert it to fat. But even then, 23 percent of whatever's left won't wind up as fat but will instead be "paid" as energy required for that conversion. And since I am fueling frequently and plentifully, I'm not losing any precious fat-burning muscle tissue—and in fact have gained muscle, which in turn also supports my caloric increase because that extra muscle requires extra fuel. Suddenly, 2,500

WHY EXTRA CARBOHYDRATE WON'T NECESSARILY BE STORED AS FAT

If, for example, you eat this "extra" slice of bread at lunch, your body will not necessarily convert it all to fat for storage. Your body exercises a number of options: it will put some to immediate use (glucose); store some in another carbohydrate form (glycogen); *then* convert what's left to stored bodyfat. Even then, all of the remainder does not end up as fat; your body "spends" some to fuel each of these processes.

Converted to glucose ⇨ bloodstream
for use as energy

Converted to glycogen ⇨ liver/muscles

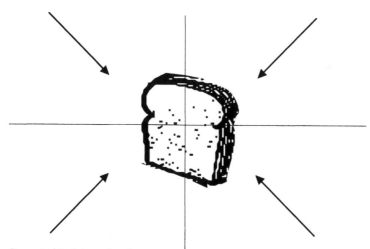

Converted to fat ⇨ stored

Burned as fuel to meet the energy
"cost" of conversions/storage

to 3,000 calories a day for a woman who's not exceptionally active makes more sense.

How anyone could consider trying a high-protein, low-carbohydrate diet for any reason after understanding this simple physiology is beyond me.

There are yet other factors, besides muscle loss, that make starving "fattening." They're detailed in the next section.

ALCOHOL IS ETHANOL. Alcohol is a carbohydrate of sorts, but not one that provides any nutrient value. It's very poor fuel. More to the point, the active ingredient in what you think of as "fruity" wine or "dry" beer is actually ethanol alcohol. Kind of a sobering thought, isn't it? But as with everything else, it doesn't mean you should never drink—just that you choose based on complete facts. Understanding what it is and what it does may not make you stop drinking, but then that's not the purpose. As with fat, the most reasonable and effective way to choose your alcohol indulgence is to keep it moderate and make it special.

Ethanol is very definitely a toxin, and your liver can process only an ounce of it every hour and a half. If you drink another ounce before it is finished processing the first, that second ounce will circulate in your bloodstream, "on hold" until the first ounce is processed.

Since alcohol is recognized by your system as an unwelcome intruder, treating and excreting it is a priority. Therefore, some other functions— including nutrient processing and absorption—are delayed or displaced. Some nutrients are lost forever. And while the second (or third or fourth) ounce is waiting, this toxin is passing through body tissues and cells.

FAT

WE DON'T UNDERSTAND FAT. Fat. While our culture incessantly talks about it, reads about it, writes about it, obsesses about it, and tries to avoid it (often unsuccessfully), there is a stunning lack of awareness about what fat is for and how it's really created. That ignorance allows Americans to do things that are totally inconsistent with the body's "system design"—ironically encouraging the body to do what they want least: be fat.

We rail against it as if it were a beastly substance with evil intent; it is our nemesis, the bane of our existence. Yet fat is not inherently a curse and does have a reason for being. It's important to understand *why* and *when* your body makes fat, because if you know which circumstances make it proficient, you can easily sidestep them. Rather than fostering a hatred of fat and blindly trying to tear it off of your body, realize that it does have its place and that—with knowledge—you can help to determine its destiny.

However much fat your body has stored is almost always an appropriate bodily response to how you eat—or, more likely, how you *don't* eat. Your body adjusts to what you do to it. You look at your fat and think "something's wrong"—but there's actually something right (just as there's nothing "wrong" when you're hungry three hours after a meal). It's how your body works.

YOUR BODY DOES USE FAT. Your body actually uses a combination of carbohydrate *and* fat for fuel *all the time.* I've said that carbohydrate is the body's critical fuel, and this is true: The body cannot run without it. However, the body uses fat as well, alongside carbohydrate, albeit in a different way.

Some people's bodies use more fat, all day long, than other people's bodies. Numerous factors affect how much of your energy need is met by fat rather than carbohydrate. Several major factors are within our power to change, though not overnight. "Fueling" is key, because how we eat (or don't eat) and how fit we are both directly and indirectly influence how willingly our bodies use fat.

How readily our bodies use fat for fuel—or, more specifically, the ratio of carbohydrate to fat used for fuel at any point in time—depends mainly on three things: your fitness level and body composition; what activity your body is engaged in at that moment; and whether you've been regularly and properly fueled.

Fitness level and body composition. A superfit athlete burns more fat—whether at rest or in competition—than the average person. Those with more muscle, those with very fit muscle (enhanced oxidative metabolism), and those with expanded cardiovascular capacity utilize fat as fuel more efficiently.

What activity your body is engaged in at the moment. The extent of your body's usage of fat for fuel at a given time depends in part upon the task at hand. There are times when fat actually will be the front-runner fuel of choice, and (more often) times when it won't. To understand when the body might favor fat over glucose, it helps to understand the strong suits of each.

Carbohydrate provides fast energy. Glucose is readily and rapidly burned for energy, and it is always present in the bloodstream at some level (either from carbohydrate food you eat, glycogen converted to glucose, or, failing that, from protein your body steals and converts). Glucose is always "on call," ready to be pulled into action.

While carbohydrate is the dynamic superhero of energy, fat is the strong, silent partner. Fat burns slowly. Slowly and quietly—but powerfully—it provides long-lasting sustenance and endurance.

Each fuel has its place. Fat is more ideal for some situations (such as a long hike or bike ride, when fuel must be doled out steadily and yet last long), while pure carbohydrate is best for others (such as an unexpected sprint). In each fuel's ideal venue it takes the lead, and the other moves to the background as the "support fuel." Either way, your body can draw on both at the same time; it's not usually an either/or proposition.

Whether you've been regularly and properly fueled. Your body makes, stores, and conserves fat under certain conditions—conditions you can avoid through the way you eat. Whether you are fueled frequently, and with quality, is crucial to whether your body uses or stores fat.

Of the three factors listed above, this one gives you the most power to encourage maximal fat usage. The others are less malleable: Your physical fitness level *is* a factor that can be altered, but that takes time—and itself requires good fueling. And all bodies essentially favor fat for long-term aerobic activity, and glucose for short-term and/or anaerobic activity.

But fueling regularly and purposefully is your chance to encourage the maximal use of fat at those times when fat is an appropriate fuel—whatever your fitness level. The way you eat can set the stage for your body to either seize or waste the opportunities it has for using fat. For example, a body "trained" by underfueling will not use fat as liberally, even during an aerobic workout, as one that has been well fueled.

"I'M ONLY TRYING TO HELP"—HISTORY REPEATS ITSELF. There is a physiological and historical logic to the fact that we store fat and to the conditions under which we do so. The environment that's ripe for fat creation is one of scarcity. When your eating habits signal that food is scarce, safety switches are tripped to make you more efficient at fat manufacture and fat conservation.

Fat was at one time so important to surviving scarcity that homo sapiens developed many different methods to ensure its efficient "stockpiling." When famine was a fact of life, the humans who survived were those who could stay "fueled" even when the environment didn't provide sufficient food for fuel.

The human body we each have today is practically identical to the model designed approximately three million years ago for a very different lifestyle. Life has changed radically, but our bodies haven't. Today, unlimited quantities of food are readily available to most of us—a situation that did not exist during the eons when the human body was evolving. We have bodies that are brilliant at making, storing, and conserving fat—at a time in history when, in America at least, that's no longer necessary.

WHY FAT? As stored fuel goes, fat boasts many advantages over carbohydrate. If you were designing the human machine for survival, you'd choose fat as most efficient for storage. There are a number of reasons for this.

More MPG (miles per gram). A gram of fat will take you more than twice as far as the same quantity of carbohydrate. Fat has 9.3 calories per gram. Protein and carbohydrate each provide 4.1 calories for every gram. Therefore, even 2 grams of either carbohydrate or protein would not provide as much fuel/energy/calories as only 1 gram of fat. Why store 2 grams and get 8 calories of stored fuel, when you can store 1 gram and get 9 calories?

Slow and steady. Fat is also efficient as a rainy-day fuel because it burns very slowly. Fat reserves by design are not depleted rapidly, even when you do "dip in" to them. A person with bodyfat in the average range could live off fat stores for two to four months, an obese person four to six months. Remember that fat is usually the background fuel. It burns so slowly that it would be virtually impossible for any of us under normal circumstances to use it all up. That's a safeguard.

No limits. Remember I said the body cannot store excess protein as protein, and can store only tiny amounts of carbohydrate as carbohydrate? Well, the body can store fat as fat—in unlimited amounts. That means no matter how much your body decides it should put away, your body will never run out of room. It will stash it somewhere. We don't always like where, but, frankly, your body doesn't care what you look like in a skirt. It is a machine engineered for self-preservation. If it runs out of fat cells to pack fat into, it will simply manufacture more fat cells.

MULTIPLE FAT-CREATION STRATEGIES. Since stored fuel is the link to life in the event of famine, and fat is the storage fuel of choice, your body actually has multiple methods of ensuring that this lifesaving padding is sufficient when you eat (or don't eat) in a way that hints of a "fuel recession." Your body will gather, save, and resist "spending" fat.

In addition to using lean muscle to create emergency glucose in response to a "fuel shortage," a poorly fueled body will also:

Make more fat. Your body can make fat out of any food you eat—even if it's not fat to begin with. Protein and carbohydrate can both be turned into fat. If eaten in ideal amounts (total daily calories about 15 to 25 percent protein, 60 to 70 percent carb) they'll be used for their own purposes rather than converted. But more of everything you eat is converted to fat if the system detects a need to stock up.

One of the few conversions that doesn't happen is from fat to anything else. Remember? Except in minimal, inadequate amounts, fat cannot be converted to glucose or glycogen or any other form of carbohydrate (only about 5 percent of a fat molecule's total weight—not sufficient to adequately fuel the brain and nervous system—can become glucose). That's why it is muscle/protein, not fat, that is used to replenish glucose levels when you're starved of carbohydrate. Neither can fat be converted to protein. Fat is either immediately burned as energy—or stored and potentially used later for energy. *Fat is fat and that's that.* And why not? A smart machine wouldn't offer any way of turning its crucial backup fuel into anything else. Fat is designed for keeps.

Store more fat. If you tell your body "food is scarce!" it will ensure that your rainy-day fuel—fat—gets stored efficiently. It creates a fertile environment for the storage of fat, encouraging the fat you eat to be stored rather than used, and more of other fuels to be converted. One way it rolls out the red carpet for fat storage is by increasing the production of lipoprotein lipase (LPL), an enzyme designed to transform dietary fat into stored fat (adipose tissue). Because of the expediency with which LPL does this, it has been dubbed "gatekeeper of the fat cell."

Studies show that LPL quantities increase significantly during periods of calorie reduction, and that it takes much longer for those enzyme levels to return to normal than it does for them to increase.

This means when you starve yourself, you actually increase the body's natural propensity for storing fat from food. When you stop starving and start eating (maybe even bingeing, because you've made yourself hysterical with hunger), your body's heightened fat-storage enzyme level doesn't dissipate immediately; the return to normal levels is a slow process. So your body remains for some time biochemically as eager to store fat as you are to eat food.

Conserve fat. Yet another way your body guards against fat loss is to be thrifty about spending it. Is a giant recession the logical time to recklessly spend your savings? Then why expect your body to freely part with fuel saved to sustain you in famine—when how you eat (or don't) suggests famine is imminent?

Thus, as a third main safeguard to prepare you for a famine, when your body senses too little fuel coming in consistently it will slow down its use of fuel to "stretch" whatever it receives and guard its stores. This usually shows up as a decline in our basal metabolic rate (BMR).

YOU HAVE SOMETHING TO SAY ABOUT YOUR BODY'S RAINY DAY. The fact that your body is greatly skilled in making, storing, and conserving fat doesn't mean it must use those skills. (You may be very good at the firing range, but having the skill doesn't mean you randomly go around shooting.) The body activates its complex fat-maximizing systems when it's signaled to do so—but we don't have to set those systems in motion.

The problem is that we do. Typical American eating patterns give false signals that hyperactivate these fat conservation systems. The main premise of starvation for "weight loss" is "my body will have to use up my excess fat if I don't give it anything else." But as you've already learned, the body doesn't run on fat alone. If it runs low on carb fuel it will relinquish fat-burning muscle tissue for conversion to glucose. You can't get your body to use fat and fat alone, because it won't. Body fat can never be converted into glucose to feed the brain adequately.

In fact, without carbohydrate, fat can't even break down properly. The fat you do lose while eliminating carbohydrates from your diet is not being burned cleanly. "Without sufficient carbohydrate, the body can't use its fat in the normal way. (Carbohydrate is needed to combine with the fat fragments so that they can be used for energy.) So the body has to go into ketosis (using fat without the help of carbohydrate), a condition in which unusual products of fat breakdown (ketone bodies) accumulate in the blood." (*Nutrition: Concepts and Controversies*, Eva May Nunnelley Hamilton et al., 1991.) Ketosis is definitely an unhealthy process for anyone, and can even cause brain damage and mental retardation in infants of women who experience it during pregnancy.

PRE-FAMINE: READY, SET. . . . Sometimes people ask why the body doesn't use fat when we starve ourselves, if starvation is what it's saving the fat for. The answer is that your body is saving fat for the real thing. Storage and maintenance occur in *preparation* for famine. You get ready, you get set—but you don't go. Real famine is a life-threatening condition, and most Americans probably won't ever be exposed to it.

And that's something to be thankful for. Your body would need to be in the midst of an authentic famine to actually begin the advanced, unnatural, and unhealthy emergency process of making fat its mainstay fuel. After three to five days of absolutely no food, your body would back off of muscle breakdown and begin digging into the fat cache it has created. The only possibility for making carbohydrate available would be conversion of your own muscle, so once the body lays off to preserve lean tissue, fat is used incompletely, as described above. This is the kind of wholesale starvation the Somalis, for example, endure.

This would be a rather dramatic and dangerous way to lose fat, not to mention miserable—and, most of all, unnecessary.

TAKING PRE-FAMINE SERIOUSLY. Shoring up for a famine is as unnecessary as actually having one. Since starvation grooms your body for fatness, a key to getting your body willing and able to use fat is reconciling your definition of starvation with that of your body.

The level of denial at which your body's red-alert is engineered to go off may not be a level you recognize as deprivation. Because of diet thinking's distorted perspective, what is devastating to your body may feel "normal." You may think: "I'm just skipping lunch." "I'm just trying to lose weight." "I'll eat later." "I forgot." "I was too busy to eat."

Many believe hunger is good, that it means "losing weight." Satiety becomes almost sacrilegious. The result of this thinking, and the eating habits that accompany it, are bodies that are always in a state of shoring up, constantly suspended in the pre-famine preparatory phase. A real famine never actually arrives. We just keep preparing . . . and preparing . . . and that's a major reason why America is overfat. Starving is fattening—and dieting, which at least half of all Americans are doing—is self-imposed starvation.

EASY, ENJOYABLE EATING SIDESTEPS FAT CREATION. Happily, to avoid sending these signals is a function of avoiding starvation—or anything close to it. That means doing something you probably won't mind at all—eating carbs steadily throughout the day (as well as that small amount of lean protein at each meal).

Even if you've trained your body to be thrifty, it can be retrained to be spendy. It just takes time—and patience. It doesn't happen overnight. You've got momentum in one direction; you've got to slow down that momentum, do a hairpin turn, and get going in the other direction. But it can be done. Given that you've got a whole lifetime, why not start now?

EATING FAT

LESS FAT, YES—NOT LESS FOOD!

Eating more fat than is used as fuel *will* also make a body fat. All but the most athletically challenged bodies will consistently use more carbohydrate than fat. If you consume more fat than the small amount your body needs, it will—surprise!—be stored as fat.

Clearly, though, a fat-fertile body is the product of much more than fat consumption alone. Just cutting dietary fat won't change your shape much. If you cut much food out with the fat, you'll train your body to get fat and stay fat. You may lose "weight"—but it will be mainly muscle.

Now you can see why "eating too much" is not the issue you think it is. Most people I teach eat *too little* to fuel their activity. Clients who claim to "overeat," it turns out, consume just a fraction of what I do. One client told me she drank diet soda all day to quiet her hunger. This is common—and senseless. Hunger is not "bad"! It's because of your meager eating—not in spite of it—that your body makes and stores more fat, and uses less. "Too much" may apply to fat or protein, but surprisingly rarely to total food volume.

YOU DON'T NEED TO ADD ANY!

There are a couple of distinctions to make when it comes to consuming fat.

The first is *source fat vs. added fat*. This distinguishes between the fat that is already naturally in food and the fat that we add to food.

Source fat is that which is already in food. The 8 grams of fat in a 4-ounce chicken breast is source fat. The olive oil you sauté it in is added fat. The 2 grams of fat in ⅔ cup oatmeal is source fat (even plain grains contain a small amount of naturally occurring fat). The fat in the cup of whole milk you add to the oatmeal is added fat.

Since most food has some source fat, it would be impossible to eat a completely nonfat diet without restricting food variety so severely that overall nutrition would be compromised. So the idea is not to eat a nonfat diet—though I've met many people who think that is the goal (or who think they already do it).

What is a low-fat diet? Let's simplify all the media-borne clutter on this and look at the facts. The U.S. Recommended Dietary Allowance suggests that 30 percent of your calories or fewer come from fat. Most disease, research, and nutrition experts today recommend 20 percent; research on several types of cancer have suggested that 30 percent is still well above the threshold that impacts prevention. Prevention diets for breast cancer, for example, are consistently close to 20 percent.

To give you a frame of reference, I now average a 10 percent fat diet (although my daily intake can vary between 8 and 20 percent of calories from fat, based on approximately 2,500 calories a day). This is lower in fat than I suggest to the average person, although it is the percentage Pritikin insisted upon, and the one Dr. Dean Ornish uses to reverse heart disease. I'm more conservative with what I recommend to our clients because 10 percent is still considered extreme by the "mainstream" health community and may seem that way to clients as well.

I definitely encourage a minimum of 10 percent, because there is still very limited data on how less might affect the body. Less, for example, may inhibit proper use of fat-soluble vitamins. And it seems sensible to me that if your body makes, stores, and saves fat more zealously when deprived of carbohydrate fuel or just total caloric intake, a too-stingy fat intake might well trigger a similar response. Still, I'd bet that if it should ever be found that eating less than 10 percent of calories from fat is "too little" for whatever reason, the negatives probably won't even begin to approach those associated with a 40 percent fat diet.

It's true that we need some fat in our diet, but the amount we absolutely need is less than one-twelfth of the average American's intake. Today that average intake hovers between 36 and 42 percent—and it's been stuck there for a long time. Having fat comprise 3 percent of your diet would be sufficient for vital functions. You could get the trace amount of fatty acid that's critical to cell life from a small bowl of plain oatmeal or a couple of slices of wheat bread. Again, though, that doesn't mean you should shoot for 3 percent, which is a minimum for survival, not a level for thriving.

SATURATED VS. UNSATURATED/ANIMAL VS. VEGETABLE

The fat our bodies do need to operate is unsaturated fat. The saturated fat that clogs our arteries is *totally unnecessary* to human functioning. So if anyone ever tells you, "Well, some butter or beef is good, because you need fat in your diet," tell them to go drink a can of Pennzoil. Eating a steak because your body "needs some fat" is like pouring 10 quarts of heavy-weight motor oil into your car, when all it needs is a little more lubrication to make it run optimally.

Saturated fat is that which is found in animal products. The fat in meat, poultry, fish, dairy products, and eggs is saturated fat. Also, tropical oils— such as palm and coconut—are saturated. These items each have different amounts of fat—some may be relatively low in fat, some high—but regardless of the amount, all of it is saturated fat.

Unsaturated fat is fat found in vegetable or plant products. That means the fat in foods like avocados, nuts, seeds, and olives is unsaturated. Olive oil, almond oil, canola oil, corn oil, sunflower oil, safflower oil, peanut oil— these are all unsaturated.

But what does "saturated" mean? How is it different from "unsaturated" fat? You parrot the words, you nod and grab for the unsaturated—but few know why.

It's pretty simple. Each molecule of fat is a chemical compound—remember high school chemistry?—and one of its "parts" is carbon. In a saturated fat, every single carbon atom has a hydrogen atom attached. Therefore, that fat is considered to be "saturated" with hydrogen. Think "soaked." In an unsaturated fat, only one (monounsaturated) or two (polyunsaturated) of the carbons have hydrogens attached. Therefore, this fat is not saturated—i.e., *un*saturated.

So, what does fat saturated with hydrogen mean to you and me? To our bodies, it means several things. First of all, the hydrogen increases the "stickiness" of blood platelets. Platelets are one of the main components of our blood, along with red cells, white cells, and plasma. Sticky blood platelets can "clump up"—favoring the formation of blood clots and thereby increasing the risk of stroke. That same tackiness is a contributing factor in the complex process by which plaque builds up on artery walls. The saturated fat itself is part of the material that forms plaque. Saturated fat has also been shown to raise blood pressure and has been linked to diabetes as well as intestinal cancers and cancer of the colon, prostate, uterus, and breast. (These happen to be America's most frequently-occurring cancers.)

It's important to know that saturated fat can be man-made as well as "natural." Anyone who has read labels will be familiar with the term "hydrogenated" or "partially hydrogenated." This refers to the addition of hydrogen to an oil that was unsaturated, so that the oil will be solid at room temperature. (A high health price to pay for being able to spread your fat, I'd say.)

CHOLESTEROL

Another strike against saturated fat is that it also increases the production of cholesterol by the body. Our bodies *produce* cholesterol, and that's an important fact that too few people realize.

People with alarming cholesterol levels go to great lengths to eliminate cholesterol-containing foods from the diet—sometimes while continuing to eat a diet fairly high in saturated fat. (Packaged and processed foods that boast "no cholesterol" still may contain saturated fat.) Or people switch from eggs (275 milligrams of cholesterol each) to a cinnamon roll with butter ("only" 31 milligrams per tablespoon). In fact, they are doing little to counteract the problem. They wonder why their cholesterol isn't going down—and then give up on making any changes at all, because "it didn't work." No one told them the whole story, so once again incomplete information is the downfall of efficient eating.

Cholesterol—like fat—is not an enemy per se. Your body produces its own because cholesterol has important functions, just as fat does. Cholesterol is a transporter of fats and thus essential to survival; it also insulates nerve fibers and cell membranes. Most of us are familiar with at least two of the five different kinds of lipoproteins that comprise cholesterol—low density (LDL) and high density (HDL). I could write an entire chapter just on the various functions of each.

But all you need to know is that lipoproteins make it possible for fat to be transported to various destinations (the liver, fat cells, muscle cells) and so the more fat you consume, the more cholesterol your body must make available to "partner up" with that fat for transporation. Excess cholesterol is part of the mixture that forms the basis for arterial plaque, and it also has the opportunity to clot your blood.

A "normal" cholesterol level is a difficult thing to determine. Medical science is still divided on the question, and part of the problem is that standards tend to be pretty lenient. Nathan Wong, Director of Preventive Cardiology at the University of California at Irvine, pointed out: "A lot of times, doctors will say a (total) cholesterol level of 200 to 250 is 'normal.' But we have to recognize that in this country, it's unhealthy to be 'normal.' It's 'normal' here to die of a heart attack or heart disease." (*Orange County Register*, November 2, 1991)

Indeed, in the 1950s, when Nathan Pritikin began his self-healing journey, his cholesterol was 300—and that was considered normal! Fortunately for him (and for millions of others who have benefited from his research and questioning), he didn't buy it. Common consensus these days is that a total cholesterol of under 200 is healthful, while another movement suggests that 150 is the desired target (since that is close to the average cholesterol level in nations with low-fat diets and low rates of the diseases that are epidemics here).

If you get your cholesterol tested, always get your HDL and LDL tested as well as total cholesterol. (This requires a blood workup done after a 12-hour fast—which is something I'd obviously never recommend doing except for this purpose. But those finger-prick tests at the mall don't do the same job.) The reason you want to know your HDL and LDL levels is because the ratio of HDL to LDL is more significant than total cholesterol. HDL is often referred to as "good" cholesterol—it carries fatty acids from your blood to the liver for processing and is protein-dense (rather than fat-dense like LDL and other types of cholesterol).

My total cholesterol (187) could probably go lower. I do eat animal (saturated) fat in chicken, fish, and turkey; if I were to eliminate those, my total cholesterol would likely drop. It's now an informed choice I could make. So can you. Some people will be willing to eliminate animal fat entirely, some significantly, some less so. Although I don't rule out being a vegetarian someday, I'm not interested right now—I like turkey sandwiches. But, *total* fat in my diet is still 10 to 15 percent calories from fat, and my *saturated* fat consumption is well below 10 percent. Plus, my HDL is 74, making the ratio excellent.

FAT IS FAT AND THAT'S THAT

All of this means that if you are going to add fat (and, remember, you don't ever need to because you will get more than enough source fat), the unsaturated oil is a healthier choice, given all the current data. Unsaturated fat will not clog your arteries, cause clotting, or stimulate cholesterol production. In fact, studies have shown unsaturated fat consumption to cause a lowering of blood cholesterol.

But this can be taken out of context, because *unsaturated fat is still fat*. While our arteries may be discriminating about saturated versus unsaturated, our fat cells aren't. *Either* kind can be stored and thus make you fat. A 40 percent unsaturated fat diet may be somewhat healthier in terms of the fat's direct effect on atherosclerosis or clotting, but it will still likely make you fat, which is not healthy. And while consuming unsaturated fats has been shown to decrease blood cholesterol levels, if you aren't eating a lot of saturated fat and cholesterol, you won't need to "put out the fire" by consuming more of a different fat to counteract it.

In addition, recent studies have shown that while the villain of the cardiovascular disease epidemic is saturated fat, cancers may be caused by either kind of fat. Breast cancer, in particular, appears to be just as sensitive to high unsaturated fat consumption. (Both diseases—and a host of others—are affected by high bodyfat as well as high dietary fat.)

In our zealous desire to eschew the dietary bad guy of the day, we often lose sight of the whole picture. While saturated fat consumption is still high in the United States, it has declined over the past several years. Why then has total fat consumption remained constant? Because as Americans eliminated some saturated fat, they replaced it with unsaturated fat.

The healthiest strategy is to eliminate fat where you can—not to replace it with a marginally "better" fat.

KNOW YOUR BRANDS

Clearly, part of fueling yourself efficiently is knowing what "brands" of fuel are available to you. The chart on the next page briefly reviews the main features of each so that you'll be better able to evaluate "dietary advice" in the future.

Now that you've got the core facts, let's take fueling one step further.

"BRANDS" OF FUEL

the Body Can Use—And How, When, and Why It Does

Think of calories as a "miles per gallon" measurement.
The number tells you how energy-intensive that fuel is—how far each gram of it will take you.

"Body fuels" differ not only by how many calories of energy they can provide per gram, but in how the body uses them, and under what circumstances. All fuels are not equal; in the same way, all calories are not equal!

4 calories per gram	4 calories per gram	9 calories per gram
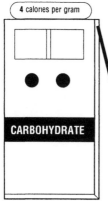	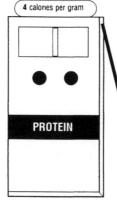	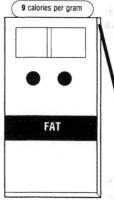
CARBOHYDRATE	**PROTEIN**	**FAT**

- The #1, immediate source of energy your body depends on.
- Easily converted to glucose ("blood sugar"), which fuels the work of most body cells and the brain and nervous system.
- Stable, relatively slow breakdown provides steady supply of fuel without erratic ups and downs.
- Body resists storing it as fat; other uses take priority.
- Tiny amounts of carbohydrate are stored, in a form called glycogen.
- Whether you use, convert, or store it, you'll expend energy (burn even more fuel) to process it.
- Complex carb foods typically are high in fiber as well.

- Not an efficient source of energy to fuel the body; not the body's first choice.
- Important for tissue repair, maintenance, building.
- Don't need much but need it consistently—small amounts regularly (such as at meals).
- Excess is stored as fat; this conversion is stressful.
- Body can convert protein (from food or your muscle tissue) to carbohydrate fuel in an emergency—but the process is toxic and harmful.

- The body's choice for "storage fuel"—the most efficient way to store energy.
- The body constantly uses small amounts as fuel, and larger amounts during extended aerobic activity.
- Only in the latter stages of progressive famine will the body use large stores just to sustain basic functions.
- Normally, the body "saves" more and spends less when it gets too little food/fuel (to prepare for famine) via several key mechanisms.
- The body can create more fat if signaled of potential fuel shortages.
- Little energy is required to turn food fat into bodyfat.

4

EXERCISE:
Increasing the Fuel Demand

We've established that muscle is responsible for burning the food you eat; as the only significant metabolically active tissue in the body, it is the largest determinant of your metabolism. More muscle, more fuel needed; less muscle, less fuel needed.

In addition to muscle mass, how much fuel you burn and how fast also depends on your activity level—how hard, fast, and often you run the machine. So your need for fuel is affected by not only the size of the engine, but also by how far the "machine" goes.

Exercise is a valuable tool for toggling your "fuel demand" because it impacts both factors: It affects the size, shape, and efficiency of the engine (your muscle mass), and it is a primary component of your activity level (and the amount you do is totally in your control).

BMR (BASAL METABOLIC RATE)

Your basal metabolic rate (BMR), which varies from person to person, is a third factor in fuel-burning efficiency. It refers to the amount of energy (fuel,

82

calories) your body needs. Sometimes research (or, more often, an article reporting research) indicates that the "energy cost" for the body at rest is 1,200 to 1,400 calories per day. But this generic interpretation is easily misunderstood. Because muscle mass size affects the amount of energy your body requires, we know that it must differ from person to person, just as muscle mass size does.

To some extent, genetics does seem to affect what that base energy "cost," or rate, is. The amount of energy your body demands (and needs you to consume), whether active or at rest, will vary even among people with the same amount of muscle. However, that variance is not as dramatic as the layperson often assumes; certainly, one's "natural" basal metabolism does not impact overall ability to be lean and fit nearly as much as some like to think. Despite what those who consider themselves too "genetically disadvantaged" to achieve fitness assume, the BMR gap between individuals may be reduced or even closed because the two factors we can change (muscle mass size and activity level) are each more powerful than the one we're born with.

Using our activity level and muscle mass as tools, each of us can affect the BMR we're given. Although BMR exists as a fuel-burning factor distinct from muscle mass and activity level, it nonetheless can be altered by changes in the other two. By increasing your lean body mass and your activity level, you can increase your BMR—just as you've seen that you can decrease your BMR by decreasing lean body mass through deprivation.

Exercise assists with increasing lean body mass, *and* increases BMR directly. Aerobic exercise boosts metabolism during the activity *and* keeps it somewhat elevated afterward. It also creates a greater demand for energy from both fat and carbohydrate than the demand your body makes if you're not exercising. Bodyfat may be "spent" by the body to meet that increased energy cost. Similarly, weight-bearing exercise (which can be aerobic or anaerobic but is usually anaerobic) helps build lean muscle tissue, which makes you a better, faster food-burner whether active or at rest.

The point here is not whether the person standing next to you was born with a faster metabolism—it's that you have the power to do something about it.

WHAT EXERCISE CAN'T DO: THE MYTHS

Covert Bailey, author of *Fit or Fat*, has referred to this as creating "a better butter burner." I dislike this characterization because it derives from and bolsters two diet-thinking assumptions. The first is that people must and will continue to eat butter and other unnecessary fats, and thus the only answer is to manipulate the body to handle it better.

The second is the fallacy that "If you exercise, you can eat anything you want," or "Exercise cancels out whatever you eat." People often expect exercise to do something, all on its own, that it simply cannot do.

Putting exercise before diet, or making it The One Solution, does not work. It simply doesn't bear out that exercise "buys" you the freedom to consume unlimited butter (or other fats, sugars, or anything else damaging to the body) without consequences. If I had to choose now, I'd eat no butter and not exercise instead of exercising and eating loads of butter.

Exercise is enormously beneficial, but it's blown way out of proportion with respect to eating. Further, basic biology, new research, and my own experience all show that not only does exercise not absolve a multitude of sins; without fuel, it doesn't do much of anything. To get the benefit of either fat burning or muscle building, exercise requires that *you start out fueled*—a critical, yet seldom-heeded distinction.

MYTH: EXERCISE AUTOMATICALLY PREVENTS HEART DISEASE

Exercise does not "clean out" your veins. Being a "better butter burner" *may* keep your hips, thighs, or tummy trimmer, but not the inside of your arteries. Exercise alone does not prevent heart disease. (Too many seemingly fit athletes have died of heart attacks or strokes.)

Exercise *has* been shown to increase HDL, which can improve your overall ratio, but to rely on that alone to manage cholesterol is a very narrow approach. It's like relying on better driving to compensate for a car without brakes or steering fluid. Exercise won't neatly "counteract" atherosclerosis if you're loading up on saturated fats, causing your liver to continually pump excess cholesterol into your blood.

Eating a high-fat diet and expecting your exercise to compensate for the resultant high blood cholesterol level or bodyfat increase is an extension of the "magic pill" approach to fitness. Exercise becomes The One Thing that you hope will cancel out your other poor habits. In the end, all the gyrations to avoid dealing with the eating part of health and fitness are not only futile, but take far more effort than it would simply to deal with eating.

MYTH: EXERCISE WILL HELP YOU "KEEP" MUSCLE DURING DIETING OR BUILD MUSCLE NO MATTER WHAT

Exercise alone does not automatically build muscle. Without the proper fuel, your body cannot make or build much of anything—in fact, if you are underfueled, your body will "eat" your muscle faster than you can build it. It takes a few days to lose muscle but months, even years, to build it back.

Yet the media and health-care and research professionals continue to insist that exercise is The Key for obesity or for "keeping it off." "The trick to stilling the yo-yo, experts agree, is exercise," said a *Shape* magazine exposé on diet companies and weight loss in March 1992. This statement has inaccurate implications: It implies that exercise is the single most important thing you can do for your health, even before consistent eating. It suggests a belief that the body can somehow magically maintain or build muscle even when it is deprived of the fuels it needs to do so. It also says it's reasonable to urge dieting (starving) people to increase their energy expenditure.

All of this flies in the face of basic biology. In fact, muscle loss from underfueling guarantees that the yo-yo syndrome will be perpetuated—and exercise without fuel will hasten, not stave off muscle loss.

Here's an example. If I am eating 800 calories a day, and I really need at least 1,200 more (mostly carbohydrate) to fuel my body's activities, there is no way any kind of exercise will allow me to maintain or build muscle. In fact, it will speed up muscle loss, because the exercise is creating an even greater need for fuel, which is not met by my measly 800 calories.

Why isn't this simple logic ever reported? If it had been, I'd have realized sooner why my five years of weight-lifting three to four hours a week never built a single pound of muscle or a single "cut" in definition. The time I wasted! As I emphasize is so often the case, just a bit of simple information was the solution: After a year or two of plentiful fueling, I was able to build 15 pounds of muscle and all the definition I wanted with only 45 minutes a week of exercise with weights. (Yes, I ate more and exercised *less*.)

The key to maintaining muscle is not exercise—*the key is eating enough!* The trick to stilling the yo-yo is not to lose any muscle, and that means not eating so little that you train your body to keep you fat and famine-prepared. They say, "Exercise while you diet and then you'll keep your muscle!" But that's not only admitting that dieting causes muscle loss—it's mistakenly asking you to exhaust yourself to save it with an effort that, under those circumstances, actually makes it worse.

Human physiology dictates that the way to keep your muscle is to not diet in the first place. Instead, eat enough fuel so your body never needs to use muscle, and so exercise is not a drain. If you want to build muscle, the key is to do weight-resistance training while eating a mainly healthy, balanced, and *ample* complex carb-laced-with-lean protein diet you enjoy.

MYTH: EXERCISE "CANCELS FAT" (OR FOOD)

Exercise does not magically negate or nullify fat—or anything else—in the diet. That many Americans make this assumption (I did!) is a perfect example of the hopeful, simplistic explanations we fabricate to justify our actions.

A March 1993 *Allure* article on exercise addicts typifies this: "It starts out logically. An indulgent midnight snack is undone with a half-hour on the StairMaster the morning after." Only in diet thinking is this "logical"! Food cannot be "undone," nor should you want to undo it. We need food, so there's no sense in trying to flush it out or eliminate it. The article goes on to complain that this supposedly sensible-in-moderation strategy can escalate into a constant quest for "damage control" called exercise bulimia. But the problem isn't just that this type of strategy can get out of control; the problem is it never worked to begin with. It's not scientifically sound.

You can't just "burn it all off"—you've seen that the way food works in the body is not a simplistic food-in, energy-out process. The body is specific about which fuels it uses for what purposes. Different kinds of exercise demand different fuels, in different amounts. Besides, exercising solely because you ate food and must "get rid of it" is like driving just because you put gasoline in the car.

There's no getting around that what you eat makes a difference. Yet you try and try to get around it anyway, hoping exercise is a possible shortcut. If you eat without purpose or precision—if you are not properly fueled—you will not enjoy exercise as much; you will not get optimal results from it; and you may in fact be wasting your time completely.

That's why I teach eating, not exercise. Too many people exercise their butts off and don't eat worth a damn. Then they wonder why it's not working, why their hard work isn't paying off. Such frustration means suffering—and sometimes quitting. Once that happens, obviously no benefits are reaped at all.

WHAT DOES EXERCISE DO?

EXERCISE BOOSTS MUSCLE QUANTITY

Weight training is the new rage, according to the women's magazines I read. Recent studies on exercisers show that those who complement *aerobic workouts* with some form of *resistance training* lose more "weight" (usually reported this way, though they mean fat) and gain muscle, too. The articles excitedly point out that weight training with aerobics seems to boost metabolism (as if it's some incredible new discovery never before dreamed of, when the simple fact is that weight training can build muscle and increased muscle means increased metabolism—this is just good old biology).

Some reporting assumes that the pairing of the two types of exercise, one performed right after the other, is relevant to or responsible for the results. There may be some special benefit to pairing the two in the same workout, and there may not. To be certain, we'd have to see studies on subjects who did aerobics a few times a week and did weight training separately (as I do) and see if they don't also build muscle and lose fat (as I have).

While the back-to-back combo might be ideal, it doesn't mean that splitting up the two types will yield nothing. The "ideal" yielded is probably marginal, if it exists at all. That's the case with most "ideals"—though unfortunately people often use them to discount their efforts. We go crazy trying to do it exactly the way the researchers of the latest study think is ideal, assume we're getting no value if we don't, and skip exercise entirely if circumstances preclude perfect adherence to every detail. Indeed, reporting often supports this kind of thinking.

But one core truth gets lost in all the hype: *any* exercise is better than none at all. Sure, it's great to experiment with your routines by incorporating the latest research, but don't overreact to unfounded emphasis on minutiae. If study subjects did 22 minutes of something, don't abandon all effort because you can only do 20. It's far more important to simply remember these basics:

EATING TAKES PRIORITY. Muscle is precious, but before you go crazy jerking weights up and down to get some, take one step back: There's something to consider about muscle even before exercise, and it's eating. Eating saves muscle *and* is preparation for building it. If you are tearing muscle apart to use as fuel and if you're not providing enough lean protein for use as building blocks to make more muscle, you cannot increase the size of your fuel-burning engine.

WEIGHT-BEARING EXERCISE BUILDS MUSCLE. The kind of exercise that builds muscle most efficiently is weight-resistance training—with free weights or circuit machines such as Nautilus®, Cybex®, or Lifecircuit®. Any weight-bearing exercise will build to some degree the muscle used—for example, running or bicycling will build (as well as shape) muscles of the legs. To achieve balanced muscle increases, and especially to fully develop the upper body, however, you need a steady program of weight training using specific machines and/or exercises with weights.

MORE MUSCLE DEMANDS MORE FOOD. How can you know if you've added enough muscle to warrant more food? A bodyfat test will tell you (provided you have an earlier number to compare it to), and you may be able to *see* added muscle, depending on how much fat you're carrying over it. But if you reach the point where you listen to your body—you fuel it and take care of it and love it and honor it, and keep it "clean" inside most of the time—you'll hear it calling for more fuel. It can be as subtle as eating essentially the same things in the same amount for a while and being satisfied—and suddenly finding you are consistently hungry even with the ample amount of food you have been consuming.

This happened to me. I "knew" I had gained muscle (and upped my carbohydrate intake appropriately) long before a body composition test confirmed that it was true. After I had gained 5 or 6 pounds of lean muscle, the breakfast and lunch I had been eating consistently began to feel insufficient. Then it dawned on me; I was feeling leaner and looking more sinewy; I had seen steady increases in the amount of weight I could lift. I must have gained muscle.

I weighed myself several times over the next few weeks and found that indeed my weight was consistently up several pounds. I knew it was not fat, because I was fueling, and the fit of my skirts and pants hadn't changed.

To feed this added muscle that was demanding fuel, I added another carbohydrate serving to breakfast (increasing from 3 servings to 4, or from about 45 grams of carbohydrate to 60) and had an extra carbohydrate serving (about 15 grams) at mid-morning snack time. It felt great, and I found I was fine the rest of the day with my previous intake. I've since made similar adjustments as I continue to add muscle.

You can experiment. It may take just 1 carb serving, maybe 2 or 3; it may work best to add it at snacks or at meals. Just remember: If you're hungry, your body is telling you something. It's good news.

EXERCISE ENHANCES MUSCLE QUALITY

Proper eating will give you the necessary "building blocks" to build not only *more* muscle, but also *better quality* muscle when you exercise. Increasing the fat-usage enzymes that are produced inside muscle cells takes exercise. The more you exercise your muscles, the more of these enzymes your muscles make, and the more efficient you become at using fat for fuel during exercise—and, increasingly, at rest as well. This means your muscles have enhanced their capacity for *oxidative metabolism*.

Since fitter muscles are better able to use fat for fuel, less of the fat you consume will be stored as fat, as more of the fat you consume is burned for energy. Further, if all of the fat your muscles demand cannot be obtained from your low-fat diet, your body will turn to stored fat to fill the need.

Also, when muscle quality improves, exercise gets easier. Regular activity stimulates the production of fat-usage enzymes so your muscles are better equipped to grab and use the fuel they need for that activity. That's one of the reasons that the more you exercise, the better you feel and the easier it is. This is part of what it means to "get in shape"; you can go harder and faster than before, and it taxes your body no more than a lower intensity of exercise once did. The muscles are improving their ability to use fat, thus sustaining energy even at higher intensity levels while sparing glucose and glycogen stores so they won't be used up quickly and leave you "low."

EXERCISE ITSELF SPEEDS METABOLISM

Our bodies use fuel even when we're not exercising—even when we sleep or sit at a desk. But the more active we are, the more fuel we use. When we exercise, we burn energy obtained from various fuels (and measured in calories) at a higher than normal resting rate *long after the exercise is over*. That elevated metabolic rate is not as high as during the actual exercise, but it is higher than if you had done nothing but sit around.

You may have read about this; it has been called the "afterburn" or the "bonus burn." To me, it makes more sense to call the burning of fuel you do during exercise the "bonus." That burning might occur for a half-hour, an hour, however long you exercise. The "afterburn" may last four to eight hours. That makes much more of a long-term difference than what you burn during exercise.

If you exercise regularly, you will have regular four- to eight-hour periods of elevated metabolism. The more of these periods you have, the closer and closer you get to simply burning fuel at a higher-than-standard rate all the time.

EXERCISE CREATES A DEMAND FOR BODY FAT AS FUEL

Remember "spot-reducing"? I do. In the 1970s, I remember reading in magazines about various exercises that would magically dissipate unwanted fat. Sit-ups would suck away my tummy fat; push-ups would trim unsightly upper-arm bulges.

A corollary fallacy, which I still not only hear from individuals but also read in many magazines and newspapers, is the notion that fat can be turned into muscle, or vice versa. One health-food store newsletter carried an article that said, "It is more desirable to turn fat and flab into toned flesh and muscles."

First of all, fat cannot be turned into anything but fat—or energy. It certainly cannot "turn into" muscle. Fat and muscle are two completely different types of tissue, and one cannot ever be turned into the other.

Second, to say "fat and flab" implies that they are two different things, but there is no such thing as "flab" distinct from fat. Flab is a meaningless euphemism—it's just fat. Third, flesh—skin—cannot be "toned." Only the muscle underneath can be shaped and firmed.

Finally, no exercise can remove fat from specific places on the body or target individual fat deposits. Adipose tissue—your stored bodyfat—is universal storage. Your personal pattern of fat distribution is chiefly a matter of nature and nurture. The only way to get your body to use any of it is (1) to eat so that your body is not signaled to hang on to it for dear life, (2) to not provide ample fat in the food you eat, and (3) to have your body burn fuel at a rate where fat is in demand. Exercise is valuable in the latter sense both because it creates an increased demand for fuel, and because aerobic exercise is a situation in which your body finds fat to be an ideal fuel.

When exercise—or when just having a big engine (muscle mass)—calls for fat as fuel, your body may signal for the release of stored fat into the bloodstream. From there it is distributed into the muscle cells to be "burned" as energy. That stored fat is released *from all over the body*. Use of arm muscles doesn't mean fat sitting atop your arm muscles will necessarily be used.

Using muscles in the thigh area doesn't mean you'll use up your "thigh fat." You can't eliminate the "tire" of fat around the middle through sit-ups. You can certainly strengthen and build the abdominal muscles beneath the fat, which helps your appearance somewhat. But those muscles will still be hidden beneath the fat, unless an overall demand for fat fuel causes bodyfat to be relinquished.

Most people find that when they lose only fat, without the muscle loss that's inherent to deprivation, fat is lost quite evenly from all over the body. This may be one reason why it seems slow and minuscule this way—because big "chunks" aren't taken from one place. It's slowly and evenly drawn from all over. Some people do tend to lose from certain places first; there are theories that male and female bodies favor different places for fat storage and fat usage. Other theories hold that fat most recently "packed away" will be broken out of storage first, with the "oldest" stored fat being the last to go.

IN SUMMARY. Fueling comes first—before any of the several factors that must be present for fat loss. Your body must be willing to part with stored fuel—and if you're not regularly, properly fueled, your body will be reluctant to spend its "savings." Then there must be a demand for fat; several factors offer opportunities to increase that demand, including aerobic exercise itself, boosted metabolic burning after exercise, and more muscle. Finally, stored bodyfat will be called on only when the diet isn't so rich in fat that bodyfat is unneeded. If fat is always more than readily available in the food you eat, your body needn't go to the trouble of breaking some out of storage. It will live off the fat in your diet and save what's on your body.

WHAT KINDS OF EXERCISE WORK BEST?

First off, let me say that my philosophy about exercise is that any kind works better than no kind at all. When people ask me how much exercise they "should" do (the universally common question, direct from diet thinking), I typically say "some."

I want to know first how much they'd like to do, or at least could actually envision themselves doing for a long time. That's probably how much and what kind would be "best"—for them.

It's not that specific kinds of exercise aren't ideal for specific kinds of results. If you're after a specific result—and you're willing to do whatever and however much exercise it takes in order to get that result—there are some general guidelines you can follow to get what you want.

FOR FAT LOSS: SLOW AND LONG IS IDEAL

Many people I talk to are still under the impression that the more they sweat, struggle, and hurt during and after exercise, the "better workout" they are getting—and the more fat they are burning. Biologically, this couldn't be further from the truth. Once again, when we examine the actual facts, the truth is the antithesis of the party line.

To explain why frenzied activity can be counterproductive to burning fat, you need to understand the nature of aerobic exercise. Most people know that aerobic exercise "burns fat" (uses it for energy), but few know what it is about aerobic exercise that makes it fat-burning exercise.

Aerobic means "with oxygen," and so exercise that makes oxygen available for fat breakdown is called aerobic. *Fat needs oxygen in order to be broken down and used for fuel.* This particular biochemical process requires the presence of oxygen. That's why muscles whose capacity for oxidative metabolism has improved are muscles that can better use fat.

Thus, in order for oxygen to be available as needed for fat usage during exercise, you have to be able to breathe. When you are gasping and wheezing and your chest hurts, and you're turning colors, these are signs that there is insufficient oxygen for the task of converting fat to energy at that moment.

What does your body do then? It burns glucose. Glucose—your blood sugar, that ready-to-use carbohydrate that's hanging out in your blood-stream—does not require oxygen for use as energy, nor does glycogen. So at times when an oxygen deficit renders fat unusable, the body uses the only fuel it can make available immediately: carbohydrate.

When you feel like you're killing yourself, but think it's all worth it because of all the fat you're burning, think again: you're probably not burning any at all. Only if you're going *slow* enough will you be able to use fat efficiently for fuel during the exercise.

What's a good way to determine if you are indeed exercising aerobically— "with oxygen"? The American College of Sports Medicine (ACSM) position statement still endorses the "target heart zone" (subtract your age from 220 to determine your maximum heart rate—the number of heartbeats per minute that would more or less kill you—and take 60 to 90 percent of that as your target heart rate. But there are a few more individualized and less cumbersome ways than doing the math and monitoring your heart rate. The

ACSM endorses these for people who are exercise beginners and/or have diseases, but they work fine for you and me, too.

Probably the simplest is the "breathe test." While exercising, notice your breathing. Is it heavier than normal—kind of a light pant—but not gasping and heaving? If so, you are probably exercising aerobically. A light sweat (rather than pouring rivers, unless it is extremely hot and humid) is another good sign.

If you exhibit the breathing and sweating characteristics described above, but still can speak to someone next to you, you're doing well. If you cannot speak, slow down. If you can sing (I mean, if you can sing just as well as you can at rest) then you might want to try increasing intensity till speaking works, but harmonizing doesn't.

For those who like checking their pulse to confirm they're exercising aerobically, 110 to 130 beats per minute is a good general target, regardless of age. This will allow the "average" (nonathlete) exerciser to burn fat while exercising. Going higher will be geared more for the improvement of cardiovascular capacity than for fat burning.

EXERCISE LONGER FOR FASTER, BETTER RESULTS

Once you know aerobic exercise can create a demand for fat and an environment that allows its use, it's common to think the way to step up fat loss—get more and faster results—is to do it harder and faster. But if you want to accelerate the process, exercising *longer* (or more often) is the key—not harder. Harder is reserved for athletes who wish to make particular improvements in speed and/or cardiovascular capacity.

If you bust your guts going as fast and hard as you can, several things are likely to happen:

▶ You probably won't be able to sustain it for very long, unless you are a highly trained athlete with a strategic purpose for going "all out."

▶ You'll probably be exercising anaerobically, meaning insufficient oxygen will be available for the utilization of fat. You'll be burning pure glucose, or close to it. If you do begin to use fat and not enough oxygen is available to complete the process, you'll be left with a by-product of incomplete fat breakdown called pyruvic acid. This gets converted to lactic acid, whose acquaintance you may have made: Its buildup in muscles is one cause of the pain associated with overdoing—what we call "charley horses."

▶ You're more likely to injure yourself, interrupting the benefits of consistent exercise.

▶ You're more likely to hate it, which means you may not exercise as often, or may not continue at all—again, reducing your overall, long-term benefits.

So the good news is that you don't have to—in fact, shouldn't—kill yourself exercising. Can you stand it? Not only are you allowed to eat, but that brisk walk after breakfast or dinner that you think you could almost deal with is actually going to do a lot more good than a gasping, sweating, aching blast of a run.

(So shame on Arnold Schwarzenegger, whom so many people look up to for fitness advice, for answering a woman's request for aerobic exercise suggestions in a September 1992 issue of *U.S. Week* with: "Bike *hard*, or run up and down the stairs, *very fast*.")

AN EXERCISE FOR EVERY OUTCOME

While longer is better for fat burning, that doesn't mean shorter is useless. Walking from the parking lot to your office or taking the stairs *will* do some good. Everything you do does some good. Recent studies show that three 10-minute jaunts are essentially as beneficial as one 30-minute outing.

I think it is most effective and empowering to think of differing lengths and intensities of exercise not as being relatively "better" or "worse" but as simply different, each with their own benefits. Long, hard, anaerobic bursts of exercise, though not ideal for fat burning, have their place—they are excellent for speed training in running or bicycling, for example. Weight training is anaerobic but does build muscle. Light aerobics—say, at 40 to 50 percent of your maximum heart rate, or with very light sweating and slightly increased breathing—is excellent for fat burning but less effective for cardiovascular capacity increases. The maximum heart rate of 60 to 70 percent is best for cardiovascular improvements but will not burn as much fat as workouts of slightly lower intensity.

This allows you to pick and choose, based on your likes and dislikes, your time, and the results you desire. I have found a very effective strategy is to combine different kinds of exercise throughout each week. This not only allows you to take advantage of all the different benefits but makes boredom less likely. Sometimes I do weight training; sometimes a quick 10-minute run; sometimes 45 minutes to an hour of fat burning; sometimes a hard burst for speed development; sometimes a half-hour of moderately strenuous aerobics to push my cardiovascular limits. There's no "right" exercise; it depends on my mood. Sometimes that means none at all. Knowing that's okay, that there's a genuine choice, makes it inviting rather than dreadful.

FUELING FOR EXERCISE

The no-eating-before-exercise myth is particularly pervasive. Maybe it's Mom's influence over us, since most people, when pressed, trace the edict back to her: "Don't swim after eating or you'll drown!" Certainly I don't recommend that you swim or do any exercise sooner than a half-hour after eating. But a half-hour is more than enough time for the body to "process" the food you've eaten to the point where moderate aerobic exercise will not upset you. You could wait up to a full hour and a half to begin exercise; wait longer than that, though, and you'll probably be exercising underfueled.

Think about it. If after three hours your blood glucose supply is mostly depleted and awaiting re-fuel, where does that leave you heading into your exercise? Even after two hours, glucose levels will be on the downswing. The body will need glucose as well as fat during the activity (both in higher amounts than if you were just sitting around) and more glucose than fat during the first 20 minutes or so—you'll be increasing your energy output just when your available fuel is getting low. You're going to run out fast— and begin drawing from other places—muscle glycogen but also muscle tissue. Doesn't make much sense to "eat" muscle for fuel during the very exercise that could help improve and build that muscle.

Logically, the body will react to "more exercise on less fuel" the way it does to general starvation. It perceives the deficit, and anticipating further and future scarcity, will pack away more stored fuel—fat—at its next oppor- tunity. Again, you're detracting the overall benefit of exercising. You may burn some fat if you exercise into fuel scarcity, but you'll inspire vigorous refilling of "fat tanks" afterward.

This can be avoided simply by eating 30 to 90 minutes before a workout. Experiment and see what works for you—the actual food that "sits" the most comfortably seems to vary widely from person to person. I find a meal works better for my energy level, but some people prefer a snack. I find anything sweet before exercise makes me thirsty, so I don't drink juice or eat fruit before a workout. In terms of timing, I've observed that I can go for a bike ride or walk even 20 minutes after a meal, while an hour wait feels best before a run.

Even after studying physiology, when I could clearly see it was scientifically inefficient to race the machine on a waning tank, the "don't eat first" belief was a tough one for me to kick. I "knew" that I would puke if I ran after eating. In fact, training for my first marathon, I ran every one of 300 or so training miles on an empty stomach, very often in the morning after 10 or so hours of "fasting"—pre-breakfast, in other words. After going on three-hour training runs, I would wonder why I came back shaking so hard I could barely untie my shoes, sometimes even dizzy and disoriented. I assumed it was part of training.

The funny part is that while almost everyone "knows" you shouldn't eat before exercise, and a good many "know" they personally would be sick if they tried it, few ever have! We urge clients to fuel appropriately before exercise, and when they do, they notice the same thing we did: never a shaky, lethargic, workout again. Never. As a result, there's a tendency to want to exercise, and to do it more—not that that's a "should," but if it occurs, it's great.

An April 1992 *Northwest Runner* article, in a heartening display of "beyond diet thinking," confirms this. (It's always refreshing to read articles that don't simply regurgitate old fitness platitudes but that actually question and examine them.) Nancy Clark, M.S., R.D., wrote: "Some athletes 'know' they have to exercise on an empty stomach or else they will suffer from an upset stomach or unwanted pit stops. Others simply hesitate to eat before they exercise because that's what their coach told them years ago. . . . If you habitually exercise on an empty stomach just because that's what you've always done, you may be surprised to discover you can achieve performance benefits with an appropriate pre-exercise energizer. . . . Research shows good results with about 300 calories of carbohydrate one hour before moderately hard exercise (*American Journal of Clinical Nutrition*, vol. 54, no. 866, 1991)."

Of course, for every enlightened passage like the one above we're buried in a hundred more espousing diet thinking. Here's one from the January 1993 issue of *Allure* suggesting you exercise on an empty stomach. It once again leaves me vexed at researchers' seeming inability to connect to everyday practices and occurrences the science in which they are steeped. Over and over I see the simplest, most obvious conclusions being overlooked in pursuit of more complex, illogical ones.

The article both quotes and paraphrases Jean-Pierre Flatt, professor of biochemistry at the University of Massachusetts Worcester Medical School. "But not all workouts burn fat with the same efficiency. A 20-minute fast run in the afternoon, for example, might not be as effective as a longer, less intense jog or walk before breakfast, says Flatt. He believes that exercising as far as possible from the last meal will mobilize fat more quickly because the body's glycogen and blood glucose levels will be at their lowest. So pre-breakfast might be the optimal time of the day, and a workout of 30 to 45 minutes most effective."

If I had the chance, I'd ask the following (and so should you when you read things like this):

▶ Can the body operate purely on fat? Does it "switch over" to using only fat when blood glucose is too low to provide adequate fuel for exercise— as it is when he suggests exercising? (If he says yes, then all of the biology textbooks I've ever read are wrong.)

▶ If insufficient glucose is available to fuel the body, can the brain and nervous system continue to function? (No—or he discredits basic biology.)

▶ Can any significant and useful amount of fat be made into that critical glucose? (No—or, again, he discredits basic biology.)

▶ Where does the body get more glucose, then? If fat cannot provide it, and you are suggesting a 45-minute walk when glucose and glycogen levels are low, where will more carbohydrate fuel come from? (The answer would be muscle/protein.)

▶ Does using muscle for fuel make exercise useful, healthy, and worthwhile?

▶ Done after breakfast, a long walk is something a person might actually want to repeat. How do you think it feels to exercise when "glycogen and glucose levels are lowest"? Doesn't that count? If it's miserable, will people keep doing it? Isn't it more important that they continue than it is to burn "more" fat during a single walk?

▶ Why do you assume that the "longer, less intense" morning walk succeeds more than the more intense 20-minute afternoon run because it took place before breakfast? You have more than one variable here. Not only is the timing different, but they are two completely different types of exercise. There's far more evidence that the *length* and *lower intensity* makes the walk a better fat burner—not the fact that it took place before breakfast. A long, less-intense walk after breakfast would surely still beat the 20-minute run—regardless of when that run took place.

▶ Even if the muscle burns more fat when you exercise "on empty," that also encourages more fat storage next time you do eat.

I would love for Dr. Platt and others who expouse his theories to talk to my hundreds of formerly inactive clients who were overjoyed to find the difference in energy and impetus to exercise that a snack or meal gave them.

I know that if I now had to exercise before breakfast, I wouldn't—period. Not just because of what I know, but how I feel.

This is a common mistake—an isolated theory obscuring logical practice. Watch out for these kinds of diversions.

THERMOGENESIS: BOOSTING YOUR "BONUS BURN"

A secondary reason to eat before exercising is to capitalize on the afterburn, also called the bonus burn or thermic effect. As I explained earlier, there is an energy cost to digestion and assimilation. Your body uses energy to break down all of those complex carbohydrates and other foods you eat, so eating actually does elevate your metabolism. This effect is known as thermogenesis.

If the afterburn of exercise increases your metabolism as well, then exercising after you've eaten bolsters the total afterburn. Why not work with your body's functions to take maximum advantage of this—given that you need the fuel anyway?

RE-FUELING AFTER EXERCISE

It's also a good idea to eat a small amount of carbohydrate after a workout (maybe not even so small, if you're an amateur or professional athlete whose strenuous physical activity exceeds an hour a day). Again, while you may want exact numbers, it's best to use your judgment and your senses. Here's a loose frame of reference: After a half-hour bike ride or 45-minute walk, an orange might suffice. After a one-hour training run or two hours of tennis, you may want to eat a large bowl of cereal and a banana, or a bagel and some orange juice. Individual needs will vary. Listen to your body.

Research has shown that the rate of muscle glycogen synthesis may be twice as high if you consume carbohydrate within a half-hour after the exercise. But this will be of most significance to the competitive athlete in terms of recovery and subsequent performance. The average person is best off simply doing what feels good.

Re-fueling after exercise should come pretty naturally if you're fueling in general, because in that case you'll always (or almost always) be eating every three to four hours. If you take care to fuel before exercise, then by the time you're done it will be nearly time to fuel again anyway. Example: If you eat a snack at 3:30 P.M., go for a walk at 4:00 P.M., and return at 4:45, it will be time for dinner soon anyway. (And it's fine to have a little something before dinner, if you feel the need right after the walk.) If you eat breakfast at 6:00 A.M. and go to the pool at 7:00 A.M., swim till 8:00 A.M. and get to work by 9:00, it's time for your snack when you get there.

However much carbohydrate you choose to re-fuel with, drinking plenty of water before, during, and after exercise is important. Though not fuel, it's something else your body definitely needs.

EXERCISING SICK

Don't exercise when you're sick. To even consider putting your body under that kind of stress when it is already stressed by illness lives in diet thinking, where you must stick to your rigid "regimen" no matter what, and where one missed workout surely spells doom for your fitness efforts.

I remember feeling that way. About eight years ago, I *left my bed* to take a long run when I had a particularly bad head and chest cold. (It was January, I think.) When I returned, I coughed and hacked for hours. What was scary was I got really hot; my face was beet-red for hours and hours and wouldn't cool off. My body was straining and struggling to deliver energy and blood to the healing projects going on inside me, and at the same time my overworked cardiovascular and muscular systems were vying for the same attention. In the name of fitness, I subjected my body to far more damage than skipping that one running session would have—but diet thinking severely distorted my priorities and logic, as it continues to do for so many.

Remember that protein is for building, maintaining, and repairing body tissues. When you're sick, the body needs protein to repair the damage; don't force your body to divert protein to muscle repair and building simply because you didn't want to skip a day at the gym.

WHAT ABOUT WHEN YOU CAN'T EXERCISE?

One of the many benefits of fueling is that your body will "hold" its fitness longer if you're not damaging or depriving it with poor or no fuel during periods of no exercise—you'll keep the muscle you "earned," instead of losing it. Thus, with fueling there need never be any "I've got to get to the club" hysteria. If you like to and *can* exercise a lot, you'll get maximum value from it all if you're fueling. It won't be just a grim race against fat. And if you exercise just a little, you'll get the most out of every little bit— so you can be really fit and feel great on minimal effort.

Feel good about what you do instead of worrying needlessly about what you're not doing. That doesn't mean it's better to stop—it's not. It's better if you exercise. There are health benefits even above and beyond fat loss and improved cardiovascular strength. But it does mean that if you really have to stop for some reason—illness, travel, short-term schedule change—you can eat in a way that will minimize the loss of benefit.

When I was taking classes for six months while working, and exercise temporarily became a once-a-week treat, I was thrilled to find that because I was "fueling" my fitness level didn't drop significantly. Of course I lost some ground in my cardiovascular fitness; I noticed that right away when I returned to it. *But I didn't gain fat and I didn't lose muscle.* Mainly, I was "holding"—not making strides but not slipping backward. And for the benefit of a time-intensive commitment that I knew wouldn't last forever, I could live with not making strides.

It felt so good to know what to do, how to handle it best—to know for sure that I was protecting what I had. And, best of all, I was still eating. Staying fit with less exercise didn't mean going hungry. That, as you can now see, would have been the worst thing—hastening muscle deterioration. It was a relief to know I wasn't mistakenly bumbling down the wrong path, thinking I was doing something good—as people do when they cut way back on eating because their exercise has slowed.

MYTH: DO A LOT OR DON'T DO IT AT ALL

Working with a core management group at one of the nation's major telephone companies, we noticed that the same thing kept coming up on people's registration forms in response to the question "Where do you feel you are most 'blocked' in getting and staying fit?" Typical responses: "Need to exercise more." "Not enough structure." "No exercise regimen." "Not enough exercise." "Not disciplined enough."

Yet these people were all walking, running, or using a stair machine two to five hours per week—more than we were at the time. Who or what gave them the idea that what they were doing is not enough? The fact that they didn't have an official "regimen," or that their exercise didn't feel rigid, unchanging, unyielding? As if creativity, choice, and spontaneity are all bad signs, signs that you are not really doing what you "should."

The bottom-line message in that thinking is that if you're not suffering, you must not be doing it right. These folks were suffering about it. How much good could their two to five hours per week be doing, when they feel guilty and wrong? The stress we place upon ourselves by worrying about eating or exercise is probably far more debilitating than any inconsistency—perceived or real—in our habits. Stress is hard on the body. It defeats the purpose of eating well or exercising.

Just as "eating less" is a nebulous recommendation, "exercising more" is a groundless, you-can-never-do-enough mind-set when whoever is suggesting it has no idea how much exercise you're already doing.

You don't need to do a lot! The myth that you have to pound yourself for an hour or more a day keeps many people from doing anything at all. When people ask how much I exercise, I say "Well, except during our short summer, about three hours." So often they say, "A day?" Heavens NO! Three hours a *week*!

People waste a lot of time exercising more than they need to. As with eating, *consistency* is key with exercise. I firmly believe it's more important to do some with regularity—whatever it is and however much—than to hit the supposed "ideal" peaks or forget it.

That choice, that never *having* to, makes exercise a joy I never knew it could be. I lost 15 pounds of fat and gained nearly that many pounds of muscle in little more than two years. Not overnight results—but I got to eat a lot, incessantly, and to *do what I felt like*. It took two years to get to a place I undoubtedly could have reached faster if I'd invested much more effort, "regimen," and "discipline." But then exercise wouldn't be the treat that it is now. Life wouldn't be as sweet.

I've been headed in the right direction the whole time—I'm just moseying my way along a path that I don't see ending. I'll be wandering and strolling in that general direction for the rest of my life.

EXERCISE IS IDEAL—AND SOME IS BETTER THAN NONE

Don't misconstrue this statement to mean that you need not exercise or should not exercise. Not true! For the record, I'd much rather you exercise than not—if I were given the choice. I think what's different about me is I respect that it is not my choice to make. I can help you understand the value and benefits, encourage you, and acknowledge every little bit you do. I know that makes more difference than telling you what you "should" do. I'd rather see you walk for 15 minutes whenever you felt like it, and really love it, than bust your gut 30 to 45 minutes three days a week because you "should."

Fortunately, some authorities have officially loosened or dismissed some of the more restrictive timing and intensity standards that probably have served more often as deterrents than they have as guidelines. I think this is wise. Not placing stringent do-or-die minimums on exercise will get more people trying it.

Fashion, fitness, and news magazines have increasingly been touting this "go easy" trend since early 1992. But after 40 years of a paradigm that has deeply engendered a public (mis)understanding, a few lines in a few magazines don't radically alter the general public consciousness. Most of the people who come to our workshops still believe *long and hard and miserable* is the only exercise that matters—just as they are convinced that they eat too much and must "cut back" (no matter how much they currently eat).

So to say that exercise isn't valuable—it definitely is—or suggest that people should not exercise is not the point. The point is that, as with good eating, people won't do it because they "should." I have presented compelling reasons to exercise and why—so people who do it know what they're getting out of it, and those who don't (or don't much), might find themselves more interested, given the benefits.

CHRIS AND THE 10-MINUTE "TRICK"

One client, Chris, indicated during a follow-up that the fueling was going fantastically. Her cholesterol had already dropped 30 points and her nurse practitioner was astonished at how much she now knew about food, fat, and her body. But Chris was discouraged about exercise. She felt strongly that she "should" be doing some, but she just couldn't "get herself" to do it. When these red-flag words came up, I could hear that Chris had backed herself into a corner.

I knew Chris had a stair machine at home, and that she had at one time played tennis regularly. Somewhere she had burned out. I acknowledged that her feelings and experience were absolutely fine, even appropriate. Then I asked her if she could deal with just 10 minutes on the stair machine every other day. She began protesting: That's not enough, that isn't good enough, etc. I calmly explained the biology again and helped her see that while more exercise than I was suggesting would produce particular results, she didn't have to want those results; she didn't have to do anything at all.

Did she want to? Yes, she said firmly. All right then: Could she do just 10 minutes? "Of course!" Okay, I said, then do that—and no more. In fact, I teased, "I forbid you to do more!" Chris called a week later; she had done 20 to 30 minutes on the machine every day—and played tennis a couple of times as well. "Sorry I 'disobeyed'—it's hard not to keep going after 10 minutes!" she gushed.

This has been my experience over and over in coaching people—with eating or exercise. Human instinct seems to be that in order to "get someone to" do something, we have to push. We can't let up, or they'll never do anything. But time and time and time again I've seen that stepping back and allowing some space, some choice, leaves people choosing wisely and well. And their experience is totally different than if I "got them to" do something.

Fueling is about fueling your body for whatever you do—including your exercise. So whether you do one hour of exercise a week or 19, fuel yourself—and that one hour will be the best hour you can do, or the 19 hours will yield the most they can yield. And one is better than none, and should be appreciated.

MORE TAKES MORE

If you want a sculpted, to-die-for body, that *will* require exercise, and more than just a little. I am intrigued by the possibility of having that kind of body, and I think of myself as being on a very leisurely ascent to that level. Meantime, I'm very healthy, I look good, and I'm happy about it.

Most people don't seem to want body-builder biceps. They just want to be healthy and reasonably fit, and they'd like to know they don't have to suffer to do it. And they *don't* have to suffer—not with exercise, any more than with eating. For those people, properly fueled exercise at 40 to 50 percent of maximum heart rate (or at 60 to 70 percent, for cardiovascular improvement) will suffice very nicely.

For those who want more and are prepared to invest in the kind of exercise that will get them there, fueling is a necessary adjunct to that kind of training, too. No matter how much I work out, without fuel I'll never get there.

FUELING AND SPORTS

Although you'd think they'd know better, I've been amazed to find that the concept of fueling for endurance and improved performance isn't common knowledge among athletes, coaches, and trainers, nor is it a common perspective or way of looking at the body among these high-performance "machines." One of our workshop participants, a former U.S. Olympic rowing team member named Ginny, cornered us after the workshop was over and said, "You've got to get this to athletes." We were stunned—didn't she learn all this as an Olympian? "No," Ginny said, "I used to go out for grueling morning training runs and rows on an empty stomach. It was a constant struggle, having the energy to keep going during training. And I had no idea that by going without meals as much as I do now, I'm slowly destroying muscle mass it took me years to build."

Larry, another client, reported that he was thrilled with the results not only for himself, but for his daughter Rachel, a rowing team member at a college in Washington State. He told us of her tortured efforts—and those of her entire team—to reduce bodyfat to levels that were satisfactory to the coach. They were constantly manipulating their diets, and Rachel was always hungry (a sign of too little fuel—not good when you're trying to achieve athletic results such as speed, endurance, and strength). Despite this, she could never get down to a bodyfat percentage that "they" wanted.

Larry wasn't sure but he had a sense that, despite all the gyrations, they were probably still giving her way too much fat and way too little food. A few months later, he called to tell us that he had passed along all of our basic recommendations and some food brand and meal ideas. Rachel had successfully reduced her bodyfat, and her entire team was "fueling." They felt great, Rachel was overjoyed that she was "allowed" to eat, and everyone was happy.

Mark told us about his niece, a high school track star, whose coach insisted she do her training runs without food or water beforehand; she was confused about why she petered out so fast and felt so terrible. Roger mentioned that his kids' soccer coach instructed them to eat four hours before a practice or game, no sooner—so by the time they played, they felt like limp rags. Another couple told us their son, a local high school track legend in Ohio, had been instructed to go without food for "a long time" before runs.

Professional sports teams could give themselves an enormous edge if they were to begin training in *fueling*—if they were willing to admit they don't necessarily know or do what's ideal.

I cringe when I see commercials in which well-known athletes are touting some high-sugar, high-fat product. It's hard for me to believe they themselves ever go near the stuff (although they'll accept thousands or millions to tell the cameras that they live on it), but even if they do live on the stuff, I hate them leaving our children with the idea that chocolate, cola, and potato chips are really what fuels their high-performance bodies. For best performance, athletes—just like the rest of us—need to efficiently and consistently fuel themselves. A high-performance race car needs to be well-cared for and optimally fueled all the time, not just the day of the race.

5

DIET THINKING

DIET THINKING IS THE CULPRIT

By now it should be at least somewhat clear that fitness failures—personal ones and cultural ones—can be traced not merely to diets and lack of knowledge about our body's needs, but to the very foundation of our thinking about the subject. While it's fashionable to attack "dieting," for example, to do so is to attack a symptom rather than to look deeper to the true cause. No one person or thing is at fault. We're all subject to systems of beliefs and assumptions through which we filter information, regardless of whether the beliefs have any factual basis. And often we're unable to step beyond a system's restrictive vision because we're not even aware we're trapped within it.

Diet thinking is one such belief system—a way of looking at, listening to, and interpreting everything we think, see, and do that's related to eating and fitness. Consumers, the media, businesses, and health educators all speak, see, and hear through its filter. Such thinking (or, just as often, *non* thinking) allows and encourages the spread of frustrating and dangerous misinformation, and obscures the truth that would set you free.

Diets don't work, yes, but no one asks how they got so thoroughly woven into the fabric of our culture in the first place. Diets never were based on anything germane; their inevitable failure could have been deduced before hundreds of millions of people wasted their time, money, and bodies. But no one ever considers that the cultural mind-set responsible for that "oversight" is the real concern, rather than the diets themselves.

Such thinking is how "weight" has managed to survive as the centerpiece of our fitness concerns for so long. Diet thinking is what enables many to remain convinced that something so irrelevant is all that's relevant—even though its unimportance is soundly demonstrated just by basic science and a close look at semantics. The fact that our cultural fixation with dieting and weight loss persists, despite mounting evidence of their failure and simple facts that undermine their every premise, reflects the stubborn foothold of diet thinking.

DISSECTING THE ANATOMY OF DIET THINKING

With some facts about your body already under your belt, and with some thoughts hopefully brewing about food as fuel and an investment in your life, you can probably begin to discern some of the parameters of diet thinking. Where previously you saw and heard through the filter without even realizing you were wearing one, you can now begin to see its shape lurking in the fog.

Chapter 2, "What's Weight Got to Do with It?," introduced you to one of the most explicit and dominant products of diet thinking. To help you become even more fluent, summarized on pages 108 and 109 are some of the key characteristics that tip you off to the presence of diet thinking.

To my mind, diet thinking's greatest flaw lies with the summary's final point—*it's not about fueling your body*. Both the goal and the means of diet thinking are several steps removed from the precise requirements of your body. A weight-loss diet may be rigid in that you must "follow" its rules to the letter in order to lose "pounds"—but it's not exacting in the sense that you provide your body with the precise fuel it needs to make it run efficiently. The two are actually antithetical. I've never seen a "diet" claim "this is what your body needs." The body's needs are not a primary concern of a diet— weight loss is. Moreover, the body's needs, if necessary, will take a back seat to getting that result.

The funny part is that eating to fuel your body based on its design, its

THE ANATOMY OF DIET THINKING

It's About Weight Loss, Maintenance, Management, or Control.

▶ Progress is measured by a number that cannot tell you a thing about health, fitness, or fatness.

"Dieter" Is a Noun; "Dieting" Is a Verb.

▶ There are "just regular people" and then there are "dieters." A dieter doesn't eat; he/she "diets."

▶ One is not a successful person who eats to be healthy, but a "successful dieter."

It's a Diet, Plan, Program.

▶ It never occurs to you to just start eating for your life and keep on going.

▶ Instead, you stop eating and "start a diet," a detour or hiatus from "regular eating" and real life.

▶ Even unstructured "healthy eating" is considered "different" and "special"—an eating "plan."

It's Temporary.

▶ It's a short-term attempt to "put out a fire"—to alter the body so you can return to living.

▶ Diets aren't meant to be lived on, just survived for the time it takes to get the short-term result.

It's Negative.

▶ It's assumed that what's good for the body must naturally be what you don't want (and vice versa).

▶ "Healthy eating" is assumed to mean limiting, reducing, losing, cutting, restricting, giving up.

▶ The focus is on what you are not, getting rid of or avoiding something, what you can't have.

▶ The mood is resignation.

▶ You're trying to fix something, not live and eat.

Your Body Is Separate.

▶ The thing you're trying to "fix" is usually your body; it's about your body, not your life.

▶ You don't see your body as an extension of you—something to cherish, work with, and care for.

▶ Endeavors are all about manipulating its size or "weight" by whatever means you're told will do it.

The Focus Is on the Micro, While the Macro Suffers.

▶ There's no sense of priorities: Endless fretting about specific vitamins and minerals, caffeine, or preservatives dwarfs concern for basic issues such as eating enough or often enough, or fat intake.

It's a "Should."

▶ There's little if any ownership, choice, sense of responsibility, or self-determination.

It's About Control and Resistance.

▶ "Control" implies rigidity, unnatural restraint, repression.

▶ You consent to constant combat with calories, food, weight, hunger, your body.

▶ It's questionable who's controlling what.

It's Got a Vocabulary.

▶ When diet thinking is operative, you're sure to see (or hear or use) words such as *have to, ought to, don't, shouldn't, fight, control, avoid, willpower, maintain, limit, portion, allowed, stick to, stay on, follow, regimen, resolve, relapse, cheat, discipline, strict, be "good," program, plan, rigorous, lifestyle, trim, thin, skinny.*

▶ The language is constructed in black-and-white, extreme absolutes: "can" and "can't," "good" and "bad," "yes" and "no," "on" and "off."

Good Things Become Enemies.

▶ Your body's source of fuel and energy—what you need to live—is mistaken for an adversary.

It's Unscientific.

▶ Theories and recommendations are premised on assumptions, not the body's science.

▶ Sources are "well, everybody knows that" or "a friend read that a scientist thinks . . ."

It's Rules to Follow.

▶ It's all "how-to"—no big picture, no context, no sense of why something works or how *you* work.

It's a Moral Issue.

▶ Eating "right" assumes there is a "wrong."

▶ Technical efficiency gets confused with moral correctness.

It's Not About Fueling Your Body.

▶ The body's precise needs are not the concern of a diet; weight loss is.

▶ To lose weight, the body's needs actually take a back seat.

system requirements, does get you great results—not weight loss, but lean-ness, health, and energy. And it achieves these not by wedging some unnatu-ral, temporary-fix tool (like a "program") into your life, but by making eating a purposeful part of your life—by directly meeting your body's needs rather than trying to trick it or take a shortcut. What could be more logical?

Now that you know the landmarks to look for, let's take a journey. On it, you'll see just how much a part of our culture diet thinking has become—like the air we breathe, it's invisible yet influences your every thought and every bite, and every aspect of your life. In the process, you'll come to recognize your own diet thinking and that of others, understand how it affects you—and learn to think beyond it.

A SHORT COURSE IN PARADIGM THINKING

Such research reflects what scientists call a paradigm shift, a funda-mental change in understanding that only occurs at rare moments in the history of science—theories clash like cymbals, and then all that was confusion suddenly comes into focus.
—*The Seattle Times*, December 29, 1991

To help you understand the insidious influence that diet thinking wields, I'd like to introduce you to the concept of paradigms.

Thomas Kuhn's *The Structure of Scientific Revolutions* details an experiment in which subjects were shown a deck of playing cards with red spades instead of black. They reported seeing black spades, because that's what they expected to see. When the "trick" was revealed, they had no trouble seeing that the spades were red. They had made the assumption based on their "playing card paradigm."

Experiments like these and countless others have shown how paradigms—a set or system of beliefs or assumptions so ingrained, so deeply etched into a culture's collective consciousness that it is invisible—filter our reality. We see only what supports our paradigms. They operate in the background, screening without our knowledge. And since it's what we call "reality," we don't question it; we take it for granted.

Joel Arthur Barker, author of *Future Edge*, has helped make paradigms a mainstream concept. Barker explains that paradigms "are invisible in many situations because it is 'just the way we do things.' Often they operate at an unconscious level. Yet they determine, to a large extent, our behavior." He calls the result the Paradigm Effect: "You are quite literally unable to perceive data right before your eyes . . . any data that exists in the real world that does not fit your paradigm will have a difficult time getting through. . . . That data that does fit your paradigm not only makes it through the filter, but is concentrated by the filtering process, thus creating the illusion of even greater support for the paradigm."

Diet thinking is a paradigm that tells people how to be fit. It operates within a cobweb of myths that literally contradict the basic physiology of the human body and the biochemistry of food metabolism. Diets, dieting, and the thinking that fertilizes them all survive because these myths are held as absolute truth by the majority. Whether or not it is true doesn't matter; it has force because it is perceived, without question, to be fact. Since you don't question it, diet *thinking* is technically a misnomer because it isn't creative, active, critical thought; it's the absence of such thinking. It's *non* thinking.

That's why when I teach the biology of how the body really works— even show the textbooks—some still cannot believe that eating a lot of carbohydrate food won't make them fat, or that starving or eating only salads won't be the best thing for getting lean, or that losing "weight" isn't the issue. The American paradigm is that those things are true. Your don't think they're true—you *know* it.

Barker calls this *"paradigm paralysis,* a terminal disease of certainty." He notes that "there is temptation to take our paradigm and convert it into *the* paradigm . . . Once we have *the* paradigm in place, then any suggested alternative has to be wrong."

CHANGING THE PARADIGM

Paradigms can, and do, change. *BodyFueling* was conceived in commitment to provoking a paradigm shift in the way we think about food and our bodies—to create new trends and dramatically alter trends already in place. Barker explains that a new paradigm (in this case, fueling) has a high likelihood of appearing while the prevailing paradigm (in this case, dieting) is still performing. That's why new-thinking ideas and language (such as "eat more; don't count calories") are being used to market old-thinking products and concepts (like "weight loss" and "programs")—and vice versa. The interest is on the rise, but what's coming out to address it is not saying anything new.

Paradigms, Barker notes, remain in place until someone—typically an outsider—challenges them. He points out that the outsider has a distinct advantage—a fresh perspective that makes new or previously unrecognized angles visible. How many times have you stared at something for ages—a picture, puzzle, a chess game—only to have someone come along and notice something so simple and obvious that you said, "Now, how come I didn't see that before?"

"Outsiders" can see most clearly, Barker says, when they are "knowledgeable about the paradigm, but not captured by it . . . They ask 'dumb' questions. They wonder about behaviors and approaches accepted by those 'in the know.' " (Like starving. Cutting carbohydrates. Counting/cutting calories. The usefulness of "weight" as a measure. The validity of "overeating.")

Though clearheaded innocence is the paradigm shifter's edge, Barker acknowledges that those enmeshed in the status quo don't necessarily appreciate this. "These people are bringing you your future. And yet, as outsiders, what is their credibility? . . . Who do they think they are?" Businesses die or lose great sums of money because of their slowness in anticipating a paradigm shift or heeding the warning of an observant "outsider." IBM and General Motors are two high-profile examples.

Certain phrases, Barker notes, are used to put the fresh-eyed observer in his place: " 'That's impossible.' 'We don't do things that way around here.' 'It's too radical a change for us.' 'When you've been around a little longer, you'll understand.' 'How dare you suggest that what we've been doing is wrong!' 'If you had been in this field as long as I have, you would understand that what you are suggesting is absolutely absurd!' "

A paradigm shifter is often someone who personally has run into one of the problems of the prevailing paradigm. It starts as just their problem (i.e., "we thought we knew how to eat; why aren't we getting results?"). "So they start to work on their problem . . . *And inadvertently they create through their solution a special example that leads to a model, a theory, an approach—a paradigm—for solving an entire class of problems.*" That's precisely how BodyFueling was born.

Barker provides strong examples of now-defunct paradigms. Because we're beyond these, they're now so clearly off-base that they illustrate paradigms better than any theoretical explanation. Barker reminds us that the people making these predictions were, without exception, experts in their field—they just couldn't see past their paradigms.

"The phonograph . . . is not of any commercial value." Thomas Edison
    remarking on his own invention, 1880

"Flight by machines heavier than air is unpractical and insignificant, if not utterly impossible." Simon Newcomb, astronomer, 1902

"There is no likelihood man can ever tap the power of the atom." Robert Millikan, Nobel Prize Winner in physics, 1920

"Who the hell wants to hear actors talk?" Harry Warner, Warner Brothers Pictures, 1927

"I think there is a world market for about five computers." Thomas J. Watson, chairman of IBM, 1943

WHY DIETS *REALLY* DON'T WORK: The Science Nobody Talks About

NO ONE IS EXEMPT FROM DIET THINKING

Clearly, general intelligence or high education doesn't prevent a mind from being blinded by paradigms. Just look at the inability of many health professionals, researchers, and educators to manage not only the health, fitness, and eating issues of others, but also their own.

Professionals specifically educated in the science of the human body have allowed (even encouraged) people to continue operating in the dark—because they are in most cases no less in the dark themselves.

I've known several morbidly obese cardiologists who are brilliant at surgically treating heart disease but can't seem to prevent it in themselves. My medical student friends report biochemistry honors students who leave class to consume beer, burgers, doughnuts, and large quantities of alcohol, even recreational drugs. ("It's as if we're studying an alien species.") I met the director of a wellness program at a large corporation who was a clear heart-attack candidate.

A number of my clients have been counselors who treat eating disorders—and have eating disorders themselves. Other clients have regaled me with stories of dieting doctors, obese dietitians, and bulimic psychologists—who, they say, shook their faith in those professions. The paradigm doesn't automatically spare those with credentials after their names; in fact, those credentials entail paradigms of their own.

In *Recalled by Life*, an inspiring book about how he became cancer-free through what he ate, Dr. Anthony Sattilaro confessed to his ignorance—and arrogance—about food and health when he skeptically abandoned his lifelong fat- and protein-laden fare: "How does one keep up his strength on this high-carbohydrate, low-protein, low-fat regimen? Maybe I needed a steak dinner to keep my strength up."

AN EASY MYSTERY TO SOLVE—FROM OUTSIDE THE PARADIGM

Thomas Kuhn, in *The Structure of Scientific Revolutions*, explains how scientific paradigms impair the "objectivity" of research, filtering the so-called "reality" that scientists can see. Kuhn found that when confronted with information that didn't fit into their belief systems, scientists distorted the information to make it fit or missed it entirely. And, of course, you don't even bother to begin studying what you don't *think* is an issue.

Thus, many professionals steeped in scientific knowledge about the body are perplexed about why "weight" is "hard to maintain." I still read and hear that researchers consider obesity to be a "mystery." Scientists who have studied the human body in consummate detail, and must know what muscle is for and what it does, watch dieters lose 100 pounds on starvation diets, gain back 100 pounds of fat, and scratch their heads, saying, "We don't understand obesity or why it's so hard to keep weight off." That's like a car expert being baffled by why pulling the six-liter engine out of a car and replacing it with a one-liter motor will cause the car to use far less gasoline.

Let's look at some select examples of the experts missing what's under their noses:

From the *Berkeley Wellness Letter*: "The researchers don't know why weight fluctuations may be a problem. One theory is that when weight is regained, fat may be more likely to settle in the abdominal area (a possible risk factor for heart disease and other disorders) . . . Or perhaps people who lose weight tend to choose an especially high-fat diet when they relapse. The researchers suggested that further studies be done to determine why frequent weight changes might account for their findings."

What about the fact (not theory) that the way people diet causes lost "pounds" to include muscle, which decreases their metabolic rate afterward? It's been known for a long time that muscle creates a requirement for fuel; the processes of muscle metabolism were clear by the middle of the century. Your body burns carbohydrate and fat to fuel the muscle. Muscle burns 98 percent of the calories we consume. Muscle size equals metabolism size. Calling for more research to discover why losing lots of "weight" through "eating less and exercising more" leaves you fatter is like undertaking more research to find out why chopping off your finger with a machete makes you bleed. It's just the way your body works!

To say we don't understand why repeated "weight" loss damages the heart is also evidence of paradigm blindness. Carbohydrate deprivation, such as is common on diets, causes muscle weight loss. The heart is a muscle. It's logical that losing muscle through chronic dieting could eventually weaken the heart. But clearly logic is irrelevant when paradigm blindness strikes— a condition worsened by the pull of a $33 billion diet industry and perhaps a thriving research industry as well.

Plus, those who translate the research you read—the media—are also stuck in the paradigm, reading into it their own biases, adopting those conclusions they expect to find, such as "eat less," "loss weight," "stick to," "willpower." New findings are crow-barred into old language. Data is both misrepresented and misheard, so that even good news ends up sounding like the same old grind.

A July 1991 *Los Angeles Times* article, printed a week after what's now known as the Yale "yo-yo dieting study" was published, exemplifies both research and reporting from the bowels of diet thinking. This particular study is just one example of science and the media together reinforcing diet thinking. But it is an especially good one because it was widely considered a "breakthrough" in the area of diet and health; it catalyzed or strengthened theories that miss the point; and it resonated with as many diet thinking assumptions as you'd ever hope to find in a single item.

Lead author Kelly Brownell, a Yale University psychologist, evaluated 3,200 men and women from the Framingham Heart Study in Massachusetts (which has shown that obesity, high blood pressure, and high blood cholesterol are risk factors for heart disease). Analyzing subjects' weight fluctuations over a 32-year period, Brownell found a link between chronic dieting (yo-yo-ing, or "weight cycling"—losing and regaining "weight" in large amounts and/or losing and gaining repeatedly) and coronary artery disease and premature death, especially in those aged 30 to 44 (the people the study also found are most likely to diet). This was independent of other risk factors such as obesity, weight, smoking, and cholesterol level.

Diet-thinking mayhem followed in the media and the scientific community. Among the conclusions to which reporters, researchers, and the public jumped:

▶ That obesity (already a known risk factor for many diseases) is healthier than repeated relapse after dieting (though the study itself did not even compare or examine which is healthier)

▶ That "thin" is a damaging standard
▶ That more research is needed

From the *L.A. Times* piece (italics are my emphasis):

> Researchers zeroing in on what makes a dieter successful over time have unearthed some *surprising* findings. . . . The next logical step for *chronic dieters?* Reduce to an *ideal weight* and stay there, Brownell said, or pick a *weight that is reasonable*—even if it is above the ideal—and *stay there*. . . .
>
> Yale's Brownell said *to lose weight and keep it off, dieters* must *identify their personal triggers to overeating*, whether it is boredom, the smell of food, depression or other factors. . . .
>
> Most important, people who decide to lose weight *must be truly ready*, Brownell said. If you're not ready, he said, it may be healthier to postpone the diet or forget it altogether. "*One way not to regain weight is not to lose it in the first place*," he said. "As silly as it sounds, that may actually be a better course. . . ." On at least one point, Hirsch and Brownell concur; more research is needed about the effects of weight fluctuation. . . . Meanwhile, he said, "Dieting should be taken seriously. It's *possible* that *dieting under some circumstances could create negative effects*."

Let's take a look at some of the diet thinking flaws here.

IT'S BIOLOGY, NOT PSYCHOLOGY!

The ways Americans manipulate the number on the scale (depriving ourselves of food, especially of carbohydrate) provokes muscle loss, a counterproductive destruction of the precious tissue that burns fuel. As you've already learned, it also causes a host of additional body reactions designed to help you better make, store, and conserve fat.

Yet the above article, and virtually all of the reporting I've seen on the subject, assumes that yo-yo dieting (and fatness in general) is a function of a psychological inability of people to control themselves. By subjecting the dieters, rather than the process itself, to endless analysis, an important opportunity to distinguish biology and "weight" from fat is wasted.

I read about this study in more than a dozen magazines and newspapers, and none ever addressed why yo-yo-ing happens in the first place. None even mentioned the biological changes caused by deprivation of food. If they did, people would realize that what they call "willpower" compounds the problem: The "better" you are at suppressing your eating, the more biologically primed you are to get fat. Being "good" makes you and keeps you fat, because the diet thinking definition of what's "good" is too little food, and the body retaliates.

Calling overfat a psychological or character issue creates three big problems.

It's a red herring for the real issue. It becomes a misleading decoy, distracting attention from the true focus: what biologically creates the fat problem—and how total miseducation about one's own body leaves one powerless to handle it.

It makes people feel bad—needlessly. Something is supposedly "wrong with you" for not keeping "it"—weight—off. In reality, not keeping fat off is your body's perfectly appropriate, biological response to dieting.

It suggests the "weak-willed" are better off doing nothing. "Experts" who emphasize psychology and who learn about the effects of yo-yo-ing without understanding or considering its biological cause as much as say, "If you're not going to be 'strong' enough to stick to your diet or keep the 'weight' off, don't do anything. Just stay fat." Staying fat is not the answer; it puts you unequivocally at risk for disease.

Also, the solution to the problem isn't arduous; it's easy. But the "good news" isn't heard because this thinking doesn't leave room for a positive solution.

CLEAR DATA, BUNGLED TRANSLATION

Once you know how the body works, dieting's dangers are hardly an enigma or a "breakthrough": continued deterioration of muscle, stimulation of fat-maintenance mechanisms, and a higher total percentage of bodyfat because of reduced muscle mass. That's all very straightforward.

Yet the conclusions drawn by researchers and reporters of the yo-yo study didn't reflect any of that. Instead of revealing why dieting (indeed, why any deprivation or undistinguished "weight" loss) would always be counterproductive, the advice that emerged suggested that for some people dieting and "weight" loss is still appropriate. Instead of saying that diets (or weight loss) simply don't work at all, they now said these would only work if the time was right: You must be in a place where you're really "ready" to lose the "weight" and "keep it off." (The difference between, or relevance of, fat weight and muscle weight was totally ignored.)

Since the initial "yo-yo research" was published in July 1991, this type of "new" cautionary advice has become the standard dietspeak in fitness and women's magazines. Instead of "don't diet" (or better yet, "don't eat too little," whether from a diet or not), they kept diets and gave them a modifier: "Only when you're sure you're ready to 'keep it off.' " This uniformly psychological response to a biological issue suggests that "weight" loss and maintenance success is all in your mind.

There is no "readiness" that will make eating less work physiologically. Biologically, you can't keep it off—no matter how "good" you are. The psychologists ignore the fact that "keeping it off" is more a function of what you took off than what you do afterward. They suggest waiting for a "favorable time to diet." But there is no favorable time to deprive your body of fuel.

Brownell himself was quoted in the March 1992 issue of *Shape*, saying, "When you decide to lose *weight* or adopt an exercise *program* you must prepare yourself *mentally and emotionally.* . . . How motivated are you compared to previous attempts to diet and exercise? . . . Do you eat when you feel lonely, bored, angry, depressed or anxious? If so, are you ready to come up with an alternative response to these feelings?" He advises *"dieters"* to "identify the *risks* and decide how best to handle them. What if you are invited to *an elaborate buffet?* . . ." (Italics added for emphasis.)

What if you are? You should eat—like everyone else. Being in what the article calls a "food-heavy environment" is not a "risk"—but notice how food is portrayed as the enemy; as always, the assumption is you'll want to eat as little as possible. Why would you need an alternative response to wanting to eat—unless you consider eating a problem, and your premise is that eating too much is the issue? In truth, why you eat and how much both pale in importance compared to *what* you eat. We need caring, educated, conscious eaters, not "successful" or "emotionally aware" dieters.

For all the difference the yo-yo brouhaha made, a year later I walked into a grocery store to see a huge headline on the cover of the February 1992 issue of *Self*: "Diet Scoop—How to Control Your Eating," and on the January 1993 *Glamour*: "Are you Dieting Wisely or Unwisely?"

It's like that old MTV ad: "Some people just don't get it."

"JUST STAY FAT": THE BACKLASH AGAINST BETTER EATING

Another reason researchers refused to conclude that diets simply don't work at all is the fear that people would abandon diets. They're wrong—and right.

What they mean is, they don't want people abandoning fat loss and health. They don't want people staying fat. But they muddy the issue by equating health and fat loss with dieting and weight loss—when in fact they are unrelated. They assume that if you give up dieting, you'll necessarily be giving up leanness. The opposite is true. "Diet only for health reasons," said Van Hubbard, M.D., Ph.D., of the National Institutes of Health. Yet the yo-yo study itself suggested diets were not healthy.

This obviously didn't leave you with many options. Those whose research indicated that dieting causes mortality also continued to suggest that not dieting also causes mortality. (And they wonder why you ignore dietary recommendations!) As a result, two distinct camps organized in light of the yo-yo data: diet and anti-diet. And since each has one good point buried in its reactionary diet thinking, I can neither fully support nor fully discount what either has to say.

The anti-diet camp has a point because dieting doesn't work, and simply loving your body is a great place to start. Their problem: They have misdiagnosed the problem as the standard of lean, when the hitch is the method used to get there. And they advocate forsaking it all instead of finding the method that works. They throw the baby (leanness, good health) out with the bathwater (dieting).

The diet camp counters, "But fat is unhealthy; just accepting it is stupid," and they too have a point. Their problem? The only solution they continue to hold out is the one that they admit doesn't work: Diets for weight loss. These methods they're recycling still aim to manipulate the weight, which is irrelevant to fat loss and health.

CHOOSING BETWEEN TWO EVILS—AND MISSING THE BOUNTY

The backlash against dieting is a leap from the frying pan into the fire— from one unhealthy extreme (dieting) to another (fatness). It's needless, because what works is neither of those. But what works—*don't diet* and *don't be fat*—is so fogged by diet thinking it's never even considered as a possibility.

A *Washington Post* headline that appeared after Brownell's study was first released condemned dieting, with "Worse Than Being Overweight?" splashed across its pages. A *New York Times* article on April 12, 1992, declared an "anti-diet revolution"—women rising up against weight loss regimes and vowing to "love themselves large." It talked about burning scales—and equated burning the scale with being fat. The message: No concern for weight must mean being fat.

Newsweek, on August 17, 1992, ran a story entitled "Let Them Eat Cake": ". . . With much the same messianic fervor they once devoted to the war against fat, some women have gone into battle against diets."

The March 1992 *Vogue* health column comes right out and says it directly: "All of this leads to the obvious question: if the majority of people regain the weight they lose after dieting, and if yo-yo dieting is risky, why not just stay fat?"

That's not what the research showed, but it left a lot of people feeling justified, even righteous, in carrying around a dangerous excess of bodyfat. There's even a National Association to Advance Fat Acceptance in Sacramento, California. True, the study showed that losing and then gaining repeatedly increased risk of coronary disease. But that's a far cry from "Dieting causes heart disease, so being fat is healthier!" That's like saying, "Since I keep falling on my face every time I stand up, I guess I'll just sit here," when simply untying your shoelaces, which have been tied to each other, would solve the problem.

In the face of the anti-diet uproar, most of the experts agree we should not deny the fact that fat is unhealthy. Leanness is healthy. Overfat (not overweight, as the misnomer goes) has been overwhelmingly shown to be a health risk. Two of every three people you know will die of heart disease, cancer, or stroke if current trends continue. All three are strongly linked to fat.

The experts' main mistake has been to continue seeing "a weight-loss diet" as the only alternative to being fat. For example, Kelly Brownell himself expressed concern with the anti-diet backlash. But the only place he could see to go back to is diets. "The pendulum is swinging away from dieting so fast that I find myself in the uncomfortable position of actually defending weight loss programs."

In the *New York Times* article, Theodore VanItallie—a Columbia University obesity researcher—called the anti-diet approach "ridiculous." He said, "It's irresponsible to encourage women with weight problems to eat what they feel like." Well, I would not encourage an overfat person to eat high-fat food. But what is over*weight*? And telling people not to eat what they feel like accomplishes nothing—except possibly driving them to eat it. Most of all, if it's "irresponsible" to encourage people to eat what they feel like, that assumes that what they will "feel like" eating will be wrong. In reality, people do also "feel like" eating all kinds of things that are great for them. Maybe they just need to know which are which. (People who "diet" would love to eat, period!)

Syracuse University psychology professor Thomas Wadden agrees with VanItallie: "People who stop dieting may get comfortable with their bodies, but I don't see them getting comfortable with an increased risk of mortality." While commenting on a study that *linked* dieting to mortality, he implies there's no way to get lean except to diet—even though every statistic says Americans aren't getting lean that way, because their diets are making them *fatter*. It's fat, not "weight," that increases mortality risk, and, as you now know, getting "comfortable" with your body doesn't preclude either eating healthily or being lean.

THE STANDARD IS FINE; THE METHOD STINKS

As fruitless as the "be fat or diet" trap is the implication that leanness itself (mistakenly called "thinness") is the problem, that our beauty standard is a supposedly impossible-to-attain lean ideal. This theory argues that it's your disappointment in failing to achieve an unattainable goal that makes you "give up" and gain the "weight" back. Others say it's a plot to dominate and oppress women; they present leanness as unnecessary, even unreasonable. They encourage you to "make peace with your body" instead—no matter its condition.

Once again, several issues are snarled into one. I certainly endorse loving your body and being at peace with it. BodyFueling is not about fighting yourself or decoy demons like "weight," or subjugating your instincts. You learn the details of your body's functions and needs, explore your body's role in your life and future, and choose whether to meet its needs. If that isn't loving—as well as intelligent and responsible—I don't know what is. What I don't sanction is the assumption that "making peace with your body" must mean making peace with being fat—and being unhealthy.

GOING TOO FAR: GLORIFYING FAT

Anti-diet advocates irresponsibly ascribe "power" to fat—when true power comes from being completely informed and exercising your choice. Naomi Wolf, author of *The Beauty Myth*, during a speaking engagement broadcast on National Public Radio in November 1991, stated that one-third bodyfat for women is "normal and healthy." Her semantics jumble the facts: 33 percent is "normal"—meaning typical, average—but *not* healthy, *not* ideal. She also stated, "Female fat is where the hormones are. It's where our sexuality is. It's where the libido is. It's female power."

While Wolf's work has many important points, this takes the diet backlash to dangerous lengths. Being misinformed detracts from power. Such carelessly vague, misleading statements for the sake of theatrics ultimately splinters the female power being claimed. To assert that there literally are hormones in the fat itself—so that people become concerned that to lose fat is to physically excrete female hormones in the process—is just plain wrong. Also, to imply that a woman needs fat to be sexual or have "female power" is ludicrous. Rather than uniting women, Wolf's theory is divisive, because it effectively promotes poor health even though poor health is, without doubt, an oppressor. There isn't much that's more oppressive than death. Where is the power in the fat of a medically obese woman (based not on appearance, but a percentage of bodyfat over 30 percent)? If the fat makes her one of the 64 percent of Americans who die prematurely of heart disease, cancer, or stroke, is that fat still worth keeping for its mystical "female power"?

If you had a broken leg and the wrong tool had repeatedly been used to set it, would you want to locate and use the right tool? Or would you say, "The heck with it. It's dumb to have your leg set anyway. Who needs a leg? Just leave it broken."

If the "tool" used on "weight" (fat) loss has never worked, should you now give up and stay fat? Or finally learn what's been going wrong and what to do about it? Don't ditch what works; teach what works! Don't bash leanness; instead, correct the unhealthy and incorrect ways people try to reach that healthy standard.

NOT JUST FOR APPEARANCES

Since being lean is part of being healthy, why knock it if people also happen to find it attractive? It's another incentive. People want to look good, and probably always will.

I agree that efforts to be lean purely for the sake of the way it looks are not to be encouraged—but that's because I think appearance alone is an insufficient motivation to have people alter their eating in any permanent way. Getting "slim" so someone will love you or hire you or not fire you is definitely unconstructive. Improvements don't last under these circumstances because there's no ownership. If it's not for you and your life, it's probably not for keeps. But eating as an investment in your life, as fueling all the things you want to do, is quite different—it brings the prospect of "healthy eating" to a whole new realm.

MEN, WOMEN, AND FAT

I also believe we're missing the point by making overfat a female or feminist issue—just as we're missing the point in diverting all our energy to eradicating so-called overeating when *underfueling* is a chief cause of high bodyfat.

Fat—high bodyfat—is a person issue and a health issue. So is the lack of education and perspective that promotes it. The damage caused by our backward, unscientific approach to eating and fitness doesn't discriminate. Both men and women in America are concerned about "weight" or diet, confused about "healthy eating," and frustrated by lack of fitness results.

Emphasizing differences also encourages the search for "special" problems and excuses. Yes, men and women have their physiological differences, but there are many fundamental needs all human bodies have—easily handled basics that are common to everyone.

Asserting that fat retention is a so-called "women's biological disadvantage" perpetuates this issue. Women are not "biologically disadvantaged." That's a claim rooted in negative perspective, not in fact. Women simply are built the way they are, and men are built the way they are. It is both demeaning and discouraging to women to say they are "set up" for failure by virtue of gender.

Disadvantaged compared to what? I hear: Men burn fat easier. Men don't gain "weight" as easily. True, men by nature have more muscle, and more muscle means more and faster fat burning. A man with 150 pounds of muscle will have a hungrier "engine" than a woman with 95 pounds of muscle. But so what? The real issue is your own body and what you can do with it.

The gap isn't actually that wide to begin with—but a woman can widen it considerably by starving herself. The average woman may have less muscle to start with than the average man, but she'll wind up with less still when she deprives herself of fuel in efforts to get thin as quickly as possible. Factor in other metabolic changes that occur during deprivation to favor fat, and you do have a disadvantaged woman. But those are disadvantages that are self-induced and *can* be avoided.

With 110 pounds muscle, I'm not so terribly different than my husband's 145 pounds of muscle. But back when I was down to 94 pounds of muscle, the gap was wider. My lean mass reached that low point because I consumed too little to fuel the activity I was doing. Sure, Robert's additional 35 pounds of muscle require more fuel, but what's that got to do with me? Besides, I get plenty to eat myself—and I know that's what I'm supposed to be doing. There's no need for martyred justifications about why I can't be fit.

We are different. We all have different body types. People do not all experience fat loss at the same rate. Even among women, there are many variables: What you've done, what you do now, what body you started with. The point is not to compete with one another. The point is that wherever you're at, you can look and feel better, and live longer—by fueling your body optimally. And the joy is that it's done by eating, not starving.

If women are at a disadvantage at all, I think it's a social one. Because women seem to be especially committed to "weight loss"—at any cost— they've been more susceptible to misinformation. In my observation, although some men are as obsessed with "weight" as women, most are more likely to shrug off what they notice doesn't work or doesn't make sense. Women seem more prepared to make sacrifices, even at the expense of health or peace of mind.

An April 1992 *Mademoiselle* article called "How I Learned to Love My Body" underlines this. In the article, author Amy Cunningham notes, "The way women care for their appearance more than they value their health is a symptom of a cultural logjam that fouls up our priorities all the time." She cites a 1983 Cincinnati College of Medicine study that surveyed 33,000 women. "Their greatest single hope as a group was to lose 10 to 15 pounds. That's above their hopes of achieving success at work, raising self-respecting kids and making the world a better place. Odds are those statistics would not have improved greatly if that same study were done today."

Whether it is society's fault that women tend to be this way I leave to other books to explore. I don't doubt that societal pressures have deeply affected the American woman's desire for the perfect figure. You could also say that perhaps men simply value themselves too highly to agree to self-abuse at any cost; if so, more power to them.

I do believe we have to stop blaming men for our bodies—for how they are naturally and for what we do about them. The fact that the man standing next to you has 50 more pounds of muscle than you does not in any way stop you from maximizing your own muscle through fueling and exercise. And it's not his fault that you never knew you could eat plenty of food and still be lean. (If there's a fault, it probably lies with the men *and* women who have long known all of what I am teaching and have not spoken up.)

If one is really interested in what will make a difference to young girls and women, militant feminist finger pointing will not do the trick. It will galvanize a certain number of women, but for what? Righteous resistance? I think it affirms and maintains victimization to stay stuck in place trying to avenge the past. Let's move on.

LEAN VERSUS THIN

Hazy, imprecise diet-thinking language helps to cloud the issue of body standards even further. Those who favor a "fatter" standard say *thin* is unreasonable; I say *lean* isn't. We're using two different words that are not interchangeable. In that sense, I agree that "thin" is a bad standard—but only because it doesn't mean "lean." One can be thin and have plenty of bodyfat.

If we eradicated all the empty, misleading words that mean something different to each individual and ultimately don't mean anything at all— thin, skinny, trim, slim, slender—we'd be left only with "overfat" and "lean." Only these are directly descriptive and, unlike the others, don't support goals or arouse concerns that serve as distractions.

The interchangeable use of these two and all the other words is rampant in the media, and it reinforces the widespread assumption that all the terms are synonymous. The February/March 1992 issue of *Health* quotes Columbia University obesity researcher Theodore VanItallie as saying, "I think a healthy leanness not only doesn't carry risks, but is probably beneficial." Then the writer goes on to say, "But confirming that skinniness really is better hasn't exactly . . ." The author uses skinniness in place of leanness, thinking she has found a perfectly sound substitute.

But people can be slim, skinny, or thin without being lean at all. One client calls it thin-fat, and reports she has been able to identify it more readily since our workshop. "I used to think anyone who was thin looked good. But now I can see the difference. There are people who are a little larger, but strong and solid—obviously lean. And there are people who are scrawny, yet if you really look, they're 'fat.' "

An acquaintance once remarked to Robert (who is over six feet tall and about 15 percent bodyfat) that she thought he looked "anorexic." He replied, "Anorectics never eat. I have food in my hand almost constantly. I consume

3,000 calories a day. Anorectics don't look like that." What he politely didn't point out is that the acquaintance has more than enough extra bodyfat to pose a health problem.

One must be careful when speaking about eating disorders and the way people look. Anorexia is not a function of how thin you are; it's about how you get there and your state of mind.

Anorexia is about *thin*, not *lean*. There is a distinction between the "lean" I am suggesting is healthy and the "thin" that clinically eating-disordered people seem to picture and pursue. Such people are not concerned about bodyfat percentages or maintaining muscle—they destroy enormous amounts of muscle in an effort to waste their bodies to smallness. Such a degree of obsession is dangerous and sometimes fatal.

It's true that some women are scared of muscle, which I think can be traced to their not understanding what muscle is and what it does. The January 1993 issue of *Allure*, in its article "Fat Gauge," quotes sports nutritionist Michelle Vivas: "I have women asking me if they stopped exercising for a year, would the muscle go away. . . . Women also ask about leaving protein out of their diets to try to reduce their muscle." Such women are clearly 100 percent uninformed about the way their bodies work, since they're not aware of muscle's critical role in achieving the low-fat look they want.

On the other hand, if any person really despises the look of muscle because it interferes with the look of "thin," I think it's safe to say their thinking is disordered. Such a person might then find my physique, for example (size 4, but decidedly muscular), to be unattractive. I love muscle because I love what I know it's doing for me—its mere existence creates a metabolic demand for fuel. If you are unable to appreciate the portion of your weight that actively works for your health and your leanness, then diet thinking has you in a lock that might mean help is in order.

Just be sure the "help" isn't in the same diet-thinking boat with you.

POOR FUELING IS NOT A JOKE

In diet thinking, food indiscretions are funny. This tends to be a subject about which people put their heads together and laugh nervously. It's as though the way food affects our bodies is all kind of a joke. You think something is "wrong" but will do it anyway, and when you laugh together about it, somehow it's all okay. "Guess I'll make up for it tomorrow, heh

heh heh!" "Better watch out for those killer cupcakes, hahahah!" "Oh, this is (heh heh, wink wink) some of that *low-calorie* cheesecake, right?"

Maybe it's because the concern is so universal that it brings people together. It creates instant rapport and camaraderie. But it's destructive, because it fans the fire of myths, misconceptions, and unhealthy attitudes, and it sanctions ignorance by glossing over it.

I happened to catch the April 28, 1992, National Public Radio coverage of the Food Pyramid's death and subsequent reprise. The lack of time devoted to constructive education, and the commentators' not-always-subtle mockery of efforts to eat healthfully were appalling to me—its only usefulness was as a perfect example of how deeply into popular culture this paradigm has bled.

The U.S. Department of Agriculture (USDA) in December 1990 officially announced revisions in the government's standard public information nutrition icon based on current research findings about diet and disease. The decades-old "four food groups" was replaced by a pyramid graphic emphasizing more grains, fruits and vegetables, and less animal food such as meat and dairy. The graphic was released in 1991, but the agriculture secretary quickly recalled it. In April 1992, the USDA released one that hadn't changed much since its initial rejection.

The segment spent a short time briefing people about the Pyramid itself, and discussing the controversy over whether the beef and dairy industries had played a role in delaying its release because the pyramid recommends reduced consumption of meat and dairy products.

Following about five minutes of discussion about the pyramid's release, NPR devoted more than twice that amount of time to a humor piece that asked NPR reporters, commentators, and listeners for commentary on their personal translations of the four food groups. Wasting precious airtime that could have been used to educate about a subject that cries out for clarification among consumers, NPR chose instead to further demonstrate that need.

Commentator Daniel Pinkwater said, "I'll tell you a little-known fact. Nature's most perfect food is pizza. It can sustain life indefinitely and encompasses the crust group, the sauce group, the cheese group, and the pepperoni group." Another commentator cited food groups as the four Fs: foam, fun, fried, and fat.

NPR editor Brooke Gladstone chimed in: "I think the best thing to do is have something green, something yellow, and something white" at every meal, which, it's noted, might include a glass of milk for the white, a pear for the green, and a piece of pound cake for the yellow. Gladstone added that for her kids, she "feels safe" if she gives them something "high in protein" that walks or crawls, and something out of the ground. But, she confesses, "I also give them a vitamin because I don't really know what I'm doing."

Here, at least, some valuable truth: A smart, successful mom who admits she is lost when it comes to this. She assumes that her children need to be well fed, while she doesn't, and she isn't at all confident that she even knows what to do for them. Based on her own rule, she doesn't: She could be giving her kids three times the protein and/or a fraction of the carbohydrate they need. A multivitamin won't help that one bit. Gladstone doesn't know how the human body works or what it needs, and her kids aren't learning it now.

As the grande finale, still another commentator claimed that the food groups are grease, salt, and carbonated beverages, explaining that how you balance these three dietary elements is to get your grease from "a hamburger or two hamburgers, or maybe two hamburgers and a hot dog, or two hamburgers and a hot dog and fried chicken," your salt "on the side by pouring it on the french fries," and your carbonation from "Coca-Cola, which cuts through the grease and the salt and everything kind of evens out there."

This is funny? This is our most high-brow and respected source for radio news? But let's face it, this is what's on people's minds. These NPR folks are bright people—the nation's best and brightest, really, the reporters and the listeners both. But their joking is the same as what I hear at parties, in grocery stores, at health clubs, even at the beginning of my own workshops.

What if a similar commentary poked fun not at poor eating but at drunk driving? ("Oh yeah, I load up and race around in my car all the time. Silly me! Ha ha ha!" or "Sure, I believe in moderate drinking! I wouldn't think of having more than ten beers before I head home from the bar! Hee hee!") People are dying at the rate of more than 2,000 a day of heart disease and stroke, and we're laughing about how the four food groups are "foam, fun, fried, and fat" or about "grease, salt, and carbonation." Our culture has completely missed the point that poor eating is as lethal as excessive alcohol consumption.

Am I being humorless? Not given the suffering that I have made it my business to see and understand. I wouldn't be considered humorless if I expressed outrage at casual cracks regarding sudden infant death syndrome, or drunk drivers who kill, or AIDS. If you're thinking to yourself, "Lighten up, Robyn," I'd say that's an indication of the breadth of diet thinking, the lock this paradigm has on our sensibilities. Even lofty public broadcasting types cannot see what's shameful about spending 10 precious radio minutes giggling about Brooke Gladstone's helplessness, instead of educating their audience about what their bodies really need.

In the end, lame jokes about self-inflicted damage through food are a flimsy substitute for the authentic lightness that comes with knowing what to do, knowing you don't have to—and knowing you want to because it's not hard and the benefits are astronomical. Brittle "humor" like the NPR report merely attempts to cover the desperation and confusion of America's relationship with food. If you want to laugh, laugh with joy at the smorgasbord of wonderful food that can fuel your life, instead of tittering half-heartedly about the food you "shouldn't" have eaten.

6

BEYOND DIET THINKING:
Looking Back at "Diets"

Every year 65 million Americans strike back at what they think is their "weight" problem, feeding a weight-loss business that topped $32 billion in 1989 and was predicted then to exceed $50 billion by 1995.

Statistics suggest that anywhere from 40 million to 80 million adults are hazardously "overweight" or that 63 percent of American adults are "over the recommended weight range for their build." Of adults currently on a diet in the United States, 71 percent are estimated to be women. About 50 percent of American women and 25 percent of American men are estimated to be dieting at any given time. It's estimated that 90 to 95 percent regain some or all of the "weight."

REGARDING YOUR "DIET DAYS" AFTER FUELING

When you stop diet thinking and start fueling, all of the premises that once validated the idea of "going on" a diet fall apart. Here are some real-life examples of what happens when diet thinking's foundation crumbles.

Pat, an energetic, cheerful, outgoing woman of 51, is candid about the frenzy of dieting she did in the 1970s and 1980s, from high-protein fads to currently popular programs like NutriSystem. "I screwed up my metabolism so bad with the high-protein things. I stuck to one for months, grim as it was. When I went and had my basal metabolic rate tested, I had slowed down so much that I was told I could only consume 600 calories a day without the excess being stored as fat."

Having taken BodyFueling ("It's the best thing I ever did"), Pat is careful now in her language. She talks about gaining or losing *fat*, not indiscriminate "weight." She is aware that by depriving herself of carbohydrate daily for close to a year, she was constantly requiring her body to convert lean muscle protein to carbohydrate fuel. Most of the "pounds" Pat lost during this period were muscle—and that loss was partly responsible for her body's overall metabolic slowdown. She understands all this now and is amazed at some of the things she put herself through—and further amazed that her physicians allowed and even encouraged it.

Pat put herself into counseling in 1989 to "de-program," as she puts it, from "the dieting mentality. I was never anorexic or bulimic, but I knew I wanted out of all of the brainwashing I'd had from these diets. Just to be able to eat food without 'knowing' I should be controlling it somehow." She laughs now about waking up to eat carrots in the middle of the night because the Weight Watchers program she was on was so adamant about her having to eat *exactly* the food they told her to.

"Diet Center seemed compulsive even to me at the time. Weighing in every day seemed crazy. Even the more nutritionally sound of the diets don't really teach you how to deal with real life, or how your body works," Pat concludes. "It's all about their food, their pills, their supplements. There's no reality attached to it at all. I know how to make choices now. I know what my body needs and why. I have a frame of reference for what's important and what isn't. I know brands and labels. I can cook and bake with no fat and no sugar. And it's all about living my life, not 'doing well on my diet.' "

A teacher in her fifties, Liz courageously shared a particularly harrowing story about dieting and health during a workshop. When we completed the biology section of the course, her eyes were wide as she pieced together a history that for the first time in 30 years made perfect sense to her.

The high-protein diets of the 1970s, which she was so proud of herself for "sticking to," despite the misery. The medically supervised fasting program. The struggle in every single instance to keep the "pounds" off (in actuality, to keep fat off after having lost pounds of muscle). And the horror of the truth behind what drove her to start all this: the doctor who told her to "lose

20 pounds and come back in a month." The doctor who told her, when she was 27, to gain only 10 pounds during her pregnancy or she would die. (She was so restrictive, she *lost* 10 pounds during that pregnancy, and her son suffered birth defects.)

Liz also revealed during our discussion about muscle loss that a recent medical examination had shown the muscle tissue around her heart to be severely deteriorated. She hadn't understood why until now. While most people can build some muscle back, it does take exercise and is not nearly as rapid a process as losing it. In the extreme case of losing 50 pounds of muscle on a liquid diet, building 50 pounds of muscle back can take a decade and a lot of work—if it is even at all possible. In Liz's case, there are no exercises to "build" the muscle surrounding the heart; the damage is done. (I encourage people to grieve the precious tissue lost due to lack of such simple education—and to know that regardless of what they have done up until now, from this day forward they have the opportunity to preserve the muscle they do have.)

Perhaps the most compelling thing of all was that when Liz came to us, after three decades of dieting, she *still* did not know anything about how to eat to fuel her body. All those diets that ravaged her body still left her uninformed and unable to buy, prepare, and eat the things her body needed. All she knew was how to diet, and how to worry about the 5 "pounds" she gained "after Thanksgiving" (which may have been water or her heavy sweater or who knows what, but which, after one weekend, were not 5 pounds of stored fat).

Connie is a 50-year-old factory worker who is inspiring in her efforts to adopt a healthy, lifelong way of eating, given her background: complete lack of education about nutrition (not that that in itself in unusual), an upbringing that insisted loads of protein is good and carbohydrate is fattening, a husband who resists changes in their diet and loves red meat, and the stress of living with both her mother and mother-in-law. Yet she has valiantly and earnestly managed to make major changes.

"I never used to eat three meals a day, but now I do," says Connie. She starts her day at 3:00 A.M. when she wakes for her morning work shift. "I couldn't believe the difference it made. I was amazed. I looked better, felt better, slept better—I was sleeping like a baby. I always used to have trouble sleeping.

"I didn't really believe it was okay to eat so much and that I'd still be all right. But I haven't 'expanded' like I thought I would if I ate that much food. I can eat the whole sandwich, not just half! My husband made me popcorn one night and he put butter and salt all over it. I literally couldn't eat it. I said, 'You ruined it!' I'm really proud that I feel that way. There's no high-fat junk in the house anymore.

"It's insane, what's out there. Everyone tells you you have to diet. You 'know' you have to. I went to a doctor about migraine headaches and he weighed me, and just based on the weight, he said, 'I can't work with you until you lose some weight.' He was totally rude."

Connie, like Pat, is a graduate of advanced dieting—participation in numerous group and commercial programs, none of which left her prepared to shop, cook, eat, or most of all think in a way that would work for life. She talks about NutriSystem: "Every week it was the same thing. 'Why did you go off? What's gonna make you go off next week?' If you hadn't lost any weight or had gained, it was 'What did you do wrong?' " The message was clear, she says: "You're on a diet now."

Chuck, another workshop participant, said about Jenny Craig, "I would get really weak. It made me mad that they gave a big guy like me the same 1,000 calories as a little guy who wanted to lose five pounds. . . . Now I have enough energy to bust my butt all day at work. Now I know my son (age two) will be healthy and know how to eat."

Jessica, a teenager, said of Jenny Craig, "You were like a specimen. You were your weight. And they were really condescending." Jessica's father, who attended our workshop with her, said later, "Jessica has gotten her eating together for the first time in her life—and your workshop led the way. None of those diet programs ever clicked. . . . It's funny, what works is so simple; people probably don't believe it can work. But learning all this cleared the confusion and brought us back to that wonderful simplicity. You're on the cutting edge, especially where the idea of personal responsibility is concerned."

Jessica's father is also a communications professional who worked with a law firm representing plantiffs in a case against a popular commercial diet company. He reported at the time that the company and plaintiffs settled out of court, and part of the agreement was that all court documents be sealed. What might they want to hide? My client Chris (of the 10-minute exercise in Chapter 4) shed light on that question when she related the story of her short-lived stint as a counselor for that company:

"They train you, sure—to sell. It was about commissions. 'Don't you want to be rich?' they'd say. We were taught that the most important thing is to get the customer to sign the contract requiring them to buy $50 to $100 per week worth of food. It didn't matter if they needed it or not. To get our commissions, the person had to buy all the food in their contract.

"They taught us how to talk to people, you know, on the phone—what to say to get them to come in. You were never to vary from the script. You weren't allowed to tell them any prices over the phone. When they came in, they got the hard sell. In exchange, we would promise them ten pounds in a week or two. Of course, there was nothing ever said about fat or muscle. It was all weight." She quit after three days.

Allure, in September 1992, published "The Allure Diet Survey," an exposé which corroborated the countless horror stories my clients have provided. At Diet Center, for example, according to the article, an *Allure* volunteer was given what amounted to a low-carb, high-protein diet including a limit of half a baked potato or a third of a cup of rice or pasta daily, as well as a glut of protein: nine ounces daily, *plus* an additional two servings of dairy protein, *plus* the recommended snack of peanut butter, of all things. She was given 18 supplements to take daily. And she was weighed several times a week.

At another popular commercial center, another *Allure* volunteer recognized the diet as basically a Weight Watchers plan and was told, "Listen, Weight Watchers is the key to life." Yet, says the article, " . . . on the *Today* show last May, a counselor for a Weight Watchers affiliate said that only one-half of 1 percent of the program's clients keep their weight off. She also said that only 5 to 7 percent of those who signed up at her center reached their goals." (Weight Watchers International, however, disavowed her statements.) At all of the commercial centers, volunteers were commanded to adhere strictly to their menus.

For this kind of deprivation and imbalance, the volunteers paid through the nose: at one commercial center, one volunteer reportedly was told she would get no information until she had "signed on the dotted line"—to pay $1,005 (registration, diet, and "Sta-b-lite" program). She was discouraged by the counselor from reading the "consumer rights notice" in the contract. So she signed. Later, she was quoted a lower price at a different branch, so she called the first center and asked for the money back. Suddenly, this center decided that her initial down payment ($502) would be enough—for six weeks of the diet, anyway, during which she was promised a loss of 17–20 pounds. Vitamins and supplements, at $23 a week, were not included, though.

At a different commercial center, another volunteer paid $185 for registration, $94 for lifestyle tapes she didn't realize were optional, $149 for a special lifetime deal, and $88.90 for the first week of food. She had to sign an agreement to buy the first eight weeks of food—another $587.

PARTICULARLY BAD DIETS

There are diets that add their own specific mutations to the basic "eat less and exercise more" paradigm, surpassing even the general scientific and contextual flaws that apply to all diets. My point in warning you about these, and passing on the warnings of others who have evaluated them, is not only to put you in a further-informed position, but also to illustrate the serious risks posed by the truly atrocious void in our education that allows them to thrive.

HIGH PROTEIN, HIGH FAT: A REVIVAL

One disturbing development is the reemergence of high-protein diets that advocate unlimited protein and even fat. *Dr. Atkin's New Diet Revolution* is just one example of recently published books that advocate this backward thinking. As you learned in detail in Chapter 3, "Fueling the Human Body: Your Owner's Manual," your body has little use for more than a small amount of fat, and uses protein for tasks other than fuel—unless you force its use as fuel. The (non)thinking behind a high-protein, high-fat diet is: "This machine ideally uses fuel A. So, let's not give it any A! Let's use only fuel B and C instead."

Unfortunately, this mind-set can be traced, in part, to the still-prevalent myth that carbohydrate food is fattening. Andrew Weil, M.D., wrote a *Mademoiselle* article back in 1988 that contained a lot of wisdom:

> People who are watching their weight often shun foods high in carbohydrate—such as potatoes, pasta, rice and bread—convinced that they turn directly into ugly fat. Instead, they load their diets with protein. . . . Complex carbohydrates have probably gained their bad reputation because of the company they keep. Most of us have learned to like our carbohydrates with lots of fat. . . . Yes, such dishes are fattening, but don't blame that on the carbo- hydrates . . . they're the body's ideal fuel, easy to break down and burn for energy. . . . They should make up the biggest part of your diet.

Five years later, this wisdom still doesn't register with many of the people I work with. Even though carbohydrate is what fuels most of the work of our body's cells, and most of the activity we engage in every day, from thinking to walking, more than half of the people I meet are still surprised to learn about its dominant role in our energy and well-being—our very existence.

The misunderstanding, even fear, of carbohydrate goes back to whether you want to lose "weight" or fat. A diet that starves you of carbohydrate will cause pounds of muscle to be stolen for fuel, and you'll lose "weight." Like the high-protein, low-carbohydrate diets of the 1970s—now widely recognized as useless and dangerous (they led to about 60 deaths after they first became popular in the early '70s)—the reprise of these strategies is all about that one little number. They are shortsighted plans to make that (meaningless) figure on the scale go down—and capitalize on Americans' uninformed quest for Another Quick Answer to manipulate it.

If you look beyond the little booby prize between your feet, what these diets really represent is the best way to get your body totally inefficient at using fat—or any fuel. Fat loss—not to mention energy, health, fitness, and a lifelong way of eating—are unachievable with such a strategy.

CAN YOU BE ADDICTED TO SOMETHING IT'S NORMAL TO NEED?

About the best thing that can be said for *The Carbohydrate Addict's Diet*, by Richard and Rachael Heller, is that it's a perfect example of what *not* to do. It's exactly the opposite of what you'd want to do for energy, health, and fat loss, given the way the human body works and uses food for fuel. Everything about modern human biochemistry runs counter to the strategy they advocate.

In my workshops now, someone routinely pipes up after we've covered the physiology of carbohydrate use: "Then isn't that book about carbohydrate addiction that tells you to cut way back on carbohydrate dangerous?" Yes.

Yet the Hellers assert that people are fat because they are "addicted" to carbohydrate. They tell you to drastically reduce your daily intake of bread, cereal, fruit, pasta, potatoes—all carbs. These are the foods that basic biology, the government's U.S. Recommended Dietary Allowance, nutrition textbooks, organizations such as the American Heart Association, research data, and the vast majority of health experts all suggest should be 55 to 70 percent of the diet that will keep bodyfat at bay and ward off cancer and cardiovascular disease; the foods most people love to eat and would be thrilled to know their bodies—all bodies—need to eat to run efficiently.

After severely restricting carbohydrates throughout the day, the Hellers endorse one main meal a day of pretty much anything you want. This is a 23-hour abstention from what your body needs most, which stimulates all of the "fattening" mechanisms your body uses when starved of its key fuel. Between-meal snacks are also severely shunned because even a piece of fruit, "eaten other than during your Reward Meal, can reverse the whole metabolic process that is emptying your fat cells."

By saying "eat anything you want" at the so-called "reward meal," you are also basically encouraged to make that meal as high in fat and protein as you want. All foods are "allowed" and in any quantity. Sample menus for other meals include "four to six ounces of pastrami" for breakfast, "two cheeseburgers (without the buns)" for lunch, and, for dinner, "How about ribs, mashed potatoes, baked beans and a large tossed salad? Dessert is up to you."

Yet consider the facts: Fat makes you fat—I mean, how can you get around it? Fat *is* fat. Consuming great quantities of it will result in the total opposite of what people really want. One client told me her sister-in-law was eating bacon and ice cream for dinner because the book said she could have anything she wanted. Another client told me her boss was thrilled because now that she wasn't eating carbohydrate, she could skip breakfast and lunch more easily. I shudder to think how many others are piecing together such motley—and downright deadly—strategies as a result of this freewheeling advice.

The processing of carbohydrate burns a great deal of energy. No matter what the destination of carbohydrate—to muscle cells for fuel, conversion to glycogen, or conversion to fat—some part is "donated" to meet the fuel demand of processing it so you can eat more of it without creating excess.

On the other hand, very little energy is needed to store fat. Since most people's bodies have a greater demand for carbohydrate than fat, most of the time, fat is less likely to be used for fuel. Fat not needed for fuel is readily stored as fat, since 95 percent of it cannot be converted to anything else.

The high-protein strategy is fattening in yet another way. The average body doesn't need much protein; 2 or 4 ounces at a serving, or 6 to 10 ounces a day, is plenty for most people. Since the body has no way to store protein except as fat, it will break down (deaminate) excess protein and convert it to fat for storage. As if that's not bad enough, on its way it leaves a toxic trail of biochemical "ash" such as nitrogen, which the body must struggle to excrete. Yet the carbohydrate addiction theory says you could eat a pound of protein at dinner (or anything you want).

Some of the protein in a high-protein diet will also be deaminated and used for fuel, to spare your muscle from shouldering the whole carbohydrate-deficit burden. Whether you use dietary protein or body protein (muscle) for fuel, the breakdown/conversion process is equally tiring and toxic. And the dietary protein your body is stealing would normally be used for the building and repair of tissue. Eating carbohydrate lets the protein you eat do its own usual—and vital—jobs.

These are all biological facts—you can find the same explanations yourself at any library. Translated, what the Hellers are saying is that the best way to lose generic "pounds" of who-cares-what-as-long-as-your-weight-goes-down is to stop eating what your body needs most for energy, health, and sheer survival. Instead, eat as much as you want of what your body needs very little of, and which it stores readily as fat.

Moreover, the Hellers suggest that one of the attributes that makes carbohydrate an enemy is that it makes you hungry for more. "Small, frequent carbohydrate meals actually feed the addiction and lead to loss of appetite control," they admonish. Your body runs on carbohydrate. "Controlling" anything that might make you want to eat more of it is rooted in the diet-thinking assumption that you always need to eat less, and so must extract from your diet anything that encourages eating.

Carbohydrates do trigger insulin production. (As you may recall, this is done to manage the use of blood glucose.) But it's normal and understandable—not "bad"—to be hungry after insulin has helped glucose out of the blood and into cells for use as fuel; blood glucose is lower again, and you need more. The Hellers call that a problem—and suggest that to avoid it you avoid carbohydrate. They are essentially offering a way to skirt a normal biochemical reaction. They define a compelling hunger or craving for carbohydrate-rich foods as "addiction,"—when in fact such hunger is appropriate, and meeting that hunger (eating lots of carbohydrate-rich foods) is what's most widely recommended for health, leanness, and disease prevention.

The result that "proves" the Hellers' theory is that they, and others, "lost weight" doing this. Sure they did. Pounds are lost. Thanks, but I'd rather hold onto my muscle tissue.

You would do well to be suspicious of any strategy that seeks to fundamentally alter, work around, or ignore the basic form and function of the body. The diet-thinking underpinning of any such strategy is the notion that you can (even should) manipulate your body for your own short-term gratification, completely displacing any consideration of the big picture that includes your long-term future and actual needs. Remember you cannot corrupt the basic design of anything without paying a price.

ADDICTS ANONYMOUS: AMERICA'S ADDICTED TO ADDICTION

All high-protein, low-carbohydrate diets promote a way of eating that directly defies the body's design and needs. You use carbohydrate for fuel constantly; it's key to your survival. It is normal, healthy, and *necessary* to eat lots of it—in fact, to have it comprise the giant's share of your fuel/food intake.

I gleefully down enormous amounts of cereal, breads, potatoes, rice, fruit, pasta. True, I've lost no "weight," but dropped 11 percentage points of bodyfat (a 44 percent drop); I'm sleek and energetic; and I haven't experienced so much as a sniffle for more than four years. You can't get this kind of glowing good health by gorging on what the body needs little of, and avoiding what it needs a lot of.

The fact is, the average American's carbohydrate intake is already too low, and fat and protein too high. The last thing Americans need is encouragement to eat less carbohydrate! The "carbohydrate addiction theory," like so many others, preys on the fact that many people don't know it's all right to crave carbohydrates. They already feel insecure and uncertain about how they eat, and so will willingly subjugate their natural desires and needs.

DIVISIVE DIVERSIONS

A new (as of June 1993) diet that introduces yet another irrelevant tangent is The Body Type Weight Loss Program. The fundamental assertion of this scheme (which through info-mercials markets a supplement program along with a diet plan) is that all human bodies are different and thus need different diets. A quiz helps you determine which of four body types you are, the point being that your body type supposedly determines what your cravings are. To lose "weight"—naturally, the purpose of the diet—you must eat or avoid certain foods based on your specific type.

In addition to being focused on weight and size, the Body Type Weight Loss Program is definitely a "thing to follow"—testimonials include such phrases as "on the program," "kept it off," and "lost 16 pounds." The premise of the diet is that by following the diet for your type, you "cure" your cravings so you don't eat too much. The physician and author who created the program was quoted as saying, "If you follow the Body Type Diet that's right for you, you're curable, you can be cured." Where's the sickness in craving food?

What I find most disturbing about this particular program, however, is that it seeks to confuse a crucial, bottom-line biological fact: all human bodies need essentially the same fuels in the same proportions. All human bodies need a great deal of energy food (carbohydrate) and far less growth food (protein) or storage fuel (fat). And all human bodies can benefit just by loosely apportioning fuel intake to those ratios.

Moreover, the claim that differing body types will always have different cravings shuts out the possibility that a "salty-craver" or a "fat-craver" can learn to love and crave carbohydrates more. Studies have shown that after 8 to 12 weeks of eating a low-fat diet, people do lose the craving for fat; my experiences and those of my clients' corroborate that. I've found that knowing what the body needs—and realizing the desire to meet those needs—usually adds appeal to the foods that fulfill them. This diet suggests that cravings are biological destiny and cannot be altered through intellect and commitment.

There's no question that in many ways each of us is a unique individual, and some of our needs differ from those of other people. But the most basic needs we have are common to all of us, and it's wise to get those handled first. There are many hundreds of car models on the road, each with their own unique features and subtle differences in performance and requirements. But all of them—except for a very few that are especially engineered otherwise—are fueled by gasoline.

TIMES ARE CHANGING, SLOWLY

You could say there are bad diets and good diets, in terms of the degree of danger they present. But any "diet" is still just that—a diet, with all the characteristics (described in Chapter 5, "Diet Thinking" and Chapter 2, "What's Weight Got to Do with It?") that doom it to physical and emotional failure.

Fueling totally replaces "diets" and "weight loss"—in context, purpose, methods, and language. Fueling is not a "better diet." It's *no diet*—just eating. There are no trendy "X Factors" and "Y Indexes." You know your body's needs, and you meet them to whatever degree you choose. By fueling your life instead of "losing pounds," and by making choices based on science instead of hearsay, you'll live happier, healthier, and saner.

One good thing about the "yo-yo study" uproar was that it helped inspire a National Institutes of Health conference in April 1992 that brought together professionals in the field to study the issues. Although the validity of weight loss itself unfortunately remained unchallenged, the national attention was a valuable first step. Diet bashing doesn't change diet thinking, but it's a start.

I don't believe diets themselves are the root problem—it's the thinking, and lack of it, that nurtured the "diet" concept—I must caution that the demise of official diets is not the end of the problem. For every person I meet who has dieted (or still does) there are two or three who wouldn't *call* what they do a "diet," but whose way of eating (or not eating) is just as inefficient or unhealthy.

In fact, while I have worked with many men and women who have suffered through the commercial dieting routine, the most common situation I encounter today is the person who is trying to "change their lifestyle"—and is totally lost. Approaching it as "a lifestyle" rather than "a diet" is no guarantee of success. Just wanting to "eat better for life" doesn't teach you how. The typical caller for the BodyFueling workshop says, "I'm trying to eat right/better/healthy, and I did a pseudo-lifestyle diet program years ago, and I have a juicer and a fat-counter, and I take vitamins, but I'm still struggling with my 'weight.' Can you help?"

Yes, I can—through providing a complete education. I know how badly that education is needed because I have heard the story above too many times to count. Americans turning away from dieting feel betrayed when quasi-healthy lifestyle efforts don't work any better than diets. Thorough, thoughtful, quality education—not "healthy lifestyle" jargon and gimmicks—must fill the void left by the demise of "dieting." Otherwise, people will continue to starve, struggle and, ultimately, give up.

Thus the end of diets is really a beginning. What a breakthrough it will be to have a generation "fueling" instead of dieting, maintaining rather than destroying their body tissue. The good news is, it's really possible.

7

OVERTURNING THE OVEREATING MYTH

After weight, the most solidly entrenched pillar of diet thinking is the notion that we must all "eat less." Because of this long-ingrained assumption, a great deal of energy is channeled into "taming overeating," which clouds the fact that the amount of food most people—especially women—consider excessive is actually required for leanness.

The biology of how your body uses food as fuel explodes the rationale for "eating less." Obviously, the volumes of food you eat can be quite *high* if it's primarily complex carbohydrate food, rather than primarily protein or fat. Secondly, it exposes extremes of "eating less" as a cause of fatness, rather than the solution. If eating less deprives you of carbohydrate, and carb deprivation leads to muscle breakdown, and muscle burns 98 percent of the calories you consume . . . well, it doesn't take a genius to see the problem here, does it?

Yet even as these basics of human biology demonstrate food quantity to be the least important issue (well behind quality and frequency), American fitness efforts remain firmly focused on how much food is "allowed"—or, to use one of diet thinking's favorite phrases, "portion control." You cut your portions, often eating infrequently or choosing poor-quality food as well, and expect positive results.

142

YOUR OVEREATING PROBABLY *ISN'T*

Diet-thinking people struggle with this. Karen, a client in her forties, said: "I've dieted for twenty-five years. I'm used to not being 'allowed' to eat more than 600 to 700 calories a day. It's hard to get used to all this eating. I look back at that sixteen-year-old who started dieting, and now I know if she hadn't, I wouldn't look the way I do right now. The joke is, when I was sixteen I didn't even *need* to diet."

People are often unable to trust even the sober black and white of a biology textbook: "I know what it says," confided one client, "and it obviously worked for you. But I can't stop thinking I should just be having a small salad." Another reported how tempting it was "just to skip a few meals" to "speed up" her results, even though we had demonstrated how that would actually slow them down. And in the *New York Times* "anti-diet" article, one woman close to tears is quoted as saying, "How can you ask me not to diet? I've been dieting my whole life. My family, everybody expects it."

When in our seminars we discuss the amount of food human bodies need to function optimally, generally three out of four participants respond to our recommendations with initial disbelief. "Are you sure I should be eating this much?" People who consider 2 or 3 servings of carbohydrate at a meal to be too much (a serving being about 15 grams of carbohydrate; 3 servings being equal to a bagel or a medium baked potato)—well, I can only imagine what they're eating. Or, should I say, not eating.

More astonishing is how many people will insist they have an overeating problem. Ruled by diet thinking, they're absolutely convinced that they eat too much *and* that this is a psychological problem. Randomly surveying the workshop registrations of 300 clients, I counted 146 who claimed somewhere on the form that "My problem is overeating" or "I'm a compulsive overeater" (self-diagnosed). When asked to describe a "typical day of eating," they list such a pittance of food that it's clear they're seriously underfueling—and many are also "overfatting" when they do eat. No one I've ever worked with who said, "I overeat, that's my problem" eats near the volume that I do.

It's because of your meager food intake—not in spite of it—that your body makes and stores more fat, and uses less. What you've been told is the solution is actually the problem—a little basic education would have made that apparent long ago. Unfortunately, as shown by the following examples, confusion and lack of education is epidemic:

From a report in the June 1992 issue of *Allure* on a recent Oxford University study:

Psychologist Sarah Beglin and psychiatrist Christopher Fairburn interviewed 243 normal women, aged 16 to 35, about their eating habits during the previous month. . . . About [9 percent] reported occurrences of what the researchers called "subjective bulimic episodes": They felt out of control with their eating, but they actually consumed very little. Many of the women were sure they'd binged . . . nearly half the women they talked to were sure they'd overeaten at least once during the month—although again, the amount of food they reported eating was not large . . . "Women are looking at their own behavior as pathological. Usually it's not," contends Beglin.

The September 1991 *Shape* reported:

Among college-age women studied over a one-year period, 85 percent believed they needed to lose weight and 60 to 70 percent reported having been on a diet, even though about 95 percent of them were already at their ideal weight, according to researchers at Tufts University School of Nutrition. . . . "Their relationship with food is one of anxiety," says Bailey [Stephen Bailey, Ph.D.]. "Women who are consuming between 800 and 1,000 calories a day don't even think they're on a diet," he says. "Restricted eating is habitual behavior for them."

NOT A PSYCHOLOGICAL PROBLEM—NOT A PROBLEM, PERIOD!

Fat is a physiological problem—no doubt in some cases having begun with a psychological issue, but in most cases probably not. To insist it's psychological takes the overfat problem totally off course. Through counseling, analysis and psychological manipulation ("behavior modification" makes you sound like a rat, doesn't it?), fat people are told to eat less when they're probably not even eating enough—when "eating less" is part of the problem, perhaps even the cause!

But this truth is clouded by diet thinking. When Americans are told leanness and health can't be achieved without addressing "deeper issues such as binge eating, food dependency, self-esteem and learning to accept one's genetically determined weight . . ." (*Shape*, March 1992), it's no surprise we assume eating is an emotional and physical land mine that has to be controlled. So we grit our teeth and starve. As a result, we get fatter and fatter, and more frustrated (as is understandable when you keep doing what you've always thought would work and it doesn't).

Jackie Berning, M.S., R.D., wrote in *Shape* magazine in April 1991: "Many doctors used to attribute the difficulty to low self-esteem and other psychological problems, but we now know there are physical factors that encourage the regaining of lost weight. . . . Rapid weight loss through restricted diet is difficult to sustain . . . because the body has mechanisms that react to starvation."

Author and educator Covert Bailey has been saying it for years. In *Fit or Fat* he points out, "There are 500-pound people who are getting fatter every day on 1,000 calories—while undergoing psychological counseling and behavior modification to convince them to eat less." Fat people are encouraged to do what physically doesn't work—and to blame their psyches when, predictably, it fails.

It's no wonder such people also don't want to exercise. Who wants to drive without enough fuel in the tank? People on diets give up exercise easily because there's little or no fuel available for the body to run at the "higher speeds" of exercise. It feels terrible, so you stop—or never start. And then you feel terrible about that. Actually, your body is being sensible, even if you aren't—it's doing what it's supposed to under the circumstances of starvation.

"THERE ARE NO CONTRADICTIONS"

It's not an anomaly that fat people eat very little and lean people eat a lot. How many times have you said (or heard someone say), "I just don't understand it. I eat hardly anything and I just can't seem to lose 'weight,' " or "I've been skipping dinner every night and I just seem to be getting fatter," or, "I can't believe so-and-so. All she/he does is eat, and he/she is thin as a rail!"

Whenever I hear these words, I think of a character in Ayn Rand's *Atlas Shrugged*, who told another, "There are no contradictions. If you think you see a contradiction, check your premises. One of them will be faulty."

There's nothing baffling about a person eating all the time and being lean, because eating all the time is an important part of what it takes! The faulty premise here is a backward generalization: "eating makes you fat" or "food is fattening." If you just look at basic biology, it's obvious. The correct sentence would read: "I eat hardly anything and *that's why* I can't lose [fat]." "He eats everything in sight and *that's why* he's thin as a rail."

A Cornell University study summarized in *Prevention* and *Parade* (the national Sunday paper supplement) confirms that frequent high-carbohydrate, low-fat eating encourages fat burning—and, regardless of quantity, does not promote fat gain:

> Cornell University nutritionists reveal that if you eat lean, you can eat all you want. . . . When a group of women switched from eating a fat-laden American diet to one in which roughly 22 percent of the calories came from fat, they steadily lost . . . about half a pound a week. While you may think this is a paltry amount, consider this: The losers ate as much low-fat food as they wanted . . . all fruits (except avocados), all beans, bread, bagels, English muffins, tortillas, most breakfast cereals, grains, pasta, nonfat milk and yogurt, lean fish, light chicken or turkey meat (without skin), pretzels, air-popped popcorn, rice cakes, angel-food cake, fig bars, animal and graham crackers, chestnuts, ices, Fudgsicles™, Creamsicles™, puddings made with skim milk and all of the new fat-free goodies (Gail A. Levey, R.D., *Parade*, November 10, 1991).

The research of Dr. Peter Vash, assistant clinical professor at UCLA and author of *The Fat to Muscle Diet*, has compared the effects of a 40 percent fat diet (the American average) with a 20 percent fat diet. Even though both diets totaled 2,000 calories, the latter group burned significantly more calories daily than the former. This shouldn't be surprising to you, now that you know carbohydrates take more energy to burn than fat does. As Dr. Vash explains: "Your body expends only six calories to turn 200 calories of food fat into bodyfat. Yet it burns 46 calories to convert 200 protein or carbohydrate calories into bodyfat." A high-carbohydrate diet gets you burning "hotter," so more food, so long as it's complex carb, is not only okay—it's an *advantage*. See how far you can get with knowledge of biology and common-sense reasoning?

OVEREATING VERSUS OVERFATTING

This makes what kind of fuel you're consuming a critical matter. Carbohydrates can be consumed in great quantities without fat gain, while fat cannot.

When I worked for a public relations firm years ago, 20 of us would gather every Monday at noon for a staff meeting. Lunch was ordered from a deli that featured triple-size sandwiches, as well as salads and soups. My standard fare was a humongous chicken breast sandwich with mustard and assorted vegetables, a bowl of vegetable, bean, or pea soup, often with a roll, and fruit salad for dessert. Almost everyone else was "on a diet" and would have either a lone pint of fruit salad, or a tiny spinach salad with bacon bits, dollops of creamy dressing, and a roll with butter.

Although my co-workers would marvel at the quantity of food I consumed, they never considered that in addition to providing sufficient fuel, my sandwich, soup, and plain roll totaled less fat than their tiny, dressing-coated spinach salads and buttered rolls. Minuscule lunches like that are not only low on satisfaction but high in fat.

It is entirely possible to consume massive quantities of food and very little fat—and by the same token to consume pitiful little quantities of food with lots of fat. And eating lots of fat definitely increases bodyfat—even more so when partnered with deprivation. Think of a large load of fat going into a machine that has been programmed to save it.

By our culture's standards, I was "overeating" for lunch, while those eating their fuel-poor mini-salads (with triple the fat) were eating "normally." But I was enjoying myself; they remained hungry. I was fueled; they weren't. I was eating less fat, and getting more food and a greater variety of nutrients.

I see this in grocery stores: overfat people in line with a cart only half-filled. They've got vegetables, salad fixings—and butter, dressing, peanut butter, whole milk, and chips. Sometimes they've got those containers of pasta or rice salad—creamy with mayo and oil. And, of course, cans of Slim-Fast. My cart might have four times as much food in it—loaded with loaves of bread; rolls, bagels, pasta, noodles, and rice; soups; fruit and vegetables; fat-free/sugar-free crackers, cookies, granola bars, pretzels, nonfat frozen yogurt; lean poultry and fish; beans, cereals, and juices. I have *never* seen an overfat person with a cart like mine. I have *never* had an overfat client who was not starving or consuming lots of fat, or some combination thereof.

"WHY DO I EAT?" WHO CARES?

How much to eat isn't all that obscures the importance of *what* and *how often*; the senseless quest for portion control also forms the basis for the pointless pursuit of reasons *why* we eat. This endless fascination with psychological motives for doing something physically necessary is universal. The question "why do we eat?" is the darling of the media, the "weight-loss" industry, and the public alike.

Since diet thinking says eating is wrong, that twisted logic dictates that if we can pinpoint emotions that make us eat, we can "work around" those feelings and thus avoid eating. This doesn't take into account, of course, that your reasons for wanting to eat might be valid—that maybe those "feelings" come at least in part (if not completely) from your body.

Since what works for leanness is to eat enough good fuel, and often enough, who cares why you're eating it? When you realize that eating is not a problem, then neither are emotions, sensations, or feelings that encourage eating. So much energy is squandered trying to manipulate feelings that "trigger" eating, to "modify" behavior that is really normal. That energy is far better spent focusing on what *kind* of eating—educating people so that when they do eat, regardless of the reason, they are in a position to make informed choices.

"I eat out of boredom, or loneliness, or frustration. That's my problem." It's not a problem! Go ahead! Feed your hungry heart! Fill the love hunger! Eat for boredom! Eat for loneliness! Eat out of stress. Eat because you and your boyfriend broke up. Eat because you didn't break up.

I eat for all kinds of reasons, all the time—but I don't eat high-fat, high-sugar items. Don't worry so much about why you eat and focus instead on eating.

EATING DISORDERS AND DIET THINKING: WHICH CAME FIRST?

I think there is a dire need for researchers and therapists of all kinds to reexamine and redefine their classifications for eating disorders. If definitions are based purely on what people eat and how much, I myself might be considered to have a disorder, based on unscientific diet thinking about what is "normal." According to those standards the fact that I eat bagels, cereal, and fruit at midnight, or an entire box of fat-free cookies while grocery shopping, might qualify me as a "binger"—even though I'm freely choosing and enjoying the food without conflict or guilt, I'm eating because I'm hungry, and I'm secure in the knowledge that my choices won't make me fat.

Compulsiveness is in the *intent*, not the action. It is the state of mind—the hysteria and mental self-abuse accompanying the eating—that makes it a disorder. A person downing a box of cookies could be being compulsive. But I'm calm and happy, enjoying myself. I know exactly what I want, and when I eat it, I'm done. No guilt, no fear.

Unfortunately, because "weight control" has so often been painted as an emotional issue, psychologists have been encouraged to assign labels and diagnoses to what might more appropriately be termed *misinformed* behavior. Remember, therapists (and other professionals) come from the same background of (mis)understanding, the same belief systems that the patients do. No one is exempt from the influence of the diet-thinking paradigm. I have been at dinner parties and banquets where brilliant doctors, psychiatrists, or other highly educated professionals said things like, "I didn't eat all day, so now I can really indulge," or "Mmm, that luscious bread looks sooo fattening!" or "I think I'll skip dinner so I can have dessert." (When I mention what I do in my business, no matter how I phrase it, they interpret it as: "Oh, so you help people lose weight/eat less/cut calories?") More than one client has recalled visiting a hypnotist to "lose weight"—and being hypnotized to "eat less and not want food."

If counselors and therapists view patients—especially the obese—through diet thinking, they're not only barking up the wrong tree, but possibly hurting their patients in the process. Research confirms that professionals do see the "fat problem" this way. *Shape* magazine in March 1992 cited a *Journal of the American Dietetic Association* article that called for major changes in the weight-loss industry (of course, my vote is to start by calling it something besides "weight loss"). It identified that research shows health professionals tend to stereotype "overweight" people as "weak-willed, ugly, awkward, self-indulgent and emotionally disturbed." If that's what they believe, what are they going to "treat"?

I believe psychological problems are created when people are mistakenly ordered to restrict their normal eating in the first place. For example, women who are eating normally (or already too little) are made to *feel* "compulsive" in the constant battle against their healthy appetites and instincts.

I think there's a desperate need for standard definitions that not only bring consistency and accuracy to the labels slapped on people by professionals, but also lay to rest the self-diagnosis that is rampant, especially among women. In my experience, the commonly self-diagnosed "disease" of compulsive overeating is nothing more in the majority of cases than people eating normally, but questioning their intake based on the skewed, unscientific standards of the culture-wide campaign to lose "weight."

If our culture got the idea that people should sleep only two hours a night, everyone who felt the physiological urge to sleep six or eight hours would then be "oversleepers." If they succumbed despite their resistance, they'd be labeled "compulsive sleepers," and might go into therapy designed to improve their willpower, to better exercise rigid control against these perfectly natural urges.

Most people who have diagnosed themselves as overeaters learn they are just fine during BodyFueling. They stop berating themselves for eating, realizing it is normal and healthy, and that it's even okay to enjoy eating at the same time that it is providing necessary fuel. They realize they weren't screwed up—just uninformed. Even people who are obese find that after decades of advice about their supposed "compulsions"—from professionals, well-meaning family, and friends—they simply need to make a few key changes they never heard about or understood.

There is every indication that eating disorders begin not in a vacuum of body standards, but in an information void about how to achieve those standards. "Liza," a client who was bulimic, spoke candidly with me about how her compulsion began: "The purpose was only to stay thin. And what I thought back then was that eating makes you fat. So I had to have all this structure to keep me from eating." What if she had learned very early that eating keeps you lean, and that starving makes you fat-fertile in a number of ways?

The black hole of education continues to encourage disordered behavior once it has triggered it. Liza injured herself again and again through compulsive overexercising after a body composition program at her athletic club told her she could lose more fat if she worked out six days instead of four and cut her caloric intake. This was downright irresponsible; anyone should have been able to tell that Liza did not need to lose any bodyfat and was obsessed with it.

Gale, an obese man, told us, "I learned a lot of things in my eating disorder treatment program. But a lot was left out, too. I didn't know how carbohydrates get used by the body, how protein gets used, and how fat gets used. Even though they gave me a pretty similar 'diet' to follow (except for snacks), without that background, it was just a diet. I had no understanding of why it works." *And he wasn't doing it when he came to our program.*

Sometimes people who've been told they're "overeaters" and have accepted that label are somewhat reluctant to remove it. They've become attached to whatever payoffs their "diagnosis" provides. One individual became quite upset during a seminar because I said her self-diagnosed "compulsive overeating" would be fine—if only she began choosing more high-carbohydrate, low-fat foods to "overeat." She insisted she just couldn't lose fat because she was an overeater.

Her description of what she actually ate on a given day was roughly half of my normal consumption in food volume—though her fat consumption was probably twice mine. She was in therapy for this "eating disorder," but was unable to see that she could make an informed decision about whether that label really fit. "Accepting" that she was an "overeater" had somehow become easier than having a choice about what she ate.

I can hand you the key to your cell and invite you to be free—but I've noticed some people would rather stay in jail.

A CASE STUDY: UNDERFUELING UNMASKED

Judy, the morbidly obese client I referred to in Chapter 1, "Fueling Your Future," went home after BodyFueling and threw out everything in her cupboards. She joined the local cooperative grocery and is taking every cooking class they offer. She has, she said, begun a new life.

> All through the years of being fat, people always tried to tell me why it was I was fat—that is, what my "issue" was. I went through life "knowing" there was something mentally wrong with me. When I did BodyFueling and learned how my body works, I saw that it was very simple. If there was anything psychological, it was caused by all of the attention on whether I was "normal" or not, on my "problems."
>
> I really didn't know what to eat, or how much, or how often, or where to buy it, or how to cook it. All those years, and no one ever talked about what my body needed and how to do it. It's always this stuff about what you're repressing and what "inner needs" you're feeding. Can you believe in all those years, no one ever talked to me about the burgers and the big fatty muffins?
>
> When you asked at the start of the seminar, "What do you think of when you hear the term *BodyFueling*," it was like bells went off. I thought instantly of making a machine go, with fuel. I realized that was what food was. It sounded totally different than anything else I'd ever heard about food.

Being obese *doesn't* mean you're emotionally screwed up. We can educate overfat people about what works. If it's done intelligently and thoroughly, without condescension and "shoulds," if their path to leanness and health isn't cluttered with imposed psychological hurdles, I can guarantee that the information will make a difference.

People love to say, "Oh, but you *can't* just approach it scientifically. People don't think that way about food. It's a very emotional issue. People have 'food issues' and you can't just approach it simply and factually. There's too much emotional 'baggage' that goes with it. People can't look at food simply as fuel."

But Judy and a thousand BodyFuelers have proven that you can. The problem is that most people have never tried. They're taught to jump to the conclusion that it couldn't possibly work for them. Who has ever considered that maybe the psychological problems show up because those who "treat" the problem are looking for it, even create it?

What did that approach ever do for Judy, obese for most of her youth and adult life? People were so convinced that, being obese, Judy couldn't possibly deal with switching from beef with mayo to turkey with mustard. It was assumed she wouldn't. She was analyzed for three decades before someone approached her about eating bagels instead of doughnuts. They decided for her.

It certainly never occurred to Judy that eating didn't have to be negative and rigidly controlled. Through all the time that friends, family, doctors, and therapists were talking with her about her "problems," the underlying message was that she shouldn't be eating and that if she was, it was a sign of psychological trouble. "I can remember all of my life being hungry. I was always hungry, but I didn't eat, because I 'knew' I shouldn't eat. I 'knew' eating was wrong," she says.

Therapists and other practitioners may protest, saying, "That's not what we meant," or "We never said that, not that way." But, my friends, you must be responsible for what you leave people with. That's what Judy heard. And you know she is not alone.

OVEREATERS ANONYMOUS

The indications are that undereating—under*fueling*—and excess fat consumption are responsible for much of America's fat problem. Therefore, the 12-step program approach of Overeaters Anonymous (OA) is probably overkill for many people who use it as a "diet" tool. It should only be used to address an actual addiction or disorder in which you really are harming yourself and cannot stop, even when you know what would work.

For many people, however, the distinction between "what would work" and "what will harm" has been blurred. Diet thinking labels harmful practices such as suppressing appetite or avoiding food as "good"; and normal, healthy ones, such as eating, "bad." So when you're doing what works, you think you need "help." If Mary is left to decide whether she is an addict, and our misinformed culture has labeled her perfectly normal carbohydrate snacking "overeating," she will try to "treat" her normal desire to eat. Perhaps her eating may even have become a little frenzied because of all of the misdirected diet programming that taught her she shouldn't eat, and that frenzy scares her. But adding more control is only going to make that worse.

Therefore, unless you've truly transcended diet thinking, self-diagnosis can't be trusted. And if you have indeed moved beyond diet thinking, it's doubtful you'll need to be in or on any kind of program.

Besides, as with any 12-step program, the assertion of Overeaters Anonymous from square one is that something is wrong with you—you're addicted; in fact, you must say so in order to stay and participate. OA also promotes the notion that you can never be "cured." You carry around forever the "knowledge" that you are an addict.

Rather than entering a 12-step program that's geared to curbing your eating, why not allow yourself the freedom to eat again? Given the coercive effect diet thinking has had on America's eating, I don't think the idea of an Underfuelers Anonymous (how to unhinge yourself from the gripping conviction that your meager pickings are "too much") is too silly.

WHAT ABOUT OVERCOMING OVEREATING?

Speaking of allowing yourself the freedom to eat again, the book and program Overcoming Overeating (OO) deserves mention because many of its tenets explode past diet thinking in an impressive manner. I don't agree with all that they say and do—obviously, I don't approve of the name, which I think is misleading. Also, OO peddles its share of diet-thinking assumptions and vocabulary. But Carol Munter and Jane Hirschmann, the women who created OO, do challenge some of the foundations of diet thinking:

WHAT I LIKE. Munter and Hirschmann are reported to be enthusiastic eaters who consume anything they want to, don't count calories or fat grams, and believe in working with the body. They point to the sense of "scarcity" created by food restriction as a harbinger of compulsiveness, and remind us that we're born with—and can regain—the natural instinct to eat for sustenance. Permission replaces discipline; no food is "bad."

WHAT I DON'T LIKE. While the means is good, the end to which it leads falls short. That is, the individual ideas that mark Overcoming Overeating's methodology are laudable, but what they're used for is limited by the boundaries of diet thinking. It's that anti-diet, only-two-options, let-yourself-be-fatter thinking—and it ends there. You abandon dieting, but then you "accept a higher 'weight' " as a result. You aren't presented with the third option—being lean by abandoning dieting, by gorging with educated precision rather than ignorant compulsion. You don't distinguish between "weight" and "fat" or between "lean and "thin," so the pursuit of health and leanness is jettisoned along with the compulsive pursuit of thinness.

A major problem with OO is that its adherents often remain confused because the power and freedom being proffered becomes entangled in the dregs of diet thinking that remain. You don't learn the biology of your body; you don't become a fully educated owner and use your newfound freedom to choose fueling. Though some do report eventually finding their way to that choice, it seems hit-or-miss.

This, from the August 17, 1992, *Newsweek*, is unfortunately typical of the reporting I've seen about OO: " 'If it's okay to be fat, why do I still want to lose weight?' asked a heavy middle-aged woman at the OO meeting." Because it's *not* okay—from a health standpoint—to be fat. And you want to lose weight because you still haven't learned that your "weight" is not just fat, and that just losing weight won't make you lean.

A 26-year-old TV producer quoted in the same article reportedly tried 50 diets before reading *Overcoming Overeating*. She insists the "program" feels great, but adds, " 'Deep inside there's a lower weight I'd like to be at. . . . though I feel comfortable where I am now and can stay here if this is where I'm meant to stay.' " I think her response is consistent with what I've noticed. There's some relief, but she hasn't broken the surface of diet thinking. There's a wistfulness, a lingering sense of disappointment and resignation about weight—no conviction that her weight really is meaningless. Her accomplishment lies mainly in what she *doesn't* do anymore. There's no joy, no sense of what she *can* do to connect eating with fueling her future.

CALORIES DON'T COUNT—
SO DON'T COUNT THEM

I hope our civilization will soon be rid completely of this archaic practice called "calorie counting." It's a retentive and diversionary extension of trying to eat less. Low-calorie diet proponents tell you calories are bad, but never even explain what they are. They're just one more thing to worry and feel guilty about.

A calorie is simply the standard unit of measurement used to measure the heat, or energy, produced when food is oxidized by the body. For the layperson, a useful analogy is that calories tell you how much "mileage" a food will give you. A food's caloric content tells you its MPG (miles per gram)—how far that food will take you.

Every gram of carbohydrate or protein will give you 4.1 calories worth of energy; each gram of fat provides 9.3. That's why fat is the choice fuel for storage. A smart machine would choose fat whenever it needed to stash away emergency fuel, because every gram of it packs more than twice the energy value of either carbohydrate or protein. If you were building a savings, would you choose to stash away nine-dollar bills or four-dollar bills?

In terms of bodyfat and body leanness, the source of your calories is what's important—so important that the number is virtually immaterial. Getting some particular total number doesn't take into account what the calories are made of—it's far more critical to get the appropriate proportions or percentages of your calories from needed fuels. To refer to calories without identifying their source makes no more sense and has no more value than to discuss weight without knowing the content of the pounds. Yet, as with weight, we've assumed that quantity is more important than the content.

Calories may come from protein, carbohydrate, and fat. The body does not use these three in the same ways, with the same readiness, or in the same amounts. You've already seen that the three behave very differently when they are digested and reach your bloodstream. For example, fat calories are stored more readily; carbohydrates burn additional calories (use more energy) to break down, offering a metabolic advantage. Protein is ideally not burned as energy at all. Calories from protein cannot be expected to serve the body in the same way as carbohydrate. They do not readily substitute for one another.

Daily calorie quotas without any regard for where the calories are coming from are ineffective for fat loss, and downright dangerous to health. To simply suggest one restrict calories to a certain number, as many diets do, is naively simplistic. People interpret this to mean any kind of calories. When I was a teenager, I figured I could eat anything as long as my calories totaled 1,000. It could be chocolate and bran muffins spaced seven hours apart (and, I painfully recall, often was just that). Just so long as I "limited my calories." Did I lose "weight"? Sure. Need I say more?

Advertising contributes to the confusion—one-calorie this and no-calorie that have left normally intelligent people thinking no calories at all would make the ideal food or diet. No one thinks to specify that no calories in a food or diet means *no fuel*—which would make it impossible to survive for any length of time. I've met bright people who believed calories were nasty little physical entities found in food—literally like raisins or nuts—which could be extracted to make the food acceptable.

Articles like "Summer Diet Plan" (Harper's *Bazaar*, January 1992) don't help. "Despite the fact that fat calories are more readily converted into body fat than other kinds, a calorie is still a calorie. And weight loss occurs only when the calories consumed are fewer than those burned. Although starches like pasta, bread and grains aren't inherently fattening, large amounts can have an undesirable effect." A registered dietitian stated for the article, "If you're trying to lose weight, you still have to limit these foods somewhat. A cup of rice has a lot more calories than a cup of plain vegetables."

It's this kind of deceiving material that leaves people trying to resist the foods the body needs most. A calorie is not just a calorie; that's ridiculous. Weight loss (including muscle) occurs when you consume less carbohydrate than the body needs. Fat loss occurs when you engage in activity that demands fuel while consuming enough carbohydrate so that you're more likely to use fat than hoard it. Either way, it has everything to do with enough grams of specific fuel, such as carbohydrate, and almost nothing do with numbers of calories.

The facts about how a calorie's source determines its destiny are part of simple human biology. You'd think it would be obvious that focusing primarily on the number alone is a sham. To merely count calories is oppressive and ultimately counterproductive. But that focus has survived for decades; even today, the health care and scientific communities continue in hot pursuit of generic calorie reduction.

Let's look at an example. Roy Walford, M.D., a physician and researcher, touts the "necessity" of low-calorie diets for health. His assertions imply that my 2,500-plus daily calories are unhealthy, even though I get three-fourths of them from complex carbs and only 10 to 15 percent from fat. Based on the "low-calorie is healthy" theory, I'd be better off eating only 1,200 calories of anything—doughnuts, steak, whatever.

Actually, if you look at the research Dr. Walford conducted to prove his low-calorie hypothesis, you can see a real leap based on diet thinking. The monkeys in his experiment ate not only a 1,200 calorie diet, but also an 11 percent fat diet. There are two variables here. Yet of those two variables, he and every reporter who covered the study pounced on the calorie limit, failing to make the low-fat percentage a prominent point. They've arbitrarily decided the calorie variable is what caused the monkeys to be healthier and live longer, rather than the low-fat nature of the experimental diet.

Other research has shown bodyfat and dietary fat to be the culprits where our nation's most fatal epidemics are concerned—and that depriving calories only lowers weight, not bodyfat. In fact, a 1,200-calorie deprivation diet stands a good chance of causing increased bodyfat. Even the government's new food labeling laws include a "Daily Value" of 2,000 calories for women and 2,500 calories for men on every label as a basic guideline. The substantial "eat all you want as long as it's low-fat complex carbohydrate" research only corroborates my experience and that of my clients.

If Dr. Walford is so sure it is the number of calories that counts, and not the 11 percent fat, that should be proven without other variables. Feed the monkeys 1,200 calories a day of protein and fat, and see if the low-calorie theory still holds. I believe that would be a better way to spend the $1 billion that has been appropriated to test the low-calorie theory on humans (which will amount to more money spent reinforcing and trying to substantiate the miserable myth that you must eat less).

According to Walford's book, personal experiences and clinical observations are irrelevant because they don't occur in a laboratory as a controlled experiment governed by all the rules of research. You can decide for yourself whether it's relevant that my clients and I eat a 10 to 20 percent fat diet, with frequent meals and snacks high in complex carbs and low to moderate in protein (15–25 percent)—but double the low-calorie proponents' suggestion of 1,000 to 1,200 calories per day. We don't trip the fat-harboring mechanisms that respond to deprivation. We've tailored suits and dresses to our fat loss. And we are healthy. I stopped catching colds and flu when I stopped trying to be active at athletics while eating as few calories as possible.

It's just this kind of research that perpetuates the overeating myth, and persuades people to underfuel. The reporting doesn't help. The April 1992 *Men's Health* had this: "How do the experts recommend we lose weight? Seventy-five percent said that *cutting calories* is Extremely Important or Very Important . . . If you cut calories, you'll cut fat." *Think!* There's absolutely no effort made to distinguish fat calories from carbohydrate calories, which only persuades people they can gorge on cake and ice cream and forego everything else. They'll eat under 900 calories because they think calories are the key—but they're still getting 45 percent of those calories from fat! With advice like, "The number of calories you eat ultimately determines how much you weigh," it's no wonder, as the article says, that "obesity is one of the country's biggest health problems."

Moreover, when told to eat fewer calories, one must ask what *is* "fewer"? Fewer than what? Generic recommendations don't take into account what you're doing to begin with. If I tell you to get "less sleep," won't you wonder how I can assert that you need less of something when I don't know what you're already getting? What if you're already sleeping only two hours a night?

The media certainly can—and typically does—make the original diet thinking much worse by botching the translation with leaps of reasoning, semantic blunders, and generalizations. Let's take another look at Walford's monkey studies, this time through a writer's perspective. An item on Walford's study in a health-food store magazine (Lauri M. Aesoph, N.D., in *Delicious!*, May/June 1992) noted: "After four years of calorie cutting, the leaner monkeys are healthy and maturing slower than the well-fed group." This reflects conjecture that the leaner monkeys are leaner because of the calorie cutting; there's no proof of this, and certainly no mention of which type of calories were cut.

Secondly, it's assumed that the diet, not the leanness itself, was responsible for the monkeys' health and slow aging. Isn't it logical that *being* lean is what made these monkeys healthier, not necessarily whatever it took to *get* lean? Finally, if the calorie-cutting was healthier, isn't it odd to call the non-calorie-cutting monkeys "well-fed"?

Walford applies the same blind assumptions to himself and others. An article in the September 1990 issue of *Self* noted that over the past five years, the 67-year-old Walford has lost 12 percent of his body weight and he recommends that "patients shed 10 to 25 percent of their weight . . . over four to six years." He makes the claim that reducing "weight" in exactly this manner "may decrease susceptibility to cancer, diabetes and cardiovascular disease, and increase your life span . . . depending on . . . how faithfully you maintain the reduced weight."

More diet thinking! What did Walford lose? What component of his body weight? If Walford is a six-foot or so male who gets any exercise at all, and he was consuming a paltry 1,200 calories a day, his loss almost certainly did include muscle. Losing 12 percent of one's body weight could be a disaster if any of it was muscle. Losing 25 percent of one's "weight," if principally muscle, could be downright deadly. Does that decrease susceptibility to disease? It's much more significant and valuable to have a 44 percent drop in body*fat* (as I have) than a 12 percent drop in body *weight*.

The reporting suggests that "low-calorie" is right for everyone. Even if "low" or "lower" actually did identify something specific, how can everyone need the same "low" number of calories? Dr. Walford surely would not dispute that muscle demands fuel and impacts metabolism—that's part of the most common and fundamental physiology of homo sapiens. More muscle means more food is needed for fuel. Since people have different amounts of muscle, that indicates that people need different amounts of fuel.

Activity level also affects how much food you need. The runner training at 60 miles a week will need more calories of fuel than the person walking three miles a week. How then can we all subsist "healthily" on 1,200 calories a day? How can a man with 160 pounds of muscle exercising seven hours a week need the same number of calories as a woman with 100 pounds of muscle exercising two hours a week? Such calorie limits are just as vague and groundless a limit as an "ideal weight."

THE CASE FOR LOW FAT, HIGH CALORIES

During my second year of fueling, I consumed 2,500 or so calories a day (about twice the low-calorie proponents' one-size-fits-all recommendation), and I didn't gain an ounce of anything except lean muscle. Of course, that added muscle meant I kept needing to eat more to maintain my new muscle. And I kept losing fat very slowly; after dropping 6 pounds of fat within six months of beginning to "fuel" this way, I lost another 10 over the next 18 months. Slow? Sure, but it was pure fat, no muscle loss—and there was no hurry because it's not like I was suffering or waiting for the end. *This is how I eat.*

"Oh, she must exercise like crazy, though." Not so. While I do bicycle everywhere for two or three months a year (summer), I otherwise do about three hours a week of aerobics—modest by any standards. I do 45 to 60 minutes of weights—*per week*. When I'm bicycling a lot, I might cycle up to five or six hours a week. But I significantly up my food intake accordingly.

Now, society considers 2,500 to 3,000 calories a day an obscene amount for a woman. Women have had it drummed into their heads that even 1,200 calories is a lot—even if they're very active. Some women swear they "gain weight" on 1,000 calories a day. (Sure, they can gain fat that way—because their underfueled bodies are fighting to store everything they eat as fat.) They—and many researchers and health professionals—assume that if 1,000 calories a day isn't working, it must be too much. So they go lower, compounding the problem.

Everything I do works to make my body burn hotter and more efficiently, and creates "permission" to spend fat when fat is an appropriate choice. I never deprive, so my body never gets a famine signal and tries to "shore up" its fat stores, and I never need to "eat" my own muscle. Dietary protein is always available to build muscle if I lift weights. I eat very little fat, so when my body does need fat for energy—during endurance exercise, say—it's more likely to "dip into" reserves of bodyfat. And processing all those complex carbs I eat raises my overall metabolism.

Am I working hard at all this? No. I enjoy unbelievable amounts of bread, bagels, rolls, rice, pasta, potatoes, oatmeal, cold cereal, soups, fruit, juice, fat-free/sugar-free cookies, cakes, muffins, and bars (baked by me or bought), homemade pizza, lasagne, calzones, manicotti (all with lowfat ricotta), Thai food, Chinese food, Cajun food—with lean poultry, fish, and seafood, skim dairy, beans, and lentils as my "garnish." I add fat to nothing. Butter and oil in exchange for unlimited, delicious, hearty food. No contest.

A November 1991 *Lear's* article by Marcia Seligson, a woman who began eating in a new way for health reasons, echoes this experience:

> . . . . We began by eating incessantly. . . . The amount of food we ingested in a day was embarrassing. . . . Though I am just as excited by and attached to food as I ever was, my preferences have changed. I can't tolerate the taste or feel of oily food any longer, and after Tom ate a chocolate cookie as an experiment last month, he got a stomachache. . . . Perhaps the most amazing result has been the end of suffering about food . . . I have a newfound sense of having more control over my body, my well-being, the aging process, and, indeed, my future.

A GREAT STUDY FADES; DIET THINKING FLOURISHES

It was interesting but not surprising that in all my reading, I saw Walford's research reported a dozen times, while I saw the Cornell study (described on page 146, in which subjects ate all they wanted of low-fat food and steadily lost fat) mentioned only twice. I've also seen mentioned only twice a 1988 study at the Stanford Center for Research in Disease Prevention, which found that subjects' percentage of bodyfat was not related to their caloric intake or to the size of their meals. Rather, it directly reflected the amount of fat in their diets. The same is true for Dr. Peter Vash's research that showed people who ate more calories of carbohydrate burned more.

Why did this research go generally unreported? Because Cornell, Stanford, and similar studies don't fit into the paradigm. "Low-calorie" conclusions do. Walford's data make sense to the diet-thinking media; they're familiar. The Cornell results, positive as they are, may well have been dismissed as implausible. Remember Joel Barker's Paradigm Effect:

> Any data that exists in the real world that does not fit your paradigm will have a difficult time getting through your filters. You will see little if any of it. That data that does fit your paradigm not only makes it through the filter, but is concentrated by the filtering process, thus creating an illusion of even greater support for the paradigm. . . . Any suggested alternative has to be wrong.

Of the two reports I did see on the Cornell experiment, both assumed it worked because participants "probably" ate fewer calories—since they ate less fat and fat has more calories per gram. But that's not what the study proved or set out to prove, nor was it the conclusion of its researchers. In diet thinking, that *would* be the only way they could have lost "weight." But now you know that they could have eaten lots more calories and still lost fat.

After reading the articles describing his theories, I checked Dr. Walford's book out of the library. I was surprised to discover that while I maintain fundamental disagreement with the low-calorie theory and the insistence on using weight as a measure, many of our concerns are shared ones. He too cautions against dieting, eating too little for exercise, and following nonsense programs. As usual, however, the media left out many qualifying details: Walford actually recommends starting out with 1,800 to 2,000 calories and going lower only if that doesn't spur "weight" loss. But the media jumped on the lowest number he'll support, and the familiar idea of "low-calorie." And, as usual, their interpretations drowned out the message of both the original research and the book that explores it.

I'm afraid research and reports will continue to be filtered by and shaped into standard, worn-out diet thinking, because that supports cultural biases shared by the researchers and writers and the majority of readers. But you don't have to join the Portion Control Patrol in its calorie-cutting frenzy. Being educated about your body and how it really works gives you an opportunity for true critical thinking—the ability to separate the facts from the mindless jargon.

Stay savvy about every detail of Chapter 3, "Fueling the Human Body: Your Owner's Manual"—maybe even check a few science textbooks out of the library to reinforce your trust in those facts, to expand your knowledge, and to deepen your understanding of the big picture. For now, those books are more trustworthy than news headlines. And if anyone ever tells you to "eat less" or "cut your calories," or that you "overeat," you'll have a few questions to ask them.

8

DIET THINKING
IN THE MEDIA

Now that you've identified the paradigm and can begin to make out its insidious form, you'll become more and more fluent in deciphering its language. You'll notice the tangled semantics and faulty reasoning. You'll start to hear yourself saying, even thinking, these things, and now you'll begin to question them.

This is good. It means that, for you, the paradigm has begun to shift. It is the difference between truly thinking and passively experiencing thoughts that got planted in your mind.

The media are collectively the single largest source of those implanted thoughts. After all, they are probably where you get most of your information—just as I did, before I tired of their interpretations and sought out bottom-line sources. I cut out the middleman and put myself in an informed position, so I could draw my own conclusions without the prejudice of diet thinking.

You can do the same, and now that you've had a baseline education, this chapter will give you the opportunity to practice.

It's important to remember that the media reflect the thoughts, feelings, opinions, and consciousness of their consumers—us. As Ralph Lauren says in a magazine ad for the American Society of Magazine Editors: "Magazines

163

are a window on America's culture." The degree to which diet thinking has permeated the media is a good barometer of the degree to which it has penetrated the culture.

It may be of interest to note that much of what follows came after all the diets-don't-work/yo-yo hullabaloo. Two or three years later, diet thinking is still busting out at the seams—the same speculative conclusions, misleading reports, and unscientific claims that prey on and fertilize diet thinking.

THE GOOD GUYS ARE OUTNUMBERED

While I have seen movement toward a more rational, fact-based approach to nutrition and fitness reporting, touting some of the same information you find in this book (or science books), I haven't found one piece yet that I would want to copy and hand out to my clients. No matter how promising it starts out, each piece sabotages its fresh perspective with a diet-thinking conclusion. This is in part because even when straining to forge a new reality, the media are still encumbered by old language, so the result is often more confusing than enlightening.

Publications I read have sporadically jumped on the bandwagon during the last few years, trading diet thinking for sense and science, but not to a uniform degree. For example, in May 1990 *U.S. News & World Report* noted: "Weight distribution and the proportion of fat to lean tissue are far more important than weight itself in predicting good health." But no groundswell of support has materialized behind such enlightened reporting—it's too outnumbered. For any item correctly explaining what works or how it works, I can find 20 or more that same day—often within the very same publication or report!—that directly or indirectly undermine it.

The truth is that a few magazine articles or quotes here and there cannot instantly alter the thinking created by hundreds of thousands of magazine articles before them that have exhorted people to diet, get thin, lose weight, count calories, cut back, "watch it," and so on. The campaign needs to be as pervasive as the misguided one of the last 40 years—and powerful enough to open the "diet thinking eyes and ears" of its public.

OLD AND NEW CLASH

One of the most confusing situations for readers occurs when one article of a publication is factually correct and semantically accurate, while the next page (or the next paragraph) presents woeful diet thinking. Sometimes the conflicting messages—the new and the old—appear in the very same headline. Remember Joel Barker's assertion that when a new paradigm appears, it will begin to emerge while the old one is still operating.

A succinct example is this tabloid cover: "Dolly Parton reveals how crash dieting almost killed her!" Then, directly underneath, another headline: "And, how to lose five pounds a week on new [something or other] diet." It would be laughable if it wasn't so serious.

When a magazine has 10 different editors and 25 different editorial assistants and copywriters, this is to be expected. Some may have the real scoop; others are operating under the influence of anywhere from mild to debilitating degrees of diet thinking. By June 1992, I could find more than a few articles that eschewed language such as "weight," "diet," "cut back," "calories," and "thin" in favor of "complex carbs," "bodyfat," "health," "snacks," "energy," and "eating." Even "fuel" was occasionally popping up as a synonym for food. But following each refreshing new thought was some throwback that made me cringe.

A good example of this old/new clash is a June 1992 *Allure* article entitled "Diet of the Mind," revealing the "secrets" of what it calls "a new breed of diet gurus." On the one hand, I found a few tidbits I felt good about. The article did mention a *Journal of the American Dietetic Association* statement that, "It is now widely agreed that obesity treatment is, in general, ineffective." Amen. The *Allure* piece, however, doesn't go on to give some of the simple biological reasons why. (I don't know if the *Journal of the American Dietetic Association* did either.)

One "guru" sounded like someone I could get behind: an L.A. psychologist who "believes that people will naturally eat the right amount of food once it loses its 'forbidden' attraction, and that the key to a successful diet, therefore, is not dieting at all." I was thrilled when I read that she has clients say, "I enjoy eating only when my body needs fuel, and only then do I eat." Then I read on to see that this mantra is used to help clients limit themselves to small portions. Ouch! Right tool, wrong purpose.

The few healthy reports are drowning in tired, worn diet thinking, swimming alongside references to "calories," "weight," "pounds," as well as elaborate psychological explanations for the biological fat rebound that occurs after dieting.

A dietitian explains that "people who want to go for a chocolate bar can instead go, in their mind's eye, to a place of peace and tranquility . . . relaxing and sending 'cleansing light' from the tips of the toes upward." What about the issue of whether or not they want the candy bar because they are hungry? What if they need fuel? People can't fuel their bodies on peace and visualizations! I think of poor Judy, hungry for 30 years, her stomach growling while psychologists told her to picture herself thin, or as a flower or a beam of light. Maybe that person should just eat a bagel! Or maybe they can eat the damn candy bar—if they have fueled throughout the rest of the day and usually do so day to day.

Manhattan psychologist Stephen Gullo, *Allure* reported, has clients listen to tapes with "pro-thin" affirmations such as "thin tastes better than a cookie." He calls this either/or concept a "positive idea," not like "the negative cliches dieters give themselves"—though I don't see the difference. Gullo also was reported to limit clients to 800 or 1,000 calories a day—now designated as Very Low Calorie by the American Dietetic Association. Worse, he calls "bread and pasta common triggers for overeating" and "restricts many clients to 100 grams of carbohydrate daily" (the equivalent of a potato plus a cup of cooked rice—or my typical breakfast).

It's the same old low-calorie diet, "stick-to-it" program mentality. It's just dressed up with some new, trendy mental exercises, justified by some thinly disguised psychospeak, and all based on the assumptions that one must "give up" food, calories, and the freedom to eat. Most of what these "gurus" do is designed to enforce that.

But what do you expect? Do you ask an English professor or a plumber or a race car driver how you should eat? Here are four Ph.D.s in psychology telling you how to handle a basically biological issue. "The problem, they insist, isn't in the body but in the head." Oh, please! Have they read about gluconeogenesis and the "protein-sparing effect of carbohydrate" lately? No, because "most of these diet meisters come from disciplines that talk more about pillow pounding than pounds." They are "helping diet-burned people understand not just what to eat but why they eat."

Why did I just eat that toast, orange, and bowl of cereal as I sat here typing at 2:00 A.M.? Because I was hungry, because I needed fuel to write late into the night, because it sounded good—just *because*. I know what fuels my body, I want to fuel my body, and I chose my snack based on that.

It's fair to note that in a three-page article, the methods of these practitioners might not be covered fully; they may have fallen victim to sound-bite journalism. It is possible that the dietitian who teaches people to visualize peace when they're hungry may also address the issue of getting enough food. But remember, I am only a reader, just like all the other readers. I cannot know anything about these people beyond what I am given to read—and neither can anyone else. What I am left with, everyone is left with.

Now it's your turn. Let's play "Spot the Diet Thinking." You may even want to use a pencil or highlighter to mark words and phrases you now recognize as diet thinking.

LEAPS OF REASONING: INTERPRETING DATA TO FIT THE BIAS

▶ The May 14, 1990, issue of *U.S. News & World Report* cites an April 1990 *New England Journal of Medicine* report in which UCLA physician Philip Kern found abnormally high levels of lipoprotein lipase (LPL)—the enzyme responsible for the transformation of fat into adipose tissue (stored fat)—in nine obese subjects who had lost an average of 90 pounds. These subjects had not only high levels of LPL, but also high levels of the genetic messenger that signals LPL production. His conclusion: "This suggests it may be easier for formerly fat people to regain weight."

(Suggest? May? This is news? Worse, *U.S. News & World Report*'s speculation is that this data is "a convincing argument for hereditary programming." Why? It doesn't say. An ordinary biology textbook says that the body increases production of LPL *after* you deprive the body of the fuel/food it needs for long periods. This indicates it's not genetic—it's the result of self-inflicted starvation.)

YOU'RE NOT ALLOWED TO EAT LIKE A "REGULAR" PERSON

▶ May 14, 1990, *U.S. News & World Report*: "Dieters don't just want to be slender, they want to stay slender. Yet simple as this goal seems, it often eludes the most iron-willed of calorie counters. The world seems to conspire against the newly thin. 'Have a piece of cake,' it whispers seductively. 'Have a Tootsie Roll.' There are office parties and baby showers, romantic dinners and family picnics, and they all come equipped with food."

(Food is "equipment" we need to survive. The occasional piece of cake is not what makes a "newly thin" person fat again! What made them thin also left them biologically primed to regain that fat. Note also the assumption that we're unable to make healthy choices in such situations. That's just not true.)

SLOPPY LANGUAGE, MUDDLED CONCEPTS

► *Allure*, March 1992: Citing Thomas Wadden, Associate Professor of Psychology at the University of Pennsylvania School of Medicine, this article notes, "An important study last year in the *New England Journal of Medicine* showed that women as little as 5 to 10 percent overweight had a 30 percent increase in risk of heart disease. That's just 7 to 14 pounds for a 140-pound woman."

(They mean over*fat*. I know that—but do others? Remember I've gained 15 pounds of muscle—an 8.5 percent "weight" gain. Am I now at risk of heart disease? No—because muscle doesn't cause heart disease. This undefined language can make women hysterical about their weight—and get them dieting themselves fatter.)

Wadden and other researchers suggest people be "taught skills to maintain weight loss, and that prevention of relapse should be a more central focus." (But "skills" are ineffective when your lean muscle has been ravaged.)

► *Health*, February/March 1992: William Castelli, Director of the Framingham Heart Study, in the article "The Great Weight Debate": "We found that one of the worst things that can happen to you is to put on weight. The real question is, is skinny better?"

(Is that the real question? I think the real questions are, why don't you say put on *fat*, so people who work out and gain muscle aren't left thinking they're doomed? And what do you mean by "skinny?" Do you know "skinny" anorexics can have 50 percent bodyfat? Is my 15 new pounds of muscle "the worst thing that ever happened" to me?)

► *Allure*, November 1992: Linda Wells, Editor-In-Chief, writes, "I've forgotten how many calories are in an Oreo, even though I still feel like a minor criminal whenever I eat one. . . . As the leader of Overcoming Overeating says, 'Maybe it's possible to become so accepting of ourselves that we may not think about being thin.' "

(Remember, though, lean and weight have nothing to do with one another. Do we want to "accept" a body prone to heart disease, cancer, and stroke?)

► *Young Miss*, October 1993, "Model Musts": Monique Pillard, President of Elite Models, says, "The ideal weight is 115 to 125, but we will take a girl who's a few pounds over if she's got potential."

DIEHARD DEDICATION TO DIET THINKING

▶ Jeffrey Steingarten, in *Vogue*, October 1991: "I've always imagined that if I could only work up an interest in those dreary high-fiber, low-calorie foods, my appetite problem would be solved. Unfortunately, nature often insists on putting protein and fat in the same package, like cows and chickens. Eating chicken without its crispy skin . . . holds little gastronomic interest." (I find it hard to believe that mayonnaise, salad oil, and chicken skin are more exciting than tomato-basil pasta tubes stuffed with ricotta, roasted peppers, garlic, and sun-dried tomatoes; or that orange-bread, pesto bagels, or spicy rice and bean burritos are dreary.)

▶ *Glamour*, December 1992: ". . . climbed on the bathroom scale the other day, after two weeks of butterless toast and a daily jog around the park, only to find the needle still stubbornly stuck on the same number when she started . . . Her life was a hollow mockery; she was destined to never be happy."

▶ *Cosmopolitan*, September 1993, "The Goddess Regime," by Cynthia Heimel: "To get in shape fast, a girl has to suffer," says the subtitle. "Lunch: calcium, kelp, chlorophyll, mineral water and a banana."

BASIC BAD INSTINCTS

▶ Jeffrey Steingarten, in *Vogue*, October 1991: "In scientific research, a high-protein lunch caused human subjects to eat 12 percent less at dinner than a high-carbohydrate lunch. This is bad news for nutritionists, both in government and on best-seller lists, who urge us to stick to pastas, grains and beans."

(Of course, this is only "bad news" based on his assumption that eating 12 percent less at dinner is better. He obviously doesn't know that much of a high-protein lunch is likely to wind up as fat, because the body can't use heaps of protein at a single sitting and has no other way to store the excess, or that digesting a high-carbohydrate lunch elevates the metabolism highest. So big deal if you eat less at dinner!)

▶ *Mademoiselle:* "Don't eat a high-carb lunch; it'll make you sleepy." (No, it won't. A high-fat lunch will, and a high-protein lunch will. Any lunch will if it's huge and you haven't eaten for more than four hours. Whoever ate a high-carb lunch and got sleepy either came to lunch starved or didn't notice how much protein and/or fat accompanied the carbs.)

▶ *Mirabella*, February 1993 (interview with singer Rosanne Cash): "She denies herself the pasta with a sigh and orders the soup and salad."

▶ *Allure*, August 1992: "The last ten pounds: it's only a dress size, but it's a nightmare to lose and requires serious strategies." (Wrong! If you lose just fat, 3 pounds is a dress size—the nightmare is losing the other 7 pounds of . . . what?)

Some of the "serious" strategies peddled by the celebrities questioned (most pictured were overfat!):

"I eat only vegetables, vegetables, vegetables, and drink gallons of water."—Alison Mazzola, editor.

"I can't eat too many vegetables because it makes the tummy big."—Maguay Le Coze, restaurateur.

"Work hard or have sex. As long as it's hard, you'll lose the weight."—Patricia Field, designer.

"I lose my ten pounds with Nikki Haskell's Star Caps. They're papaya and garlic, and they're fabulous."—Beverly Johnson, model.

"No starvation here: That's declassé. Instead, the goal is 1,200 calories a day for women and 1,400 to 1,500 for men. 'We really believe in feeding people.' "—Yvonne Nienstadt, Health Director of Cal-a-Vie spa in Vista, California.

(That's feeding people?)

▶ *Us* magazine, January 1993: "I figure I have another year that I can eat anything I want. When I see myself drastically gaining weight, I'll start the whole diet and workout thing, but for now I'm going to live it up."—Milla Jovovich, model and actress.

STAY IN CONTROL

▶ *Ladies Home Journal*, November 1992 ("Oprah" cover story): "Overeating—the most common addiction. We're in control of our lives—why can't we control our eating?"

▶ *Mademoiselle*, October 1992, "Diet News": "Sometimes, it seems the biggest difference between a thin woman and an overweight woman is willpower. One has it, the other doesn't."

▶ *Parade* magazine, November 10, 1991, "Our Food Survey": "Cumulatively . . . 489 million pounds were gained, 630 million lost. That's a lot of willpower in action. And most dieters (72 percent) have done it the hard way—through portion control."

▶ *Mademoiselle*, January 1993: "If you don't keep track of your meals and snacks, the exercise sessions you make and the ones you miss, who will? That's why, when it comes to maintaining your shape, the best security measure may be a daily journal . . . keeping careful notes on what you can eat, when you work out and how you feel can help you take control." (They call this the "post-holiday recovery plan." Note how eating at the holidays is treated like a sickness!)

▶ *Glamour*, January 1993: "Take control now . . . focus on weight maintenance and prevent your weight from becoming a problem. Don't let your weight get out of control."

"I'LL TRY ANYTHING" DRAMA

▶ *Allure*, August 1992, Eileen Ford, co-founder of Ford Model Agency: "At a certain point, you have to parade around naked in front of a mirror and say, 'It is mind over matter, and my mind will control this matter.' I make myself eat a carrot or a whole head of celery before every meal because it cuts down my appetite. But mainly, the last part of weight loss is mental commitment. If you say, 'I'll just go off the diet for a week,' that's doom."

▶ *Cosmopolitan*, 1992, issue unknown: "Sure, genes help, but even top models have to work at their figures! . . . but I do adore eating, so choose high-protein, low-fat bingeable foods . . . take lecithin and bee-pollen pills (from health-food store), to burn fat, and go on a popcorn and Coca-Cola diet when desperate to lose weight (like right before the Paris fashion shows)."

LANGUAGE THAT LANGUISHES: THE DREARIEST DIET THINKING

▶ *Berkeley Wellness Letter*, October 1991, University of California: "Any diet program must teach skills to maintain weight loss and prevent relapse. A diet isn't over when you've shed your excess pounds—it's just beginning."

▶ *Cooking Light*, March/April 1993: "Do we know what actually works, and what makes some people keep the weight off? John Foryet, Ph.D., director of the Nutrition Research Clinic at Baylor College of Medicine, feels the main differences . . . are psychological. He profiles a 'successful loser' as one who incorporates lifestyle modifications."

▶ *Parade*, March 14, 1993: "Almost all experts agree that keeping slim is the hard part . . . Some of the reasons lie wrapped in biological and psychological mystery." But what scientists do believe, says the story, is that "You may have been born to be fat . . . You may have accrued a lot of fat cells in childhood . . . Everybody around you is overweight and consumes lots of food . . . You have mental or emotional problems . . . You have a false image of how you look . . . and therefore feel free to eat."

"BREAKTHROUGHS" AND "MYSTERIES" THAT AREN'T

▶ *Mademoiselle*, October 1992: "Dozens of studies now suggest that people . . . may overeat certain foods because their brains have lower than normal levels of serotonin and other mood- and appetite-regulating chemicals."

(A clear case of overlooking the obvious—that they're ravenous because they're starving themselves—in favor of complex theories.)

"Cookies, ice cream, pasta, bread, potatoes—these are the foods many women tend to cut out when they're dieting, and they are all carbohydrates. They are also the foods many women report craving, and the foods they binge on. Fearing weight gain, women may struggle to avoid these foods altogether. During such carbohydrate-craving periods, these women may eat and eat. . . . Carbohydrate cravers need this type of food to maintain serotonin levels and keep their moods balanced, research suggests. . . . 'People eat carbohydrates because they produce a calming, tranquilizing effect,' says Dr. Judith Wurtman."

(No! Read a biology textbook! "Carbohydrate-cravers" aren't special— they're human! Everyone needs carbohydrates—and not just to balance moods, but to survive! We eat them because we run on them; if your body doesn't get them, it will beg for them! How can you do research about carbohydrates and overlook this?)

This same article enthuses about how women can "cure" their cravings by eating carbohydrates, citing the example of one woman "suffering from obesity" who showed great improvement in how she looked and felt after Dr. Wurtman "added carbohydrates to her diet."

(Why is this treated like a new breakthrough?)

▶ *Self*, March 1992: "Diet Resistant Fat: No matter how little you eat or how hard you work out, it just won't budge." (An accurate statement would read: "Fat: As long as you eat too little and work out hard, it just won't budge because that's how the body works.")

CALORIE UNCONSCIOUS

▶ *Allure*, January 1993, "The Last 5 Pounds": This piece begins by saying that women who think they need to lose five or ten pounds probably don't—

but hastens to offer a way to do it anyway: "Simply start weeding out calories," says Helen Roe, a registered dietitian. . . . A combination of the following tricks can add up: Nix the dressing on a salad at lunch and lose two pounds. Hold the mayo on a sandwich and drop another pound and a half. Pass up a glass of wine and watch a pound disappear. Have an egg-white omelet instead of a regular one on Sunday and lose three pounds in a year. Consume one Fig Newton instead of two and drop another three quarters of a pound. Accompany this with a touch of exercise and the weight will fall off."

(This is inanely simplistic. Even if merely cutting "calories" did magically shave "pounds," it could only be relative to whatever else you do. Merely passing up something, with no attention to what else you eat, cannot make fat drop off your body.)

▶ *Delicious!* magazine, November/December 1992, "Ten Tips for Lifelong Health": "Here, Charles B. Simone, M.M.S., M.D., shares his plan to strengthen immunity. Simone is a medical oncologist, immunologist and radiation oncologist in Lawrenceville, NJ. 1. Maintain a healthy weight. 2. Decrease the number of daily calories."

▶ *Mademoiselle*, September 1993, "Sizing up a Serving": " . . . common sense says it's how much you eat that really matters. . . . If you're dieting, these distinctions are crucial. . . . Most people don't realize how big the portions they're eating really are," explains the registered dietitian and American Dietetic Association spokesperson quoted in the article. "It's important to be aware of what a serving looks like, so you can't pretend you're eating fewer calories than you are."

(Obviously, common sense is meaningless when it's defined within diet thinking.)

LYING IN WEIGHT

▶ *Allure*, December 1992: "As a writer, I make truth my business, and yet I'll admit right now that I have never told anyone how much I really weigh—not my husband, not my best friend, not my mother, and even when my life depended on it, not the hot-air-balloon pilot or the man who ties the bindings on my skis. I am a reasonably attractive, big-boned, tall, athletic, muscular woman and I have struggled with my weight every day since my first conscious memory."

DIET THINKING ON DRUGS

▶ *Elle*, October 1992, "Diet Pills: Popping off the Pounds": "If pharmaceutical labs have their way, a new generation of diet pills will soon be on the market. What if a pill could artificially increase serotonin: would you feel full, even while eating less? That's the premise behind dexfenfluramine, manufactured by Interneuron Pharmaceuticals Inc. According to Richard Wurtman, M.D. [professor of neuroscience and co-founder of Interneuron] . . . patients treated with dexfenfluramine eat less and significantly reduce their intake of carbohydrates."

(As if the idea of trying to restrict carbohydrate, create fake fullness and "treat" one's desire to eat as if it were an illness isn't backward enough, the drug trials suggested that so-called "success" required pill-popping forever; after losing weight through a therapy of pills, overuse and "behavior modification," patients were weaned from the pills, only to find that the weight returned.

Does this sound like a life? Anti-fat pills? Why not just know how fat—and everything else—works, and eat accordingly? Can it really be worse than drugs and "behavior modification"?)

▶ *Allure*, October 1992, "The New Diet Drugs": "In a survey published earlier this year in the *American Journal of Clinical Nutrition*, 50 top obesity researchers concurred that a new generation of diet drugs, many of which are now being developed or tested, will take a vital role in helping the very overweight achieve and maintain weight loss . . . A substance called acarbose blocks digestion of complex carbohydrates and reduces body weight in animals . . . Atkinson thinks the concept could work and hopes scientists can eventually develop a drug for humans that does what acarbose does for animals."

(Why is time, effort, and money being spent to block the digestion of our most needed fuel?)

NO HELP AT ALL

An article by Jane Kirby, R.D., featured in *Glamour*, July 1993, offered a recipe for blueberry muffins containing 9 to 14 grams of fat per muffin—with this excuse: "It's hard to lower the calories and fat in these muffins and still produce something deliciously light and delicate." This gets an "F" for effort.

SHORT TAKES

▶ *Reader's Digest*, November 1992: "10 Ways to Lose 10 Pounds."

▶ *Glamour*, January 1993: "Zap Holiday Fat!"

(You were fine all year, and then the pie you ate on Christmas Eve made you fat? It's as if the starving/dieting/fat eating you did all year wasn't an issue, or your body actually discriminates between holiday fat and other fat. And it implies that not only was the creation of the problem short-term and temporary, but the solution will be, too—just a zap!)

ADVERTISING

Advertising, as long as it's been around, has been a great mirror for American attitudes and trends—and for what's considered important to people, since smart advertising speaks to people's desires and priorities. There are plenty of TV ads airing, as of this writing, that make a clear case for my observation about people's priorities and their current level of knowledge:

Cases in point:

▶ The 1992 Olympics advertising, which hailed Snickers and M&Ms as "the official snack food of the U.S. Olympics." Come on! You know most superathletes don't touch the stuff—and those who do are inhibiting the potential of their performance. Those candies are loaded with fat and sugar, and there are undeniable physiological consequences to consuming them that affect one's short-term performance as well as long-term health.

▶ "Don't eat Wheat Thins because they taste good," says Sandy Duncan. "Eat them because they're baked, not fried . . ." (but still loaded with hydrogenated vegetable oil. A box has more grams of fat than one-and-a-half Big Macs. And, yes, people do eat a whole box of crackers—which is fine if they're fat-free.)

▶ "Such a great mother!" exclaims a woman to her friend, upon seeing the friend's selection of JIF—*low-salt, low-sugar* JIF. She watches salt and sugar, but peanut butter gets 80 percent of its calories from fat—nearly three times the U.S. RDA for fat and four times the increasingly favored 20 percent. It's fat, not salt, that kills Americans—and there are leaner protein sources.)

▶ A winter 1991 Fun Foods ad asserts that "there's no way to make oatmeal taste good" and that "the only alternative has been a bowl of sugar."

(This brainwashes kids and moms into thinking it's hopeless to make fresh, whole food taste great in healthy ways. They say the only alternative (until their product) has been hopeless junk. Their product? Microwave meals—all loaded with fat.

▶ "The choice is yours" claims an ad for the BIO/SYN nutrition bar. "You can burn either fat or carbohydrates as an energy source."

(It's not either/or; you're constantly using both. And the choice *isn't* yours. You can change the ratio over time through good fueling and muscle increases, but you deciding so won't change what your body will use tonight—and neither will eating a sports bar.)

"Sorry, high carbohydrate and carbo rich energy snacks make it **impossible** [their emphasis] to burn stored body fat. In fact, you'll tend to store even greater amounts of fat with a high carbohydrate diet, regardless of the amount or intensity of exercise."

(This contradicts human biology and recent studies. In fact, they even come right out and admit their claims fly in the face of established science: "Most exercise physiologists say 'That's impossible.' We call it good science.")

▶ Ultra Slim-Fast: "The healthy way to lose weight." "Give us a week—we'll take off the weight." "You can't find a lunch with less fat."

▶ First-of-the-year advertising is always a field day for diet thinking. Last January I opened my Sunday papers to supplements like these: "NEW! The weight loss plan for chocolate lovers. Nestlé Sweet Success. Same low calories as other Diet Shakes. And the great chocolate taste only Nestlé can deliver!" As if all that's important is "low calorie," and that you get your chocolate!

A Klondike® Lite ice cream bar ad showed a calendar with "Diet starts today!" scrawled across it in red. Kellogg's Special K: "Save 93¢ for your '93 diet." An ad for Sun Chips "multigrain" snacks doesn't tell you they're about 50 grams of fat per 7-ounce bag. Milky Way II—25% Fewer Calories: "Now it's 25% easier to keep your New Year's Resolution." (Quick math tells you: 25 percent of 20 grams of fat is 5 grams. That's 5 grams fewer than the standard Milky Way—15 instead of 20. And let's not forget the sugar and corn syrup.) Another coupon circular advertised cigarettes, cocoa cereal, and cold medicine—causes and cures, all on the same page.

Keep in mind that the material quoted here is just a microscopic representation of what's out there. I could go on. I have stacks of books, newspapers, and magazines piled around my office with highlighted assumptions, misleading semantics, and unfounded speculation. I get tired of tearing out magazine pages. I would probably have a neater office if I saved things that didn't have diet thinking in it.

It's your turn now.

9

BODYFUELING DAY TO DAY:
Eating for Living

The biological picture of what's going on inside your body gives you a fairly explicit map to what kind of eating will provide optimal energy, longevity, and leanness. For example, you can see that the *frequency* of eating is crucial, *quality* of fuel is a close second—and *quantity* is hardly an issue at all if you eat mostly complex carbohydrates and very little fat.

But if you're like most people, you'll want some tools and parameters to put these blueprints into purposeful, everyday practice.

FUEL PROFILES

In BodyFueling, I provide "fuel profiles"—estimates of carbohydrate and protein intake ranges—for each workshop participant. I provide these not as restrictive guidelines about food intake, but rather to ensure that people eat enough. These are meant to be a foundation or starting point for meeting fuel needs—not a be-all-end-all thing to "follow," "stick to," or "stay on."

One individual's fuel profile varies from another's based on activity level

177

and lean body mass. As you know now, your activity level and the size of your lean body mass are the most significant factors in your basic need for fuel. However, your need for fuel may change daily—as well as over the long term, as you gain muscle and/or increase activity level.

(That's yet another factor that makes "being on a diet" ridiculously disconnected from the reality of living. Typically, diets insist you eat essentially the same amounts every day. If you listen to your body and respond to its variable needs—say you want toast and a whole banana instead of "half a medium banana"—you've "blown it" because you have not followed it to the letter of the law. Faced with meaningless restrictions your body and mind rebel.)

The quantities I've listed on page 181 will help you start to get a sense of how much food your body needs. But everyone has individual needs, and myriad factors influence the need for fuel/energy from day to day. You might need one less or one more serving of carbohydrate (or two) at any given meal or snack, depending on not only your unique physical makeup but also that day's requirements—activity, exercise, stress level, and so on. Thus guidelines here are general, not gospel. Imagine I am handing you a plate and saying, "Here is about what your plate should look like; nudge it around a bit from there"—not "Here is what your plate *must* look like—don't stray a bite."

Don't jam down more than you can swallow just because it says so here (or anywhere); similarly, don't deny yourself an extra slice (or two) of toast because your profile doesn't indicate it. You are an individual, and your body knows best. It will tell you what it wants—if only you begin listening to and taking care of it again.

Because diet thinking is so ingrained, because you are programmed with "less" and "stick to," I must reiterate this: It's not critical to watch quantities exactly—not nearly as critical as the frequency with which you eat and the quality of what you're eating. The only critical aspect of quantity is eating enough carbohydrate.

Why give numbers at all? I'd prefer not to. I'd be inclined to simply teach you how your body works, guide you in developing a lifelong vision, and help you make the connection that you'll need your body to fulfill that vision. I'd rather say, "To have that body and that health, eat lots of complex carbohydrates and small amounts of lean protein daily, and don't add fat unless it's precious to you."

I have two reasons for providing numbers, rather than simply leaving you with what I've just said. One is that Americans like numbers and rules—

and although I've done my best to stay away from them wherever possible, I've found people get a little crazy if I'm too general in the "how to" area.

The more significant reason is that diet thinking has left you with no sense of what "a lot of carbohydrate" or "a little fat" looks like. Most people's idea of "a lot of food" isn't. For most people, the fuel profile represents more than they are currently eating. If I didn't give parameters, most people wouldn't eat enough.

The only time not to trust your body is if at first you find you're not hungry for anything or not hungry for long periods of time. This is a physiological reaction to underfueling, common to people who have starved themselves for many years. If you haven't eaten breakfast for 20 years, your body may have stopped asking for any a long time ago—*but that doesn't mean you don't need it.* And remember, not eating breakfast because you'll get hungry for lunch is diet thinking—it's *good* to be hungry for lunch (and a pre-lunch snack, too!).

Eating regularly does make you want to eat more—but that's not bad! You've learned that when you eat carbohydrate, insulin is produced—and insulin does bring blood sugar down. (However, that's not an arbitrary reaction—it's allowing that glucose to be oxidized for the energy you need!) When blood glucose drops, you want to eat more. This is supposed to happen. You could interrupt the normal sequence of events by not taking in fuel at all—but why? Your body will just get its carbohydrate fuel by destructive means.

At breakfast, for example, if your fuel profile indicates several servings of carbohydrates but you are certain that you cannot take any solid food after decades of not eating till noon or later, start out slow. You might want to start out with a banana (or half, if you can't even finish that) or some juice or a few bites of toast. Do that till you feel you can eat the whole banana or the whole slice. Add bite by bite until you're getting at least 2 servings (or 30 grams) of complex carbohydrate each morning within an hour of rising— the sooner the better!

Breakfast is crucial, because your blood glucose is never lower in any 24-hour period than it is upon arising. Your last snack, even when you're fueling, is likely to have been a few hours before bed, and then you sleep for hours. When you wake up, you've consumed no fuel for anywhere from six to twelve hours. Get up and start your busy day without addressing the near-empty tank, and before too long you'll find yourself in an energy-sapping, muscle-eating, metabolism-slowing fuel deficit.

The charts that follow will provide you with some guidance in assessing your fuel needs. The ranges shown are fairly broad, but they will give you a frame of reference to start with as you begin to incorporate the basics of fueling. Better yet, skip the gram-counting approach entirely and go to page 185 for "My Recommended Easygoing Alternative."

With the carbohydrate ranges as wide as they are (to account for varying activity levels, even among people with similar muscle mass), you can see that it's not terribly important to know exactly what your muscle mass is. I don't even like to distinguish between men and women; both need enough carbohydrates to fuel their activity and lean mass, and as those factors increase, so will a person's fuel need. Just about any man or woman could conceivably require between 3 and 10 servings of complex carb at each meal. Most people will be somewhere in the middle, and your body will tell you better than anyone else can what specifically works in that range. If 5 servings make you feel as if you'll burst, that tells you something. If 3 servings leave you ravenous, that's pretty simple to interpret, too.

Unlike carbohydrate, protein requirements are "fixed" numbers and *do* differ for men and women. The generally larger, more muscled male body will require a little more protein (but not as much more as some men believe!). If you're ever hungry after fueling and want to add more food, add carbohydrate, not protein. You'll rarely need more than what's shown on page 181, which is consistent with U.S. RDA guidelines.

Interestingly, while the government's Recommended Dietary Allowances offer explicit quotas for protein as well as all kinds of vitamins and minerals, and suggest a specific limit for fat, past editions of the National Research Council's *Recommended Dietary Allowances* offer no specific quotas for carbohydrate—which is only our most critical fuel! However, most nutrition texts specify at least 300 to 400 grams of carbohydrate daily for the moderately active person—and more for those who exercise more than one hour daily. The FDA's new food labeling scheme will for the first time include a recommendation for carbohydrate—though indirectly—by suggesting 2,000 to 2,500 calories daily and 65 percent of those calories from carbohydrate. That's 325 to 400 grams daily. (As a frame of reference, most "weight loss" diets "allow" about 100 grams or less of carbohydrate daily.)

If you were to believe the media's portrayal of the average American "overeater," you'd think this fuel profile would be license for many people to go hog-wild and push the ranges to the upper limits. I've found just the opposite to be true. For most people, diet thinking has made it tough to imagine eating beyond the low end of the profile—no matter who they are or what activity they're doing. If you're in that place, start at that low end and go from there slowly, paying attention to your comfort level.

FUEL PROFILE

▶ **DAILY CARBOHYDRATE INTAKE:** 275–500 grams is a broad general range. (One serving = 15 grams carbohydrate.) Where you are in the range will depend on how much lean tissue you have and how much exercise you do. For example, someone who is 90 pounds lean and exercises an hour or two a week will probably have carbohydrate requirements at the lower end of this range, while someone with 160 pounds of lean tissue who exercises seven hours a week will probably find their needs hover at the higher end of the range.

▶ **DAILY PROTEIN INTAKE:** Protein is a *fixed* amount because our need for it as adults does *not* vary much (with the exception of pregnant and lactating women). It is also different for men and women. U.S. Recommended Dietary Allowances for protein are 46–50 g. for women, 60–65 g. for pregnant/ lactating women, and 58–63 g. for men. (One serving = 6 grams protein.)

▶ **DAILY FAT INTAKE:** You *need not* take in added fats for fuel. The fats listed in the fuel profiles below are not to be *added*; you'll most likely get close to the amounts shown just by eating the proteins and carbs also listed. Fatty acids occur naturally in predominantly carbohydrate and protein foods, and will provide the tiny amount required daily. An intake range of 20–65 grams daily is a fuel-smart ideal.

Remember that the above are ranges and averages; they are not meant to be followed rigidly! The rest of this chapter details ways to find your own best place within these ranges, based on your individual and changing needs. See page 182 for examples of how to assemble a meal based on your fuel profile.

Women

BREAKFAST	LUNCH	DINNER	SNACKS
12 g. PROTEIN	12–18 g. PROTEIN	12–18 g. PROTEIN	30–75 g. CARBO.
60–150 g. CARBO.	60–150 g. CARBO.	60–150 g. CARBO.	0–10 g. FAT
0–15 g. FAT	0–15 g. FAT	0–15 g. FAT	

Men

BREAKFAST	LUNCH	DINNER	SNACKS
12–18 g. PROTEIN	18–24 g. PROTEIN	18–24 g. PROTEIN	30–75 g. CARBO.
60–150 g. CARBO.	60–150 g. CARBO.	60–150 g. CARBO.	0–10 g. FAT
0–15 g. FAT	0–15 g. FAT	0–15 g. FAT	

ASSEMBLING MEALS USING THE PROFILE

Lean proteins and complex carbohydrates are the foods represented in the profile on page 181. Below are the most familiar of the fresh-food sources of protein and carbohydrate. For packaged foods that also fill the bill, see Food Brand Recommendations, pages 198–199.

Each protein food in the amount listed represents what I call a serving (about 6 to 8 grams) of protein. Each carbohydrate food in the amount listed represents one serving (or about 15 grams) of carbohydrate. So, for example, if you wanted to assemble a meal for a profile of two protein and four carbohydrate servings, you would:

Choose 2 from the Proteins

1 oz. chicken or turkey
1½ oz. most fish
1½ oz. fish or shellfish
1 cup nonfat or 1% milk
1 cup nonfat/low-fat yogurt
¼ cup cottage cheese
   (1%, nonfat or dry curd)
1½ oz. nonfat cream cheese
2 oz. low-fat/nonfat ricotta
¾ oz. low-fat or nonfat hard
   cheese
2 oz. Quark cheese spread
1 egg (or 2 whites mixed with
   one yolk)
1 cup fruit yogurt
1 cup lentils (combine with grain
   for complete protein)
1 cup split peas (combine with
   grain for complete protein)
½ cup beans (combine with grain
   for complete protein)
or any other low-fat item with 6
   grams of protein

And 4 of the Carbohydrates

1 slice bread
1 small roll or cocktail bagel
⅓ regular-size bagel (one whole
   makes 3 servings)
⅓ cup oatmeal (dry)
½ to 1 cup cold cereals*
   (average; check package for exact
   grams)
¼–⅓ cup fat-free granola
1 fruit
4 to 8 ounces fruit juice
   (unsweetened)
1 large wheat or corn tortilla
1 cup fruit yogurt
½ cup couscous
⅓ cup rice or barley
½ cup pasta; 1 pasta tube
   (manicotti)
⅓ baked potato (one whole is 3
   servings)
1 small red potato
1 cup lentils
⅓ to ½ cup beans
or any other low-fat item with
   15 grams of carbohydrate
*All foods in amounts listed are
   cooked except oatmeal

Most foods are primarily protein or primarily carbohydrate (or primarily fat!). A few protein foods do contain significant carbohydrate, and vice versa. Such foods will appear on both lists. For example, fruit yogurt (not sugared, of course) at breakfast will give you a good dose of carbohydrate and protein.

In terms of protein requirements, the average man needs 18–24 grams per meal, not to exceed 63 grams per day. (Recall that excess protein is stored as fat—and the conversion process is toxic.) A woman rarely requires more than 12 to 18 grams per meal, except during pregnancy and breastfeeding (when the U.S. Recommended Dietary Allowance rises from 44–50 grams to 60–65 grams). Snacks shouldn't provide significant protein (unless your meals don't).

This doesn't mean you should never eat a 4-ounce chicken breast if you're a woman. As with every aspect of fueling, the key is consistency! Too much protein on Monday won't matter. Too much every day is another story.

Familiarize yourself with what foods are mainly protein, mainly fat, and mainly carbohydrate, and try to know visually what 1 cup of lentils or 3 ounces of fish really amounts to. It's a good idea to invest some start-up time weighing and measuring—just long enough to get adept at visualizing your "fuel supply."

FRUIT

"One fruit," as listed on the carbohydrate side on page 182, generally refers to one whole fruit (i.e., one apple, pear, banana, orange, nectarine), with the following exceptions:

strawberries = 1½ cups
cantaloupe = ½ the melon
pomegranate, mango, papaya = ½
honeydew = ⅛–¼ of the melon
peaches, kiwi, plums, mandarins = 2 each
other berries = 1 cup
grapes = ⅔ cup

For fruit juice, 1 serving is 4 to 6 ounces of orange, pineapple, and other "sweet" ones, 6 to 8 ounces of grapefruit and apple.

Juice is almost as good as fruit for getting carbohydrate into your bloodstream, although you miss the fiber, and it may not provide the physical or mental satisfaction of having (chewing) a snack. You may also find that because juices are often more concentrated than the fresh fruit, they trigger a "wilder" insulin surge. This can quickly strong-arm the blood glucose out of the blood and leave you needing something more substantial (which is fine as long as you do get something more substantial). However, juices are convenient—and may be less conspicuous than a chewy bagel in a professional situation. They certainly beat having nothing.

VEGETABLES

Most vegetables, unless specified, simply don't provide enough carbohydrate to count as adequate fuel. Like anything without much carbohydrate value, vegetables aren't worth much *when it comes to energy*. No matter how many vitamins and minerals it has, if it's low in carbohydrate you'll be short on fuel.

I certainly don't want you to give you the impression that you should skip vegetables because they're not fuel-dense. Eating plenty of vegetables is good—they provide important vitamins and minerals, and I recommend piling some on at least one meal a day. Think of them as richly nutritious garnish. Just don't try to subsist on vegetables alone, or you'll be short-changing yourself on fuel. Aside from potatoes, peas, and a few others, it would take more vegetables than most people are willing to eat at one sitting to provide enough carbohydrate fuel for a meal. For example, you'd have to eat 5 pounds of lettuce-and-tomato salad to equal the carb fuel in two slices of bread. It would take 9 cups of broccoli to provide the carb you'd get from a baked potato and a dinner roll. You're likely to fill up or get tired of these before they add up to significant carbohydrate.

There are a few veggies and legumes that do count as carbs and/or protein (i.e., they provide significant grams of carbohydrate or protein when eaten in a standard portion). These are noted on the appropriate lists above, under protein and carbohydrate. In general, however, a roll, cereal, fruit, or fat-free/sugar-free snack bar or cookie is a much smarter snack than celery sticks. If you like celery sticks, have them—but eat them along with some more substantial carbohydrate.

WALK, DON'T RUN: MY RECOMMENDED EASYGOING ALTERNATIVE

Use of the preceding fuel profile, in conjunction with at least a bit of aerobics and weight training, is likely to yield the most progressive fat loss. That's only because if you monitor the number of grams of protein and carbohydrate you take in, you ensure a degree of precision in meeting your body's needs—and the better you fuel, the better the results. But please remember that this means relatively fast—not "fast" in fast-weight-loss terms. Fast "weight" loss is exactly what BodyFueling is designed to avoid.

I know authentic fat loss is a goal for many of you, but rather than driving aggressively toward that goal, why not coast? Just let your now-informed instincts guide you. I've drawn up the fuel plate below as an alternative to using the fuel profile. Instead of watching portions, you simply stay aware of protein and carb *proportions*. You're not counting and measuring—but you're still fueling and moving in a healthy direction.

Use the fuel-smart "plate" to plan your own plate's carb-to-protein ratio at each meal:

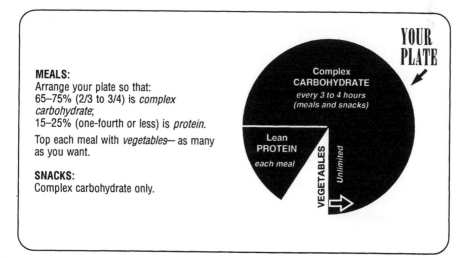

MEALS:
Arrange your plate so that:
65–75% (2/3 to 3/4) is *complex carbohydrate*;
15–25% (one-fourth or less) is *protein*.

Top each meal with *vegetables*— as many as you want.

SNACKS:
Complex carbohydrate only.

YOUR PLATE

Complex
CARBOHYDRATE
every 3 to 4 hours
(meals and snacks)

Lean
PROTEIN
each meal

VEGETABLES
Unlimited

Also, it's far less complicated to know what foods are complex carbohydrate and which are protein—eating a lot of one and a little of the other—than it is to remember serving numbers and to count grams. You'll prefer this route if you feel as I do that the more details you have to "follow," and the more numbers you have to crunch, the higher the cost to your sense of freedom. The fuel profile numbers provide a frame of reference for those who want to be sure they're on target. But watch the tendency to use it against yourself, to try to "follow it" or "do it right." Remember, this is *eating* we're talking about, not a "plan." These are guides, not gospel.

Simply eating the appropriate proportions of carbohydrate to protein, keeping fats to a minimum, and fueling with carbohydrate frequently is a giant step forward for most people. And it still works—unless you're in a hurry and counting the days till fat loss, which is diet thinking anyway.

It's possible to relate to the Fuel Profile outside of diet thinking too, and not use it merely as a short-term fat-loss instrument. But the flexible "rough-estimate plate proportion" approach is more natural—like real eating in real life.

Coming full circle from where we began this book, it's important to remember that you have your whole life—probably a longer one if you eat this way. Stay focused on fueling what's important to you. I'd rather see you eat well and often, be reasonably accurate, and enjoy it than fuss with small details or seek perfection. Take time to carve out a basic way of eating that works for you, because your patience will be amply rewarded, both in mind and body.

"Darlene" is an example of someone who squandered the opportunity to begin a leisurely "coast" toward ever-improving fitness, then wanted to race to a short-term goal at the last minute. She did our workshop but applied what she learned in only a limited way. A year later, she called us two weeks before a trip to Hawaii, hoping we'd endorse her plan to go on a high-protein crash diet to whip her body into shape for the beach.

No! She could have been enjoying a hearty, plentiful but specifically fuel-smart way of eating for 12 months that would have her where she wanted to be right now—no "crashing" necessary. Instead, she blew it off for 12 months, and now wants to do something that will damage her body's ability to burn food and fat during and after her vacation—damage that's only partly alterable, and then only with a good deal of work.

Even though it wouldn't have meant deprivation to start fueling and just keep fueling, it was hard for Darlene back then to look ahead 12 months. Why change if she wasn't going to see the results next week? That's the way America thinks. But there's simply no substitute for a year-round way of eating that works—for all the vacations, for the rest of your life.

There are good reasons to start fueling even if you won't see results next

week: It is what your body needs, based on its fundamental design. It is also
the way virtually every disease-prevention study suggests you eat (though I
don't know why we need studies to tell us that eating according to how the
machine works will be good for the body, or that defying its design will
harm it). It will feel good. And you can "turn it on" and forget about it—
leave it on.

LISTENING TO YOUR BODY

When I began fueling, I counted grams to ensure I was getting the appropriate amounts of everything daily. But as my own transformation progressed
from ordinary "I'll try this for a while" thinking to the joy of consciously,
purposefully, and lovingly investing in myself, I relaxed. My vigilance soft-
ened till I was using the "easygoing alternative," eating as much as I felt
like I needed—as long as each plate resembled the proportions of the "plate
chart" above.

Understanding carbohydrate use by the body reassures that you have a lot
more leeway than I'd imagined. I began to count on my body to tell me
what I needed and when I needed it. I found my body would cry out for
some carb just shy of every three hours—like clockwork. I didn't need to
watch the clock or "stick to" this plan I had given myself. My mind knew
the basic parameters; my body was smart enough to bend them slightly.

Interestingly, my sense of my needs never took me far off the original
profile. But the experience is more freedom and flexibility. In other words,
I don't have to eat 4 servings of carbohydrate every single day at lunch. I
could have 3 some days, 5 or even 6 on other days. And I routinely began
to eat at least 3 carb servings at snack times, instead of one or two—especially
as I added lean muscle.

I also measured things at first, and that fell away too after about a month.
But it was a valuable exercise, because I became intimately familiar with
serving sizes. I can tell 2 ounces or 4 ounces of chicken at a glance. I can
"feel" whether a slice of turkey is a half-ounce or 1 ounce. I can eyeball 1
cup of pasta or 2 cups of rice. And because of that I can go to a buffet and
instinctively assemble a plate that is consistent with my fuel needs.

As months and years of fueling go by, you can look forward to making a
fine art of "sensing" your body's needs, and you'll probably trust that sense
more and more. Some days my snack is a nectarine, others it's a loaf of bread.

Why? Probably a bunch of reasons, some of which modern science may not be able to account for.

I *know* when I'm done eating. It's a deep certainty; something goes "thunk" into place. Until I get that "thunk," I allow myself to keep going. I don't (usually) judge it, no matter how big the amount or how weird the craving (say, eight slices of toast). I always reach a point where my body says, "Ahhhhhhh. There." And then I really don't want any more. I have to think there was a reason my body said keep going. It certainly isn't going to hurt me (I don't butter the toast, of course).

If I tried to stop myself after the third slice of toast, based on some arbitrary standard, I'd be uncomfortable and dissatisfied. Why draw a line, and based on what? Is four slices too many? Five? Says who? It's the idea that you should be done, based on some predetermined portion "ideal" not customized to you, that drives you to lose touch with what you really need.

A DAY IN THE LIFE

My typical day from morning till night goes something like this: **Breakfast**—⅔ cup of (measured dry) oatmeal and a handful of raisins, two slices of toast with either 2 ounces of chicken or turkey, an ounce of low-fat cheese or a cup of yogurt. **Snack** might be a bowl of cold cereal with Rice Dream® nondairy beverage, or a bagel, or a few slices of toast, or toast and fruit, or a roll and a fruit, or fat-free crackers and fruit, or homemade muffins/cake/cookies, or some low-fat, no-sugar mini-donuts, or fruit juice, or fat-free toaster tarts. **Lunch**—couscous or soup with bread, or leftovers (rice and beans, pasta and cheese), or a sandwich (turkey, chicken, tuna, low-fat mozzarella and tomato, low-fat ground turkey-breast burger), and some fruit, low-fat/fat-free chips, and/or fat-free cookies or more cereal.

Dinner—anything from bean-and-rice (or bean-and-nonfat-cheese) burritos; to turkey and Spanish rice; to Chinese chicken with rice and vegetables; to homemade pizza, lasagne, or manicotti; to spicy Cajun rice with prawns; to Indian ginger-curry couscous; to spaghetti and turkey balls; to homemade bean (or split-pea or lentil) soup and fresh bread; to seafood stew; to Cornish hen with garlic and grilled red potatoes; to pasta topped with chicken or ricotta and roasted vegetables and garlic; to baked potatoes topped with cheese or stuffed with shrimp; to turkey burgers with tomato, lettuce, and low-fat chips; to chicken-breast/low-fat mozzarella/broiled red pepper sandwiches with garlic "fries" (baked potato sliced and "sautéed" in a non-stick pan); to turkey-ball subs with peppers, onions, and zesty tomato sauce

. . . (I could go on, but it probably makes more sense just to do a cookbook). **Afternoon and evening snacks** can be the same as morning, or nonfat, fruit-sweetened frozen yogurt.

What might your day look like? Here are just a few examples of how you can "build" a meal by pairing enough grams of carbohydrate with enough grams of protein. The sample breakfasts below are based on the profile of someone who wants to get 12 grams (2 servings) of protein and 60 grams (4 servings) of carbohydrate. Remember, this is just to get you started—not the breakfasts you "should" eat!!

SAMPLE BREAKFASTS: 12 G. PROTEIN, 60 G. CARBS

Option 1: 1 slice toast + 4 oz. low-fat/nonfat ricotta; ⅔ cup oatmeal + 1 cup nonfat yogurt, 1 cup blueberries

Option 2: 2 slices toast with 1½ oz. nonfat mozzarella; ⅔ cup (measured dry) oatmeal

Option 3: 2 eggs cooked any way (without oil or butter) + 3–4 slices toast (*depending on number of grams carb per slice*)

Option 4: 1 large bagel, 1½ oz. nonfat cream cheese + 1 cup "oatios" + 1 cup nonfat milk

Option 5: 1 bagel, 4 oz. Quark® nonfat cheese spread (or ¼ cup cottage cheese) + 1 orange

Option 6: 2 English muffins with 1 egg + 1 oz. turkey breast (or lean turkey/chicken sausage)

Option 7: 1 potato ("fried" in non-stick skillet with spices) + 1½ oz. low-fat mozzarella + 1 slice toast

FUELING AND DIETARY FAT REDUCTION

While eating lots and lots of carbohydrate food, the smart fueler will want to avoid fat wherever possible. That's easy today, because thousands of new low-fat and fat-free food products have been introduced during the last couple of years.

Fat moderation is much more approachable than total fat elimination

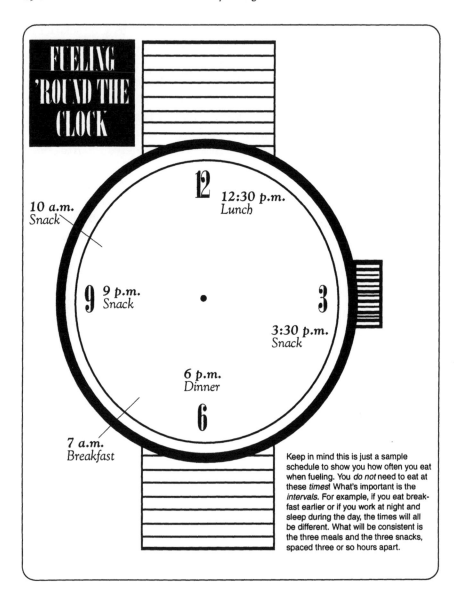

FUELING 'ROUND THE CLOCK

10 a.m.
Snack

12:30 p.m.
Lunch

9 p.m.
Snack

3:30 p.m.
Snack

6 p.m.
Dinner

7 a.m.
Breakfast

Keep in mind this is just a sample schedule to show you how often you eat when fueling. You *do not* need to eat at these *times!* What's important is the *intervals.* For example, if you eat breakfast earlier or if you work at night and sleep during the day, the times will all be different. What will be consistent is the three meals and the three snacks, spaced three or so hours apart.

(which is virtually impossible anyway, unless you completely eliminate most foods, which is definitely not healthy). One strategy many people find useful is to organize your fat intake around only your most cherished favorites. Walk away from added fats and fatty foods that don't turn you on. So maybe the Chocolate Decadence every Friday night stays, but the mayo in your tuna goes because it isn't worth the cost, and all-fruit jam replaces butter on the morning toast quite painlessly. Maybe sugar-free, low-fat ice cream or frozen yogurt is perfectly satisfactory four of every six times you eat frozen dessert. You work it out.

Be able to spot high-fat/all-fat items at a glance. Read labels and learn the fat content of foods that tend not to be labeled. I've created (see page 192) a complete guide to "hidden fat detection" (and sugar too!), and I've included a method for determining the percentage of calories from fat contained in food (see page 193). You may *choose* to eat fat at times, but you have no choice if you don't know a food is loaded with fat.

It is possible to get too rigid about fat consumption. If you tended to be obsessive about calories, you may find yourself doing the same with fat grams. Try to remember there's no one thing that makes you fat, no one day of indulging. And the purpose here is not to keep you "inside the lines," following orders, but to have you *make conscious choices based on facts and your future*. In the end, your future probably speaks louder than a dollop of dressing.

It's less important that you avoid a single food that has 2 more grams of fat than you think it should than it is to consistently incorporate all aspects of fueling into your life. And as long as you're keeping the fat content between 10 and 30 percent of total calories (or 20 to 65 grams daily) and the protein to 15 to 25 percent of total calories (or 46 to 63 grams daily), you can probably eat more food than you're eating now—or thought you could.

GUIDE TO FAT & SUGAR DETECTION

ALL FAT (100% or close to it)

Butter
Oils
Margarine
Butter-substitute spreads
Mayonnaise
Salad dressings

VERY HIGH IN FAT

Beef (even extra-extra lean)   Coconut/coconut
Pork   milk and cream
Duck   Tofu (regular)
Bacon   Lamb/mutton
Hard cheeses   Hot dogs
Whole milk (4% milkfat)   Ham
and milk products *(cream,*   Avocado
ice cream, 4% cottage cheese,
whole-milk cheeses, whole-milk yogurt)
        Nuts, seeds, and nut butters
        Chocolate/carob (powder's OK)

NOT NECESSARILY OBVIOUS SIMPLE SUGAR "ALIASES"

Dextrose   Corn sweetener
Sucrose   Cornstarch
Maltodextrin (from corn)   Honey
Corn syrup   Maple syrup
High-fructose corn syrup   Molasses

SUGAR NOTES:

Fructose is a sugar in fruit. It is more complex than processed white sugar, but concentrated fruit juice may produce similar effects.

Lactose is a sugar found in milk. It produces a mild to severe allergic reaction in some people.

A *maltose* is a complex sweetener. Rice syrup and barley malt are two man-made examples. Maltoses also occur naturally in some foods.

COMMON SOURCES OF HIDDEN (NOT OBVIOUS) FATS

The following are foods to be conscious about— read labels and check fat /sugar content. For most foods listed below, I say "many" (not "all") because there ARE exceptions in those categories— more and more all the time. The point is to be educated enough to make informed choices.

Commercially baked cakes, cookies, candy bars

Many commercial breads and rolls

Commercially baked muffins *("oat bran" or not)*

Many frozen yogurts

Many "natural" yogurts

Many chips (potato, corn, etc.)

Salads (with dressing, mayo)

Many "diet" foods (from snacks to frozen meals)

Many "health food" snacks, meals

Many granolas and granola bars

Many canned soups, chilis, beans

Many packaged and processed foods

Many sauces and gravies

Label Euphemisms

"Natural," "lite," "healthy," "organic," "vegetarian," "low cholesterol" do not necessarily mean a food is healthy— not by fueling standards! In particular, it may be high in fat or sugar.

"Low cholesterol" (or no cholesterol) doesn't mean low in fat. Low-cholesterol foods *may* have saturated fat, which causes your body to produce cholesterol.

PERCENTAGE OF CALORIES FROM FAT

1 GRAM OF CARBOHYDRATE PROVIDES **4** CALORIES WORTH OF ENERGY
1 GRAM OF PROTEIN PROVIDES **4** CALORIES WORTH OF ENERGY
1 GRAM OF **FAT** PROVIDES **9 CALORIES** WORTH OF ENERGY
    (THAT MEANS 2 GRAMS IS 18 CALORIES, 3 GRAMS IS 27 CALORIES, 10 GRAMS IS 90 CALORIES)

Once you know that <u>each gram of fat has 9 calories</u> there are only two things you need to know about any food to figure out the total % of calories from fat:

* How many *total* calories in the serving of food
* How many <u>total grams of fat</u> in the serving of food

\# OF CALORIES FROM FAT = **NO. OF GRAMS OF FAT** × 9 (cals. per gram)
% OF CALORIES FROM FAT = **NO. OF CALORIES FROM FAT** ÷ **TOTAL CALORIES OF ITEM.**

If a food has 90 calories and five grams of fat, you know that 45 of those 90 calories are fat calories (because five grams of fat × 9 calories for each gram = 45 calories total). That means it gets *half* or *50%* of its calories from fat (45 ÷ 90).

TRY IT:
One cup of whole milk (4% milkfat by volume) has 8 grams of fat and 150 total calories.
What percentage of calories are from fat?
8 grams fat × **9** cals. per gram = 72.
72 of its 150 calories are from fat.
Divide **72** by **150** total calories = **.48** (i.e. **48%**)
Whole milk gets **48%** of its calories from fat.

HOW TO USE THIS
This is useful for spotting foods that are composed mostly of fat, or contain too much fat. The idea is that if you are aiming for a 15–20% fat diet, but eating lots of foods that are 40–100% fat, it will pose a very interesting challenge to maintain the overall percentage.

*HOW **NOT** TO USE THIS*
Bottom line is *how much total fat you take in*, not what percent fat your foods are. For example, oil is 100% fat, but if you consumed only half a tablespoon, you would be adding just 7 grams of fat to your day's intake. If you ate enough of a food that only gets 10% of its calories from fat, you might add many more grams than that!

A much easier way to do this (instead of running around with a calculator) is simply to choose foods with less than 4 grams of fat per serving.

10

FROM THE SHELF
TO YOUR TABLE:
A Practical Guide

BUYING FOOD

Fueling efficiently is easiest when you have fuel—good food you like and want to eat—readily available at all times. That means a well-stocked kitchen. Fueling tends to fall apart when the cupboards are empty and you think your only alternatives are vending machines and burger barns.

I recommend grocery shopping only once a week and buying all the food you need for the entire week—instead of "running to the store" three or four times and spending more time and money, all told, than you would in a single larger trip. (This also saves you the frustration of always standing in line.)

A once-a-week grocery jaunt that gives you everything you need also takes much less time—and will be much cheaper—than eating out even once during the week. The price of one dinner for two at a decent restaurant is the same as my weekly grocery bill for two. While this may not be a concern for you, it is for many people. If you hear yourself complaining about the high price of food and your strained budget, look to see if most of it's being spent in restaurants rather than the grocery store.

Grocery shopping is further frustrating when you spend the time and money and still don't wind up with what you need. Ever get the packages on the kitchen counter, stare at them blankly, and say, "Where's the food? What can we eat for dinner?" The grocery list on page 197 should help. Barring truly unruly cashier lines, and after your initial frenzy of label reading, it will get you in and out of the store in about an hour. More importantly, it's designed to start you connecting your eating to your shopping, in advance, without a lot of complicated planning.

The idea is to think in terms of buying fuel, and how much you'll need, so you get it all. Look at each item and think *seven days*. If you're shopping for a week, you want to buy one week's worth of the items each family member will be eating. For example, you'll need seven nights worth of dinner proteins for yourself (or 14 for two of you, etc.). You'll need seven yogurts, if yogurt is one of your morning proteins. You'll need enough dinner carbs for a week, so buy enough rice, pasta, and potatoes for you and whomever else. If you always snack on fruit, you'll need 21 fruits. If you'll be eating primarily sandwiches for lunch, you'll need seven portions of deli meat or tuna, or whatever, sized for you, and at least a few loaves of bread.

For your convenience, have foods packaged in serving amounts. For example, if you need 4 servings of protein for dinner and seafood is one ounce per serving, buy 4 ounces (¼ pound) of fresh-cooked shrimp and you have one prepackaged dinner to top pasta and veggies, mix with rice, or stuff a baked potato). If you'll be eating 2 ounces of turkey for lunches, you can have the deli wrap 2-ounce servings of turkey (though this is not the most environmentally conscious solution—it's better to simply eyeball one-eighth of a one-pound package).

Buy in bulk. It's not only cheaper, but generally healthier and more environmentally responsible too. Oats in the cardboard "tin" or in little packets is up to three times more expensive than bulk. Bulk food is generally plain; bulk rolled oats, for example, are not "maple and brown sugar flavored" (which means "loaded with all kinds of sugar and artificial maple flavor"). You can add what you want when you serve it. Many groceries and most co-ops carry bulk items. Small health food stores tend to be pricier, though they are good sources for alternative brands or bulk food if your local grocery chain doesn't carry them.

PACKAGED FOOD

While it's nice to have fresh food, there are probably times you can't—or won't. I eat fresh, whole, raw, and fresh-cooked food when I can. If I can't, though, you can bet I'm going to eat something!

Rather than avoid packaged food entirely—which is unrealistic for many of us—it's a healthy compromise to identify and choose from the growing number of packaged foods that are low fat and low sugar (or no sugar or fat added). On pages 198 and 199 is a list of brands that specialize in this new breed of packaged foods. You should be able to find many of them in well-stocked grocery and health food stores.

These new products include what I call "healthy 'junk' food." That means that, at worst, they may not be loaded with nutrients that contribute to your health, but neither are they loaded with stuff that detracts from it. Sometimes I get more carbohydrate than I really need from such snacks, but that's about the worst of it.

LABEL READING

To keep it simple, there are two central issues to contend with when reading food labels.

▶ What *does* it provide? (Does it have the fuel I need?)
▶ What *doesn't* it provide? (Is it high in fat and sugars?)

Information about protein, fat, and carbohydrate content is usually given on package labels in grams. It's important to note that all information is for the manufacturer's (arbitrary) idea of a serving—*not* for the whole package. You'll see this confirmed by the statement "nutrition information per serving; X servings per container." For example, if the label says 12 grams of protein, that's "per serving." If the manufacturer says there are "3 servings per container" then the whole package provides 36 grams of protein.

Keep in mind that their "servings" don't have anything to do with what I'm calling a serving. Some cans of soup say "2 servings per container," when you might easily eat the entire contents. It's fine to eat the whole can of soup even if it says "2 servings per container," and the same goes for other foods. Rather than try to follow various labels' "serving" guidelines, just make sure

GROCERY LIST

PROTEINS

chicken (boneless, skinless breast or thighs)
turkey (whole, breast, fillet)
chicken/turkey sausage or ground meat *(lowfat/no skin)*
fish/seafood
sliced deli turkey, chicken
tuna
beans, lentils, and dried peas
eggs

CARBOHYDRATE FUEL

rice (raw/bulk or packaged—*no oils, sugars*)
pasta
couscous
quinola
beans, lentils, and dried peas
baking potatoes, sweet potatoes, small red potatoes, white/new potatoes
soups or instant soup/couscous/rice & bean cups

oatmeal, rolled rye, barley, bulghur wheat, other whole grain hot cereals
oatios, flakes, bran, krispies or other plain cereal *(preferably unsweetened)*

breads
rolls
bagels or mini-bagels
English muffins
(For breads, be sure sugars/oils are low on ingredients list.)

DAIRY PROTEINS

yogurt (plain nonfat, unsweetened, or fruit-sweetened)
milk (skim or 1%)
cottage cheese (1%)
fat-free cream cheese
fat-free/low-fat hard cheese (less than 4 grams per oz.)
ricotta cheese (*lowfat*, not part-skim)
nonfat Quark®

Milk Substitutes (soy milk, Rice Dream)

FAVORITE FRUITS: _____
_____
_____
_____
_____
_____

FAVORITE VEGGIES: _____
_____
_____
_____
_____
_____

CONDIMENTS

Jam
Spices
Salsa
Mustard
Tomato sauce

SNACKS (mini-fuel-ups)

fat-free/alternative-sweetened cookies
fat-free crackers and chips
fat-free toaster pastries
juices
bagels
rolls

FOOD BRAND RECOMMENDATIONS

Here are some examples of favorite food categories in which there are many alternatives to traditional high-fat and high-sugar foods. These are not the only kinds of food that offer so many choices, nor are the brands listed the only fuel-smart ones in their categories. Not all brands listed may be available in all parts of the country— but the point is not to limit your eating to these brands anyway. The point is to recognize that no matter what you like, there are plenty of healthy and tasty alternatives. Read labels and ingredients so that you can recognize versions distributed in your area.

PACKAGED/INSTANT RICES

- **Nile Spice**'s Rozdali rice
- **Lundberg**'s RizCous *(couscous-like grain made from rice)*
- **Near East** flavored rices
- **Konriko** flavored rices
- **Casbah** rices, taboulis, couscous mix
- **Fantastic Foods** rices, taboulis, and couscous
  (Watch for fat in some varieties, or fat in cooking directions.)

INSTANT SOUPS & MEALS

- **Nile Spice** instant couscous and soup cups
- **Fantastic Foods** soup or rice-n-bean cups
- **Casbah** instant soup cups

CANNED SOUPS, CHILI, BEANS

- **Health Valley** fat-free soups and chilis
  (CAUTION: Health Valley has regular— not fat-free— soups.)
- **Hain** 99% fat-free soups
- **Swanson's** 1/3-less-salt chicken broth
- **Shelton** turkey chili
- **Bearitos** vegetarian chili and refried black beans
- **Hain** refried beans
- **Rosarita** refried beans (low-fat or fat-free!)

NONFAT/LOW-FAT YOGURTS
(NO SUGAR OR HONEY)

- **Dannon** *Light* w/Nutrasweet® *(all their others have sugar)*
- **Continental** nonfat yogurts
- **Alta-Dena** low-fat/nonfat yogurts and yogurt shakes
- **Cascade Fresh** fruit-sweetened low-fat and nonfat
- **Knudsen's** fat-free yogurts
- **Stonyfield Farms** (nonfat variety)
- ANY brand plain nonfat

CHEESE/SPREADS

- **Kraft** Philadelphia fat-free cream cheese
  (not the "reduced fat" kind; it's FAT FREE!)
- **Quark** nonfat spreadable cheese
  (spreads like cream cheese, tastes like sour cream)
- **Frigo** TrulyLite low-fat mozzarella
- **Healthy Choice** fat-free cheeses
- **Alpine Lace** fat-free cheeses
- **Precious** Lite ricotta cheese
- *** Gardenia** low-fat ricotta cheese
- *** Frigo** TrulyLite low-fat *or* fat-free ricotta cheese
  (The three ricotta brands above each make "part-skim" also, which is only slightly higher in fat, still better than whole-milk ricotta.)
- **Kraft** Free fat-free cheese singles
- **Guiltless Gourmet** oil-free nacho cheese dips

COOKIES, BARS, TARTS

- **Health Valley** fat-free cookies
- **Health Valley** fat-free fruit bars and fruit bakes
- **Health Valley** fat-free granola bars
- **Frookie** fat-free cookies
- **Frookie** fat-free fig Fruitins
- **Nature's Warehouse** fat-free cookies
- **Nature's Warehouse** fig bars and raspberry bars
- **Auburn Farms** Jammers fat-free cookies
- **Auburn Farms** Toast-n-Jammers (toaster tarts)
- **Tree of Life** toasted almond fat-free cookies

Those below do have some fat and/or molasses/honey— but less than other "health food" cookies.

- **Frookie** Animal Frackers
- **Small World** animal cookies
- **Pride o' the Farm** cookies
- **Health Valley** amaranth graham crackers or oat bran grahams
- **New Morning** graham crackers
- **Mi-Del** graham crackers

CRACKERS AND CHIPS

- **Health Valley** fat-free crackers
- **Tree of Life** fat-free crackers
- **Frookie** fat-free crackers
- **Premium** fat-free saltines
- **Lifestream** fat-free crackers
- **Auburn Farms** fat-free 7-grainers
- **American Grains** "Poppers" low-fat potato chips
- **American Grains** Tortilla Bites (corn/bean chips)
- **Guiltless Gourmet** no-oil tortilla corn chips
- **Basically Baked** tortilla chips
- **Bearitos** oil-free tortilla chips
- **Barbara's** Amazing Bakes (try Pesto flavor!)
- **American Grains** Rice Bites rice chips
- **Guiltless Gourmet** no-dill quesa sauces and bean dips

COLD CEREALS

- **New Morning** Oatios
- **Barbara's** cold cereals
  (CAUTION: her cookies/treats are higher-fat "health" food, but the cereals are good fruit-sweetened alternatives)
- **Nature's Path** Manna-Grain oat bran flakes, Heritage Flakes, Millet Flakes, or Heritage–Os
- **Health Valley** cereals (a wide variety)
- **Health Valley** fat-free granola
- **Erewhon** cereals (hot and cold)
- **Arrowhead Mills** cold cereals
- **Kellogg's** Nutri-Grain cereals
- **Post GrapeNuts**/Grape-Nuts Flakes
- **Nabisco** Shredded Wheat or Shredded Wheat n' Bran
- **Perky's** cold cereals
- **Golden Temple** Granola
- **Kashi**—puffed or cooked
- **Lifestream** cereals

ALL-FRUIT JAMS

- **Cascadian Farms**
- **Harvest Moon**
- **Polaner's**
- **Welch's Totally Fruit**
- **Sorrell Ridge**
- **R.W. Knudsen**
- **Smucker's Simply Fruit** (*not* their "low sugar")
- **Nature's Conserve**

JUICES

- **Nice-n-Natural**
- **Cold Mountain**
- **Heinke**
- **R.W. Knudsen**
- **Santa Cruz Natural**

NON-DAIRY MILK SUBSTITUTES

- **Rice Dream** 1% fat milk beverages
  (CAUTION: Their frozen desserts are higher in fat than their milks.)
- **Health Valley** 1% Fat-Free Soy Moo
- **Edensoy** or **WestSoy** *Lite* soy milks
  (Many soy milks are as high—or almost—as whole milks.)
- **White Almond** beverage

FROZEN DESSERTS
GROCERY

- **Star's** nonfat/fruit-juice-sweetened frozen yogurt
  (NOT their ice cream or regular yogurt)
- **Stonyfield Farms** nonfat frozen yogurt
- **Cascadian Farms** fruit sorbets
- **Nouvelle Sorbet** fruit sherbets

SOFT-SERVE/SPECIALTY

- **TCBY** soft-serve nonfat Nutrasweet®-sweetened
  (their regular has sugar)
- **Alta-Dena** nonfat *(the best!)*
- **Gise** lactose-reduced low-fat frozen yogurt
- **Vitari** or **Fruitage** all-fruit soft-serve
- **Baskin-Robbins** Sugar-free ice cream
  (The fat-free has sugar; the Light has more fat and sugar than either.)

the food provides appropriate amounts of protein and complex carbohydrate. Be conscious of added sugars and fats as well, and you're most of the way there.

To determine total "fuel value" for the whole item, multiply the number of protein or carbohydrate grams "per serving" by the number of servings in the whole package. The can of soup with 2 servings per container and 16 grams of carbohydrate per serving has 32 grams of carbohydrate total. Remember, you want to be sure you're getting *enough* carbohydrate and protein. It's easy to spend too much time worrying about what might be in your food that shouldn't be, but fueling is far more dependent on what to eat than what to cut.

As for fat, try for 3 grams or less per serving on most packages in your cart to help keep your overall fat intake modest.

I recommend you at least start with this simplified approach, which will cover the most important issues, rather than fuss with the rest of a label. A government mandate for new labels, which are required beginning May 1994, seeks to ease some of the confusion people experience. My concern is that they will make matters worse. The new labels contain even more information than before—much of it not fuel-related. Unfortunately, when the labels were signed into law, no educational funding for programs to help people make sense of them were passed along with it.

My own belief is that those who designed this new label shouldn't have been so quick to add all that data, but instead should have chosen to educate people about the information already there. I've seen too many highly intelligent people express total helplessness about the old labels.

Newly standardized serving sizes were supposed to become more realistic, but a March 1993 *Berkeley Wellness Letter* label sample showed ½ cup for macaroni and cheese. (Who eats ½ cup of macaroni and cheese?) At 13 grams of fat per ½ cup, that's 52 grams of fat if you eat 2 cups.

It's also easy to foresee the havoc that the new Percents of Daily Values will create. That's the percentage of recommended daily quotas a serving of a food provides—if you're eating 2,000 calories and if your goal is 30 percent of calories from fat. Just when people are learning about recognizing "percent of calories from fat," these labels switch to "percent of daily value," a totally new concept. For example, in the macaroni-and-cheese label, the ½ cup is said to be 20 percent of your total daily fat intake. You might glance at that and think, "Oh, good, this food is 20 percent fat." But this doesn't mean it gets 20 percent of its calories from fat. It gets 46 percent of its calories from fat (see page 193 if you're not sure how I arrived at that), which *is not* 20 percent of the daily fat intake recommended if you eat 2,000 calories a day. If you ate 2 cups, you'd have used up 80 percent of your daily fat quota!

I also can't imagine why the labels list calories from fat (which requires further calculation to determine percentage of calories from fat). Why not simply state the percentage itself?

And all that's valid only if you eat 2,000 calories a day. All the numbers become meaningless to the masses of people trying in vain to subsist on 600, 900, 1,200, or 1,500 calories. Nor do the numbers work if you wish to eat the less than 30 percent of calories from fat now recommended by many health experts, or more carbohydrate than the 60 percent assumed by these daily values.

CURRENT SAMPLE LABEL

Nutrition Information Per Serving

Servings per container: 2 *(so multiply everything by 2 for total grams)*
Protein   **4 grams**   *(× 2 = 8; whole container worth 8 grams =*
                 1 protein serving)
Carbohydrate **14 grams** *(× 2 = 28; whole container worth 28 grams =*
                 2 carb servings)
Fat   **2 grams**   *(best if this number is less than 4)*

TIPS ON READING INGREDIENTS

What if no nutrition information is given on the label?

1. You can choose a different brand. (See Food Brand Recommendations, page 198.)
2. Sometimes, just ingredients tell you enough to make a wise choice—and to guess carb/protein value.

"LEADERS" ARE LARGER. Ingredients are given in *descending order* of "appearance"—that is, a food contains more of the first ingredient listed than anything else and less of the last ingredient.

• Serving sizes were supposed to "get real." This sample (the one critiqued in two popular health newsletters) suggests 1/2 cup of macaroni and cheese as the serving size. Who eats 1/2 cup of macaroni and cheese? The 4 servings that make up the whole container is probably more realistic— which means you have to be label-savvy enough to multiply every piece of info given by 4. The total fat for a measly half-cup (13 g) is high enough, but if you eat two cups (the whole box), multiply by 4—that's 52 grams of fat.

• Includes sugars that occur naturally as well as added sugars (like corn syrup). So foods like yogurt, milk, and fruit juices will appear high in sugar. (Source: *Nutrition Action Newsletter*, March 1993)

• No explanation of how this relates to anything else on the label, how people can use it and to what purpose. Believe me, people don't know!

NEW SAMPLE LABEL

FDA-approved labels that will begin appearing in May 1994

Nutrition Facts

Serving Size: 1/2 cup
Servings per container: 4

Amount Per Serving

Calories 260		Calories from Fat 120
		% Daily Value
Total Fat	13g	20%
Saturated Fat	5g	25%
Cholesterol	30mg	10%
Sodium	660mg	28%
Total Carbohydrate	31g	11%
Dietary Fiber	0g	0%
Sugars	5g	
Protein	5g	

Vitamin A 4%	Vitamin C 2%	Calcium 15%	Iron 4%

* Percents (%) of a Daily Value are based on a 2,000-calorie diet. Your Daily Values may vary higher or lower depending on your calorie needs:

Nutrient		2,000 Calories	2,500 Calories
Total Fat	Less than	65g	80g
Sat Fat	Less than	20g	25g
Cholesterol	Less than	300mg	300mg
Sodium	Less than	2,400mg	2,400 mg
Total Carbohydrate		300g	375g
Fiber 25g 30g			

1g Fat = 9 calories
1g Carbohydrate = 4 calories
1g Protein = 4 calories

This is still needlessly high, in my opinion. 65 to 80 grams of fat may be 30 percent of a 2,000-2,500 calorie diet, but it still takes me three days to consume that much fat in my 2,500-calories-plus. I'd have to work to find that much fat I'd really want to eat. Besides, 30 percent is not "ideal"— it's a maximum.

• Should show *percentage* of calories from fat. That's what virtually every source has urged you to learn about and use for years. (The U.S. RDA recommendation for fat is 30 *percent* of calories or less; the latest disease prevention research indicates 20 percent or less.) Simply giving calories from fat forces people to divide calories from fat by total calories to get percentage of calories from fat—if they even think to do it, or know how.

• "Daily value" is an entirely new concept about which people have no information other than what's on this label. The fact that a *percent* of Daily Value is used will likely confuse people, because the "percent" that's been the focus everywhere else is "percentage of calories from..." Thus, when people see the "% Daily Value" for total fat as 20%, they may assume without thinking that the food is 20% fat.
  That's not what this means. (The food gets a whopping 46 percent of its calories from fat—well over ANY recommendation or even the national consumption average—and this isn't shown.) It means that a half-cup of this food uses up 20% of your daily fat allotment if you're eating the exact number of calories considered a Daily Value.
  Which leads us to the final flaw: Every "Percent of Daily Value" is based on either a 2,000 calorie or 2,500 calorie diet. While such generous recommendations are good, their mere mention on a label won't pierce the diet thinking of a person who "knows" he must eat 600, 900, 1,200, or 1,500 calories a day. And for those people—indeed, anyone not eating exactly 2,000 or 2,500 calories daily—all of those "Percents of Daily Values" become useless.

BOTTOM LINE: This label adds a lot of information without explaining it *or* clarifying existing information. No uniform education system or package will accompany the release of this label (as of this writing).

HONOR SIMPLICITY. Try to choose foods with a maximum of 10 (or so) ingredients. (You needn't be fanatical about this. It's just a guideline that helps you to avoid those foods with 96 multisyllabic ingredients.)

FATS AND SUGARS SHOULD TRAIL THE LIST. Whenever possible, choose foods with no sugar or oils/fats added. If they are added, it's best if they are in the second half of the list (i.e., if there are 10 ingredients, sugar or fat should show up among the last five listed.)

GUESS GRAMS. You can probably make fairly accurate guess of a food's "fuel value." For example, if a bagel is 45 to 50 grams carbohydrate (worth 3 carb servings), a roll the same size probably is too—unless it's loaded with sugars or fats. Also, if oil is the last of 11 ingredients, total fat is likely to be low.

If you remember the above guidelines when selecting food, you'll be able to make an educated choice about whether an item suits your nutritional needs. Look at the following sample labels that came from four different loaves of bread. Examining their ingredients will give you an idea of the differences that can exist between similar products.

OK	Whole wheat flour, wheat gluten, malted barley, molasses, canola oil, salt, yeast
BETTER	Whole wheat flour, sourdough starter, rye flour, canola oil, salt, yeast
BEST	Whole wheat flour, rye flour, water, sea salt
YUCK	Enriched flour, malted barley flour, ferrous sulfate, niacin, thiamine hydrochloride, honey, high fructose corn syrup, sodium caseinate, partially hydrogenated soybean oil, cornstarch, soy flour, soy protein, cornmeal, vinegar, yeast, sugar, yeast nutrients (calcium phosphate, ammonium sulfate, potassium iodate), dough conditioner (sodium stearoyl lactylate)

FOOD MARKETING

MYTH: If it says "healthy" or if it's sold in a "health food" store, it must be good for you.

FACT: Foods that are called "healthy" or "health food"—as well as those labeled "natural," "organic," and even "diet"—can be loaded with fat and sugar. Take a stroll through the aisles of any health-food store or co-op and you'll find numerous foods that don't even meet the U.S. RDA for percent of calories from fat: high-fat cheeses, nut butters, whole dairy products, oils and toppings, dressings, chips, crackers, cookies, canned and packaged products. Many are labeled "natural," "unrefined," "unprocessed," "organic," "low-sodium," "wheat-free," even "low-fat," or "diet," but it's wise to remember that these terms can be misleading. For example, fat and sugar are "natural." But are they healthy? Earthquakes are "natural," too.

Like any other form of advertising food marketing is designed to sell products. There are companies that are committed to and concerned about health, and who actually make food with that specific purpose, and label it accordingly. But for the most part, you need to read and think, not just react. Don't toss it into your cart just because the brand name has the word "healthy" in it.

Again, the new label laws aim to regulate the worst of the subjective, relative terms—such as "lite"—but some remain. The biggest problem with these is not that they're false, but that they bank on you leaping to favorable conclusions based on a single claim. "No sodium" isn't a lie; it just doesn't guarantee it won't also have 12 grams of fat per serving. And it doesn't inform you that no studies have ever proven conclusively that salt causes hypertension, and that a high-fat diet and obesity do. It's hoped that you'll make the leap from "low-sodium" to "no need to worry about anything else that might be unhealthy about this food either."

They're not wrong for trying to get you to buy their food—that's their purpose and it's a perfectly legitimate one. (This is a capitalist country.) But you have a different purpose—fueling your body and being healthy—so you need to be educated enough to read beyond the bright label banners and know that a food with "no cholesterol" could still get most of its calories from fat, and that a food with "no fat" can still be loaded with sugar and corn syrup.

For every food like that, there is a different brand that does it better. I firmly believe that; it's been my experience with nearly every food I like.

"There's always another brand" is my motto. If you find low-fat yogurt that's got sugar, or no-sugar yogurt that's high in fat, don't settle for it. There are great pure-fruit, unsweetened, or juice-sweetened nonfat and low-fat yogurts. The same goes for frozen desserts, cookies, crackers, cereals, spaghetti sauces, and soups. And much more.

"HEALTH FOOD" FOR THOUGHT

Is food that's not considered "health food" actually "sick food"? Why do all the major grocery stores in which I've ever shopped have a "nutrition" aisle? What am I supposed to think about what's in the rest of the store? All food should be health food. If it's not, it shouldn't be classified as food.

Here are some tricky examples of "health foods" that started bad rumors about what healthy eating means:

TOFU. There are low-fat varieties, but most get more than half their calories from fat, sometimes 7 to 10 grams per serving (and you're likely to eat more than one). Many tofus leave you no better off than beef (except at least tofu fat is unsaturated). Choose lower-fat brands (if you still want it).

SOY MILK. Again, there are lower-fat soy milks, but it's often assumed that soy milk is "automatically" healthier. Not true—unless you're allergic to cow's milk. Check labels for those with 2 to 3 grams (or less) of fat per serving.

MUFFINS. Unless you've made them yourself and know for sure how much oil, sugar, and eggs went into them, muffins are not an automatically healthy choice. Most, in fact, are little more than greasy cupcakes: Bakery, convenience-store, and other commercially made muffins are almost always loaded with fat and sugar. And their timing—typically in the morning, after a 7- to 12-hour fast when your body most needs good fuel—is awful, making them a bodyfat-raising as well as energy-poor breakfast.

GRANOLA. This cereal mix somehow got associated with "health nuts" and "earthiness," but it's usually high in fat and sugar—more so than even kids' cereals. There are good low-fat and fat-free brands available now. Granola bars are mostly the same—some are excellent, but unless specifically stated otherwise the traditional "old-style" granola bar is likely to have as much fat and sugar as a candy bar. Better to have a candy bar instead and really satisfy yourself if that's what you crave, so you can be done with it and eat some fuel!

SALAD. This can be a disaster too. Unless there's some lean meat in it and you accompany it with some carbohydrate, it contains no fuel or building tools to speak of. It can be as empty as a candy bar—and, with dressing, even higher in fat.

To equal the fat in one salad with only 4 tablespoons of regular blue cheese dressing, you could instead eat ALL of the following: 2 pints of Stars espresso mocha chip nonfat frozen yogurt, 4 large bagels, 12 cups of rice, 2 instant tomato minestrone couscous cups, 1 cup of raisins, 5 apples, and 5 baked potatoes.

"DIET FOOD." Many frozen diet dinners are a travesty; you can have three times the volume with less fat—and for less money, too. I've seen something called a "diet bar" in health-food stores—it's a tiny little candy with 15 grams of fat. It's possible to eat three huge meals and not get that much fat!

Have you seen the little crunchy diet snack that comes in a bag the size of your palm? It promises to "keep you full for hours" and costs almost a dollar. And it has 10 grams of fat per bag. First of all, why would I try to stay full on a measly bag of chips? Secondly, how could that handful keep you full for hours? Third, why would I spend a dollar for them—when I could buy a half-pound of beans, a half-pound of rice, and some tortillas for that dollar and stuff myself full on burritos for a whole week—and still get less than 10 grams of fat?

Ultra Slim-Fast frozen chicken fettucine dinner

12 ounces   12 grams of fat $3.12 (1992, Seattle, Wash.)

2 cups pasta, 3-oz. chicken breast with tomato sauce, garlic, peppers and spices

22 ounces   8 grams of fat $2.26

The frozen meal costs 38% more for 50% *more fat* and 55% of the volume. Less food and *still* more fat—that's the Ultra Grim Past!

THE SO-CALLED "HIGH COST" OF HEALTHY EATING

MYTH: Healthy food is more expensive than "junk."

FACT: If you're not buying trendy foods from small health-food stores, good fuel is cheap and plentiful. Junk food that doesn't even provide fuel has far more potential for blowing a budget.

Eliminating the following from one grocery or "warehouse savings" trip will trim about $65—enough for another week's worth of groceries for two! One pound of butter, a can of shortening, a six-pack of beer or bottle of wine, a bottle of salad dressing, three large bags of chips, a 5-pound "brick" of cheese, one box of sugary kids' cereal, a jar of mayo, a case of soda pop, 1 pound of sugar, a dozen muffins, a pint of cream, a can of beer nuts, a jar of nondairy creamer, a bottle of cooking oil, two frozen dinners, two candy bars, and a week's supply of Slim-Fast. (I have seen carts like this—no kidding.)

That same $65 could buy the following at my local grocery store (early 1993): 2 pounds ground turkey (100 percent breast), a half-pound of cooked shrimp meat, a half-pound of chicken, six loaves of bread, two boxes of fat-free crackers, a jar of all-fruit jam, eight fresh bagels, 12 bananas, eight oranges, two apples, two red peppers, carrots, broccoli, snow peas, two baking potatoes, mushrooms, two onions, six bulbs of garlic, six different spices (in bulk; enough to fill six regular spice jars), one can of broth, a pound of oatmeal, a box of cold cereal, two cans of tuna, a box of instant rice, a half-pound of bulk brown rice, a pound of bulk rye flour, a pound of bulk black beans, tortillas, one carton of Rice Dream® nondairy beverage, ricotta cheese, low-fat mozzarella, six flavored yogurts, one large plain yogurt, 2 pounds of pasta, one jar of pasta sauce, a half-pound of bulk raisins, and one box of fat-free cookies. Not bad!

We usually spend $70 to $80 a week for two of us, and that covers breakfast, lunch, dinner, and snacks. On average, $10 a day feeds both of us—lavishly. (Remember, I'm talking about two people who together consume 5,000 to 6,000 calories a day.)

While you may never think beyond your moment at the cash register, there is also the high cost of not eating healthy to be considered. What about the cost of developing, delivering, and buying high-tech health-care services? It's food for thought.

COOKING

It's hard for me to imagine "rules" applying to cooking any more than to eating. Rules not only abdicate choice and responsibility, but in the case of cooking they inhibit creativity. Though you could hardly call it a rule, the most specific guideline I would ask you to observe is to cut loose and experiment wildly with all the foods you know are great fuel.

The "Mix-n-Match Meal" diagram below may help you do just that. "Preparing healthy meals" can be as simple as pulling together a meal from those two lists—kind of like choosing from a Chinese menu!

THE MIX-N-MATCH MEAL

CARBOHYDRATE A	B PROTEIN
PASTA (wheat, amaranth, corn, quinoa, or rice)	CHICKEN
BAKED POTATO	TURKEY
RED POTATOES	FISH (snapper, cod, sole, tuna, etc.)
RICE (white, brown, wild, basmati, etc.)	SEAFOOD (shrimp, scallops, clams, etc.)
BREAD	BEANS/LEGUMES (lentils; black, red, etc.)
COUSCOUS	LOW-FAT SOFT OR HARD CHEESE
BARLEY	GROUND TURKEY (100% BREAST)
QUINOA	TURKEY/CHICKEN SAUSAGE (low-fat)
SWEET POTATO	

Amounts will be based on what you know works for you either roughly duplicating the fuel-smart plate or using the fuel profile. However you do it, if you're fueling you'll be eating a *lot* from column A and a *little* from column B.

Vegetables, condiments, and spices are your C list. Spices are great things. By varying spices and vegetables (or fruits), you could conceivably make at least nine different ethnic dishes out of chicken and rice: Indian, Cajun, Mexican, Spanish, Hawaiian, Italian, Ethiopian, Chinese, or Japanese. And that's just chicken and rice! Imagine what you can do with all the other carbs and proteins. Remember: vegetables, nonfat condiments and spices have little or no fuel value—they're there for vitamins/minerals (vegetables) and flavor (spices and condiments).

A few additional caveats:

▶ You need not add oils, butter, or margarine to your food. I have prepared many packaged foods that call for a teaspoon of butter or margarine or oil, and not used any; we've never found that the food suffered for it. If you *must*, absolutely *must* cook with oil for some reason I haven't thought of, use a smidgen of unsaturated (not animal or tropical) oil such as olive oil, safflower oil, sunflower oil, or canola oil. (My trick is to pour a dime-sized or smaller dollop into a nonstick skillet and smear it with my fingers to coat the pan—good for stirfry.) While unsaturated fats, if not used by the body for energy, will still be stored or used as fat, at least they won't help coat your arteries, predispose clotting, or stimulate cholesterol production.

▶ Feel free to experiment with various sauces. Don't forget that tomato-, mustard-, and yogurt-based sauces will be lowest in fat, though there are substitutes for just about anything, from fat-free nacho cheese sauce/dip to fat-free gravy.

▶ With regard to "following" recipes: Don't worry about doing it "right." Experiment—it's fun! Forget the teaspoons and tablespoons. Go nuts with the nutmeg. If it says green onions and you like red, so be it. Trust your intelligence as well as your creativity.

EATING OUT

MYTH: You can't fuel yourself well if you travel and eat out a lot; it's just too hard. There aren't enough options.

FACT: You have four options, as I see it—all the freedom in the world. Like everything else, it's a choice you make.

1. Don't go (save time and money).
2. Go and ask for exactly the fuel you want.
3. Go and have whatever they offer (because you fuel most of the time).
4. Go to places that cater to fueling.

Try eating out less. Besides not being as healthy (usually), it takes more time than doing it at home—and costs a lot more money. Salmon with potatoes and vegetables costs $6 to $9 for two at home. The same two meals at a decent restaurant would cost at least $30 to $50—and probably won't be prepared as healthfully. A sandwich at an average deli costs more than a loaf of bread and a pound of turkey meat.

I prefer my own cooking these days. Recently we considered dining out for a celebration—and realized we couldn't think of anywhere we'd want to go or anything we could order that we'd enjoy more than something we prepared at home.

If you do go out a lot, it's still well within your reach to sustain good fueling. If you choose meals that are simply prepared and avoid obvious fats, you can eat pretty much anywhere. Don't hesitate to ask for what you want, and ask several times if you have to. It's your body and your money. Be pleasant but firm. When I get two tiny red potatoes with my chicken, I sweetly ask for four more—no oil, please—and another basket of bread. I've never been refused (and if I was, I wouldn't go back). Then I take half of the monster protein portion home for tomorrow.

Be specific—and very conscious about whether what you've asked for is what you get. Don't trust someone else to decide how much gunk it's okay to put into *your* engine. I was having lunch at an open market with a friend last summer. We both ordered sandwiches from a deli stand. I ordered a turkey club with lettuce and tomato, mustard, no mayo. My friend ordered the same, and told the person behind the counter, "Just go *light* on the mayo with mine."

I groaned inwardly. "Go light on . . ." or "just a little . . ." are invitations for not getting what you want. One person's light/little may be your over-dose. Most don't know, and many don't care, what's going to be optimal.

I watched the guy closely as he made my friend's sandwich. He used the same amount that he had on other peoples' sandwiches before she ordered—at least 3 teaspoons, at 15 grams of fat apiece. One hundred percent fat.

It's one thing if you love mayo—if it's your favorite and you consciously choose to eat it. But if it's not your heart's desire and you really could do without it, it just doesn't make sense to bury your food in it.

11

BODYFUELING IN PROGRESS:
Navigating the Path

Now—with awareness, information, background, context, and everyday tools—you are fully prepared to begin fueling your body, and your life, if you wish to do so.

As you begin to fuel, and as the experience blossoms from "trying it" to living it, you may find yourself at any of a number of crossroads I've found to be common along the journey from diet thinking to fueling. At these points, you may be presented with opportunities to either slip into diet thinking, or continue forging your own path of fueling.

If you stay grounded in the scientific facts, and if you continue to question your own nonthinking as well as that of others, you will become increasingly facile at recognizing diet-thinking traps that sidetrack happy fueling, and more adept at simply stepping around them. In the following pages, I'll address the issues and concerns that crop up most often in my work with people after they have begun fueling and provide some guidance on navigating this new path and maintaining the true spirit of fueling.

FORGET "PROGRAMS"

I very purposely do not call BodyFueling a program. The purpose of BodyFueling is to provide vital education and to instill a sense of choice and responsibility—the opportunity to make informed, inspired decisions moment to moment, forever. I am more interested in you *living your life* than in you "doing my program" or "sticking to my plan." That approach is doomed to fail regardless of the content.

I have yet to see anything else that adequately addresses this insistence upon assigning a special temporary status to something as basic as eating. Even as the concept "eat more" begins to climb out of the pit of diet thinking, it is forever being presented as a "program," "plan," or "diet."

"Programs" are one of the telltale markers of diet thinking, as I mentioned when I introduced you to the fundamentals of diet thinking in Chapter 5. This point deserves a reprise here, because I've noticed the "how-to" or getting-into-action part of eating differently is where Americans are most vulnerable to programitis—the tendency to automatically lunge for a highly structured Thing to Begin Monday that has an End. You "go on" a program that will stop when you return to "normal" eating—which implies that whatever you do on your "program" isn't normal. It rarely occurs to you to simply begin eating differently, and have that become what's "normal" for you.

Fueling is just that: eating differently, eating knowledgeably and efficiently—but when all is said and done, it's eating. You completely forego a life held together by a string of short-term "plans" and "programs." If you intend to fuel your body and think you're "starting the BodyFueling program," you're not only mistaken; you've missed the point completely.

As much as anything else, "successful" fueling depends on how you're approaching it: what you're doing it for and why. You can be doing things that add up to fueling, yet it can feel like a diet and be just a plan. For example, I talked with four clients who had once been on a "diet" that espoused many of the *technical* aspects of fueling: high carbohydrate, plenty of food, etc. But to all of them, it always was a "plan," a "program." What made it a plan, I wanted to know? Why wasn't it just "the way they ate"?

"It got boring," one said. Why were they doing it? "To lose weight, of course." Aha. Anything else? "What else is there?" another revealed.

They didn't learn why the diet's recommended way of eating worked. They never thought of that way of eating as "fueling" or even "caring for and investing in" their bodies. They never connected that investment to the full length of their lives and their profound desire to live actively and productively. There was no partnership between them and their bodies, and no sense of responsibility. They were just "on the plan." And not long after, not surprisingly, they were "off the plan."

"I've been trying to follow it," some of my own clients will say of BodyFueling a few weeks after a workshop. Don't! I reply. Just eat! Eating, fueling, sustenance is not about "following" anything. It's a basic necessity as well as a pleasure—not something you "go on" until you get to a goal and then "go off." Eating is no different than sleeping or breathing—they're each critical to life. But "programs" *make* it different.

Fueling is a journey, and there is no ultimate destination. On a path, you are not seeking the end; you expect to be moving always. This is the inherent opposite of a weight-loss diet, which is about waiting for, and hurrying to, The Result. Also, to suggest that there is one single place to "get to" suggests there is a limit to how fit and healthy you can be—that after a certain point, you simply cannot reach any further or develop any more. There is no evidence of such a limit; it exists only in your own mind. By targeting a "destination" you want to reach, you have created an end to the road. What made you think you had to stop there?

The program mentality is in part responsible. By relinquishing your power to its rules, you allow the program to determine what you can and cannot do. Americans expect their eating to be regulated—by someone other than themselves. Near the end of a class, people will ask, "Is XYZ allowed?" I respond, "Anything is allowed."

The question is not "Can I keep eating XYZ" but "Can I . . . and still get what I want? And how much do I want what I want?" When you're simply eating, or fueling, there's no such thing as "Can I have this? Is it allowed?" Of course it is. You can eat Butter Blinkies all day and night if you like. You just won't be as fit and healthy as you will if you fuel. It's your choice.

After fueling her body happily for six months and losing several dress sizes, Ann went on vacation to Hawaii for two weeks and gave herself total permission to eat whatever she wanted. (This is part of fueling your body, not the antithesis.) This is what she observed:

"I fully expected my clothes to get tight by the end of two weeks—and I was prepared for that; it wasn't going to be a problem. I know that the way I eat now will always be to fuel my body, and I would do that as soon as I returned.

"But the amazing thing is, nothing happened. I indulged myself fully every day, and at the end of the trip my latest new clothes, which were already getting loose again before the trip, were looser still. So I got a whole new take on fueling. My body isn't just responding directly to good fuel. Its handling of food—all food—has altered dramatically. It's now more efficient at processing, whether I'm fueling optimally or not.

"And it's a miracle to have approached this whole trip the way I did. I've never before been able to look at eating as simply the choices I make each day. It would have been 'off the diet for the trip' and 'on the diet after the trip.' The way I look at it now is as new and important as the way I eat."

CONSISTENCY, NOT PERFECTION: YOU CAN'T DO IT "WRONG"

Since lives aren't perfect—and I think few would argue that they're meant to be—then eating, if it is a seamless part of your life, is not meant to be perfect either. If you're not focused on "staying on" or "sticking to" something, then an occasion when you don't fuel (i.e., you miss a snack or meal, eat a very high-fat food, or don't eat enough) is hardly an occasion to flagellate yourself.

It's not being perfect that will do it. It's being relatively *consistent*. Rarely is a path perfectly straight, unwavering in a single direction. It moves all over the place. "We fail to realize that mastery is not about perfection. It's about a process, a journey . . . the master is the one who is willing to try and fail and try again," says George Leonard in his book *Mastery*.

The benefit of being extremely stringent and hating it, as opposed to being moderate and enjoying yourself, will be marginal to nonexistent. There's a definite law of diminishing returns—it's not healthy to be pinched and miserable, nor to drive yourself crazy trying to find the perfect food with just the right number of grams of fat. And as I discussed in the chapter on exercise, the healthiest thing to do is what you'll do, not the ideal that you won't ever achieve.

You can fuel at any moment. No one can ever take that away from you. And every moment is new. Every day is new. Not fueling doesn't mean anything—except that you didn't fuel just then.

I CAN HAVE IT—I DON'T *WANT* IT

Knowing you don't have to be perfect has a surprising way of bringing you closer to perfection than you ever thought possible. One day, while wandering downtown streets in search of a snack (a rare occasion in which I was unprepared), I discovered that none of the high-fat, sugary treats Americans are supposed to love held any appeal to me. It had been ages since I'd indulged in anything "nuclear," as my husband calls such "treats." I was "due." I had my choice of anything.

But I didn't want a headache or a sugar buzz or that fatty-food sluggishness. I wanted lots of tasty food that would give me energy to keep walking around. I chose Macheezmo Mouse, a local healthy-fast-Mexican-food place, and had brown rice with salsa, low-fat cheese, and a tortilla. That's what I wanted.

At a friend's birthday party at a fine restaurant, where only the desserts were richer than the entrées, I reaffirmed that my idea of "treat" no longer fits with even the idea of "treat" I would still endorse (even encourage) for most people. Some people call it suffering or denial to pass up this kind of food; to me, it was actually suffering to eat it. Good fueling is my treat. The biggest treat I can imagine is to feel healthy and energetic and know I am nurturing my precious body.

After the creamy pasta and chocolate cake that night, I felt leaden and had a headache. I wanted to wash that food out of me. Not because I feared "gaining weight" (or fat) from it—I know that doesn't happen in an evening—but because it didn't feel like it was serving my body. I craved plain, wholesome food—fuel. Next morning, my big bowl of oatmeal, toast, and plain chicken felt more sensational than ever—pure, clean, and tasty, and a welcome relief.

Don't despair if you're not at this point yet. It doesn't start with me (or you) ordering: "Okay, start desiring foods that fuel you—now!" It's a process, one that starts with you knowing what foods fuel you, realizing you want and need to be fueled and healthy, and then giving fueling a chance. Let yourself be charmed by how you feel after doing it for a while.

I wasn't always this way, either. Anyone who knew me years ago knows that I was a dessert queen. Because I wasn't thinking about health, life, and high performance—I just wanted to stay "thin" that week—I'd do anything I thought would "allow" me to "get away with" living on ice cream and chocolate. Now that I know how my body works, doing those things is unimaginable.

Think about the concept of "treat"—it should be something that makes you feel good, right? Ever wonder why then we term it a "treat" to consume things we know make us feel and look less than wonderful? Would you say, "Yea, I'm going to celebrate by stabbing myself in the face with a sharp object?" No, but you often say "Yea, I'm going to 'treat' myself to that [name of favorite garbage food]" when you know your body will protest.

Sure, some of those things taste good. Some of them also give you head-aches, make you depressed, drain your energy, add bodyfat, cause drowsiness or jitteriness, or whatever other reaction to sugar, fat, and alcohol you experience. Rather than say "I shouldn't" as if you don't hold the power to make an informed choice, the question you can ask yourself at every banquet table is: Will it taste good enough to make the "hangover" worthwhile? If yes, go ahead. Just indulge consciously and selectively. If you pass it up, it won't be because you couldn't have it, but because you don't want to.

Once you're informed, it's all a matter of choice. What's most important to you?

SOCIAL COMMENTARIES

In this diet-thinking world, it's still conspicuous when someone is choosy about what they put in their bodies. Few people can imagine actually think-ing before they stuff whatever's in front of them into their face. Fueling with precision isn't recognized as a willing act of self-love and a natural way of being around food; it's assumed to be some temporary, rigid plan. We never consider that being selective could be a natural way of life.

Therefore, if I pass on a meal or dessert because I deem it inappropriate fuel or not worth the cost, sometimes people will automatically demand, "Are you on a diet?" No, I say, it just didn't look good to me, or didn't seem worth it. I try not to preach and, unless asked to make recommenda-tions, stick to modest personal statements such as, "I just like to be discerning about what goes into my body." I do the same when people ask, "Are you hypoglycemic?" because I'm eating a snack. (To eat frequently is considered so odd, it's assumed something is wrong.) I usually reply, "No, I'm not hypoglycemic—I'm human. This is how often humans need to eat."

"TOO BUSY" TO EAT

MYTH: I'm too busy to snack (or to eat a healthy lunch instead of a burger and fries).

FACT: You're a powerful, successful, active, busy person who has accom-plished far greater things in your life than managing to swallow a banana at

10 o'clock in the morning at your desk, or bringing leftover pasta and rolls, or going the extra five minutes to the deli that serves sandwiches and soup. You're too busy *not* to snack. You're too busy to have that "lag," that fuzzy feeling mid-morning or mid-afternoon. You're too busy to eat the muscle tissue that represents your strength and stamina and metabolism. You're too busy to shorten your life.

Saving a minute now by not eating could cost you a lot later. (It's the same as saving a few minutes by not putting gas in your car—then running dry in mid-commute.) Statistical odds are that the alternative to high-carb, low-fat snacks and meals may be a disease much more time-consuming and unpleasant than remembering to take a bagel with you to work. A coronary artery surgery costs $30,000 to $40,000, takes about six months to fully recover from, and doesn't cure you. It's a matter of pay now—with a modicum of effort—or pay later with poor energy and health.

MAKING SURE IT HAPPENS

Almost nothing is more important than fueling your machine frequently throughout the day. That means snacking as well as eating three solid meals. Sounds like fun after decades of misguided starving, yes?

Having food with you everywhere is a habit that can be developed. (You weren't born taking your keys with you every day.) The best defense is to keep good fuel handy—in the office, at home, in the car, at your mother's, etc. It can be as simple as a slice or two of bread or an apple. If it's taste and variety you're after, flavored or seasoned rolls and bagels, homemade muffins (bake several dozen and freeze), exotic fruits or juices may do the trick.

Plan meetings and appointments so that you have time to eat beforehand. Try not to schedule meetings that last more than three hours without breaks. Take a few minutes each night to look at the next day's schedule and figure out what you will need. Prepare your food the night before. Plan breakfast, and pack lunch and snacks so they're ready to go.

I have clients who have schedules or work you'd think might make it tough to wedge a snack in. But they do it. They keep six-packs of fruit juice under the seat in the car; munch a banana or small box of raisins on the way to the next appointment.

Some get bolder and begin to demand that life around them conform to what they know are the body's requirements for good performance—*every* body's requirements. They denounce meetings that go for hours without a break, or that take place in steak houses, or that present giant boxes of danish as the only sustenance. They begin to educate people around them about how the body works—and why the current situation doesn't. It's ignorance of the body's needs and nonthinking that keep our world inconsistent with those needs. If whoever schedules the four-hour meeting realizes that it does matter—and it's not a matter of being a wimp, but a matter of being human—that person may be inclined to make changes too.

I'll fuel myself anytime, anywhere. I will whip out a bagel or banana no matter where I am. I will stuff a sandwich into my mouth while facilitating a workshop. (Admittedly, it fits with the subject; I'm not suggesting that an executive do this while giving a speech to a conservative group. But, then again, I'm not assuming he or she can't, either.)

I don't leave the house without food any more than I would leave the house without keys or wallet. It's simply that much of a necessity; what happens if I'm caught short without food is just too branded in my consciousness. I take food even if I don't think I'll be away from food for a full three hours; there are traffic jams, changes in plans. If I am caught without food at snack time or mealtime on some rare occasion, I'll go to the nearest grocery store and get some.

Sometimes people laugh at Robert and me because anywhere we go—to our own workshop, another class, a concert, a meeting, shopping—we always carry a cloth sack packed with provisions. For road trips, the back seat is piled with bags of sandwiches, rolls, fat-free crackers and cookies, fruit, and juice. (And our trusty five-gallon water jug; for shorter trips we take a one-liter bottle.)

Once Robert was stuck in a snowstorm. It took him nearly five hours to make a trip that normally takes less than 30 minutes. But he had food and water with him. While others cried with frustration at the wheels of their cars as day turned into night, Robert was calmly munching in the middle of the dark, snow-blown freeway.

I wouldn't think of leaving it to chance, fate, or other people to be responsible for me being fueled. I wouldn't think of placing myself in a position where I am forced to rely on the limited selection at a roadside fast-food place, if one does appear on the horizon. I am simply that committed to my body. It's very matter-of-fact: It's *my body*. What could be more important? What else can get done if I'm not fueled?

I'll even eat dinner before going to a banquet, wedding, or conference, or other preplanned, one-choice sort of meal. If the only choice is beef, with pasta and vegetables swimming in oil, butter, and cheese, I can pass and just munch on a roll or two. Conspicuous? Embarrassing? I don't care. To me, it's ridiculous to be more concerned about decorum than the condition of your own body. I will not ingest garbage that doesn't interest me just to be polite. I'll eat garbage once in a great while, but I choose the time and place, and I choose the garbage. The food I'm willing to indulge in outside the bounds of good fueling usually comes at dessert, not in the form of a steak or a stick of butter.

If the wedding dinner or banquet is good fuel, I eat it. Yes, I'll have had two dinners, one at home and one at the party—but remember the forgiving nature of carbohydrate. It won't hurt to do that on occasion. Most people would never eat two full dinners, thinking that would be the ultimate downfall. But they will commonly and unthinkingly skip meals and snacks or accept greasy garbage they don't really want—which is something I'll never do. Priorities change when you understand the design of the machine.

WHAT ABOUT THE REST OF THE FAMILY?

Parents sometimes say to me, "Kids have to have junk, though, don't they? They want it, I mean, you know. . . ." Often they trail off, suddenly uncertain about something they've always accepted without question.

I cannot count the number of times I have seen a child not old enough to speak in a grocery cart chomping on a frosted doughnut or bag of jelly beans, or leaving a fast-food restaurant clutching a cheeseburger. They didn't ask for that food; it's what they were given! As soon as toddlers have teeth, many parents are plying them with their own favorite nonfuel, assuming the child will want ("need") it too. They're not thinking that what they feed the child represents an investment in his or her future. And it's just as important an investment—in my humble opinion, far more important—than a college fund.

Later, yes, the kids will ask for it—because it's all they know to ask for, and possibly also because by then they experience a physical addiction to it. The assumption that children come out of the womb craving packaged pies and french fries is ludicrous. Our bodies were not designed to "ask" for those kinds of foods; most of human existence has been without them. Chinese children don't ask for cupcakes. Indian children don't demand fried chicken nuggets or moon pies.

It *is* possible to fuel your children with the same commitment with which you fuel yourself. Parents like our cousins or one set of friends may be fairly rare. Both couples puree fresh fruits and vegetables and cook rice, oats, and other grains for their babies. (No throwaway jars that cost more than fresh, contain as much corn syrup as food, and wind up in landfills.) The child among them who is old enough to chew gets a fruit if he wants a snack, not a brownie, and he will not see the inside of a fast-food restaurant till he is old enough to pay for it himself. And they are the happiest, most glowing little children I have ever seen.

Most of my clients find inspiration for family-wide transformation in the opportunity to pass on a positive and accurate legacy to their children. While many worry at first about what the rest of the family will think of fueling— or any changes at all—those who are clear about the advantages and determined to make the switch simply do so. Just as you can find time for a snack if you really perceive its importance, you can manage to make fueling work in a family context if you're serious about it.

Most find their families quite adaptable, merely needing a chance to learn—just as you did—that healthy eating won't limit them to a few leafy greens, textured vegetable protein, and beet juice.

One family who read an early draft of *BodyFueling* proceeded to eliminate fatty and sugary foods from their cupboards. After several months, however, they allowed the children a "treat"—some high-fat potato chips. After eating them, the son complained, "Mommy, I don't feel so good. Those chips gave me a stomachache. I think they're too high in fat." When I heard this story, I almost cried. It's simply such a condescending lie to say children, given the chance, aren't capable of this.

Some bluntly don't care whether the family objects or not: "When I put the pieces together and realized what our careless eating was costing us in every way, both now and later, I didn't care what they thought," said a single mother (who was initially aghast when a comparison revealed how much more time and money she spent on fast food than simple, tasty "fuel" meals at home). "I told them, 'This is what we're going to eat; I'm not making anything else,' and, well, they ate it!

"If they want sugar and fat, they'll have to get it somewhere else. And if they do eat those things at friends' houses, or buy them with their allowances, they're still going to get far less of it overall because they're not getting any here! And you know, they're making the choice. They're learning it's up to them." Bravo.

RESULTS: STOP DIGGING UP THE GARDEN!

Fat loss can be a result of fueling—one result, not the only result. Other benefits and advantages you'll see and feel when you begin fueling your body in the way it needs include:

▶ More energy and vitality
▶ Muscle gain (or at least maintenance)
▶ Strength
▶ Better workout performance and stamina
▶ Longevity
▶ Less illness and reduced risk of disease
▶ Time savings
▶ Cost savings—to you and others
▶ Ease of food preparation
▶ Enjoyment of cooking
▶ Less confusion
▶ An end to worrying about "weight"

Fueling isn't merely a "fat-loss tool." It's what your body needs for overall optimal functioning. More and more I find people recognize this; they want to "eat better" for all kinds of reasons. While many people are concerned with fat loss, a growing number of basically healthy and lean (or almost-lean) people are seeking input for more energy, disease prevention, athletic performance, or general knowledge and improvement. Most eventually conclude that health, strength, and longevity are paramount—and they realize that, conveniently, leanness will be an unavoidable corollary of all those.

Still, fat loss remains a focal point of interest, even when people begin to loosen their grip on "weight." As I've explained, tearing your eyes away from the prize you may expect a month from now, and instead gazing way out into your life, is the hardest thing for most people to do. You can't resist the urge to dig up the garden to see if it's grown. You watch the pot to see if it's boiling. You can't see the forest (your life, your health) for the tree (this minute).

The amount of concern I've witnessed about the speed of fat loss is a monument not only to lack of understanding about the body's capabilities, but also to diet thinking. One woman who called just to inquire about the workshop wanted to know if I could explain why she "hadn't lost any fat yet" since she "cut down on peanut butter" one month earlier. Another caller complained that "the high-carb thing" didn't work for her because "I start out losing fat, but then I hit a plateau and can't lose any more."

"Plateau" is definitely a diet-thinking word; it implies that there is something wrong if your body doesn't respond without end to your pushing and shoving. It doesn't consider that, if fat loss slows or stops, your body is giving you a message, and knows better than your one-track, fat-loss-crazed mind whether it really needs to do what you think it needs to do. "Did it ever occur to you," I asked this woman, "that you didn't need to lose any more fat?" "Well—no," responded the woman.

Perhaps the most striking example of nonthinking in this arena was "Leah," a burger and milkshake lover in her late thirties who exercised like a nut, underfueled, and "overfatted." At the end of her workshop, she announced that she wasn't sure if she could "motivate herself" to make changes in her diet if she wasn't going to see immediate results. Momentarily stunned by the shortsightedness of this thought, I then pointed out how nonsensical it was: "If you don't make any changes, you'll never see those results. Never is a lot longer to wait than however long fueling might take." "Hmmm—you've got a point," she said slowly.

"And you can stop going all day without food," I added. "In fact, you'll need to, to get the results you want. I'm not telling you to starve. I'm encouraging you to eat more, more often. How much 'motivation' do you need for that?" Leah couldn't answer.

Americans have wanted the fast fix for a long time, and it's that very practice that caused a lot of us to starve for quick "weight" loss, unwittingly programming our bodies for future fat gain. Now you cry that it isn't turning around fast enough. It can be turned around, but it does take time. You cannot underfuel, overgrease, and under- or overuse your body for 20 years, then put a bit of good "gas" in one day and expect an instant race car.

I think it seems like it takes so much time because your mind takes time to change, not just your body. Your body is a machine; we know pretty much what it needs and what it will do if you're good to it, and roughly how much time it will take to do it. (We know it won't take 10 days, and we know it won't take 10 years either.)

"But that's not good enough!" you cry. Why not? Your mind is slower and more stubborn than your body. Ten to 60 years of diet thinking is harder to lose than any amount of fat. My clients, bless every one of them, have shown me this.

Christine: "I'm doing pretty good. My cholesterol is down from 250 to 175 and when my doctor asked why, she couldn't believe how much I knew. But I wish I could eat less."

Jean, leaving the workshop for a long road trip, refusing our offer of fat-free cookies and muffins: "No, thanks. I have celery sticks with me."

Lisa, one *week* after the workshop: "I'm doing okay, I guess. I haven't lost any fat yet."

The rate at which people lose fat (best measured by appearance and the fit of clothes) varies widely. It depends on how efficiently and impeccably you begin to fuel yourself now, how inefficiently you've done it before and for how long, and what your body's natural tendencies are. The more abuse your body has taken—the more starved it's been—the better trained it is to save fat instead of spend it. You can retrain your body—but that means nurturing it, not further assaulting it.

It may take a year, maybe even two or three, to lose all the fat you want to. But what a year! You're not sitting around suffering, waiting for the pot to boil. You're eating. Plenty. An increase in energy, if you haven't been fueling efficiently before, is an immediate result you can enjoy. If you really do plan to care for yourself from now on, to eat efficiently and give your body what it needs—and if what it needs turns out to be lots of great stuff—you may well ask yourself, "What's my hurry?"

After I began fueling, it took me six months to lose 6 pounds of fat, and then another two years to lose 10 more. Results like that are wonderful physically—it was a major boon to my health and appearance. It was clearly pure fat loss; it was steady in that direction, even though slow. And it really just happened as a result of fueling my life and investing in my health and energy—not in an all-out effort to harvest cosmetic benefits.

No one can promise you that you will lose X amount of fat in X amount of time. How could they? You are an individual, and they can't tell you exactly what you are going to do from now on, any more than they can tell exactly where your body is now. There are a few things I can promise you, though.

If you fuel yourself, you'll always be headed in the direction you want to be going. Your whole life will become that never-ending path, getting better, fitter, and healthier continuously. You'll notice landmarks, milestones—but none need mean you're "done."

You'll have fun. You'll be eating, not dieting; living your life, not "on a program." You'll be eating a lot of food. It may even mean rediscovering food and eating.

You'll enjoy peace and confidence. That's what comes with knowing that any biology book you get your hands on will confirm that the amounts and proportions of food you consume are just what you need.

I firmly believe that without a perspective that goes far beyond next month or even next year, it's unlikely you'll transcend the paradigm of diet thinking. I also believe that superstition about a watched pot not boiling. So stop lifting up your shirt every day to see if your belly's gone. It won't disappear any faster than it appeared. Appreciate the changes inside that will show up in what *doesn't* happen 30 years from now, not just in what *does* happen two weeks from now. Live your life and forget about manipulating your thighs. It will come.

HEDGING YOUR BETS FOR FAT LOSS

If fueling isn't meeting your fat-loss expectations, and you've determined those expectations are reasonable, you may not be fueling completely. In one-on-one work with clients, I have yet to come across a single person who, after a closer look, actually was consistently fueling in every regard—frequency, quality, and quantity—and not seeing fat loss, if fat loss was needed. These are the six most common roadblocks people encounter:

1. Too much protein. If you've thought you were fueling consistently, but believe you're not seeing reasonably progressive fat loss (loosening of clothing after eight weeks), this is one to check. You've learned that excess protein at any one sitting will be converted to fat. But it can take time to adjust because the world is so protein-crazy. Most restaurants still seem determined to give you twice as much protein and half the carbohydrate you need (though it would be far cheaper to give us what we actually use!). Even you—or whoever prepares your food—may not be quite certain what 2 or 3 ounces of chicken looks like. Find out!

2. Not eating often enough. I can't count how many times during one-on-one work people swear they fuel by the clock, only to have a food diary three days later reveal, "Gee, I didn't realize I was going seven hours without food there."

Frequency is number one—to keep your body burning "hot," give you energy to be active, and preserve precious lean muscle. So why do you find it so easy to put it last? Habit, for one. Say you've pushed through every day without eating for the last 20 years. Now you know all the ways your body conspires to pack fat away in that fuel deficit. But that doesn't make frequent fueling an instant habit. Only you can.

3. Hidden fat. Often a client will be certain he/she has dramatically whittled dietary fat. When I check out the fridge, I hear "No kidding! I had no idea that had fat in it." Look! Or, "But it's olive oil (or margarine); I thought it was 'less fattening.' " When it comes to fat loss, fat is fat.

4. *Too much carbohydrate.* This is the least common trip-up, because it's difficult to gain fat by eating complex carbohydrate (and it's still more important to eat enough of this stuff). Still, if you regularly eat more than a serving or two above your fuel needs, the body may begin converting the excess to fat—or using it as fuel in lieu of stored bodyfat. You might be "misusing" a food that is much higher in carbohydrate than you think (one client was eating lots of pomegranates every day, unaware that one packs the carbohydrate power of three or four peaches), or eating lots of simple carbohydrate (sugar). Refined sugar is a biochemical accomplice to fat storage, and the short-lived, ultimately exhausting energy surge/crash it creates may drive you to chase it with more of the same—or worse.

5. *Not much activity.* Exercising "more" does offer benefits if you provide the fuel your body needs to sustain added activity. If increased activity makes you hungrier, do add carbohydrate. Adding two hours of exercise per week, then going hungry when appetite increases correspondingly, will only backfire.

Increasing exercise for more progressive fat loss and/or muscle gain doesn't mean you must triple your output. Chronic exhaustion is a tip that you may be adding too much. Go slow; increase in increments. And remember: Longer is better than harder/faster for fat burning.

6. *You may not need to lose fat.* If you're not losing fat, you may not need to. When someone who clearly has excess bodyfat to lose complains, "It isn't working," we start exploring the other five snags listed above. But when an already-lean person seems overly focused on fat loss, I know there may be other issues to deal with first. When Sarah, for example, glumly reported that she hadn't lost any fat yet, bells went off. First, it was only two weeks since her workshop; second, she was already undeniably lean, though it took a good bit of discussion for her to grasp this.

I've observed that the body is a pretty evenhanded machine. If you fuel 50 percent, you'll have a 50 percent kind of body. But that doesn't mean fueling only half the time is bad. Fueling is not morally correct—just scientifically accurate. You don't have to fuel; you don't have to want to. You're entitled to eat exactly as you please. But only fueling will give you all the benefits with none of the negatives. When energy and leanness are more important to you than whatever takes you off track, you'll fuel.

IF FUELING DOESN'T FEEL GOOD

If fueling doesn't work, or if it doesn't feel good, something is wrong. This is the way your body is designed to use fuel, so if it's not using it or using it well, then the machine is malfunctioning. An example: A client found she could not tolerate any carbohydrate whatsoever. She had long avoided it because it made her so uncomfortable, but when she learned her body needed it, she tried to integrate it back into her diet. She felt constantly nauseous and achy and had great difficulty digesting.

Tests revealed that, because she'd had her stomach pumped as a young woman due to poisoning, she had suffered significant liver damage. She was then able to begin treatment to heal her liver so that she could feed her body the way it was intended to be fed.

THE ULTIMATE TRIUMPH: MORE FAT, NO FEAR

A little bit of bodyfat fluctuation is normal and natural, and is nothing to worry about if your eating remains consistently fuel-hearty and low-fat. I've noticed I do gain fat in the winter—but my response to it is radically different than it would have been a few years ago. That's thanks to the big-picture context of fueling for life, coupled with the knowledge that reducing bodyfat slightly again will not involve anything resembling starving or suffering.

As I believe would be the case for most anyone, it is nothing short of a miracle to me that I can observe my body getting a bit fatter and, rather than launch into a frenzy of "eating less and exercising more," simply shrug and say, "Well, it'll come off when spring comes," and continue to fuel and do whatever exercise I feel like. This calm knowing is what thrills me most about fueling. I think if the truth were told, it's what people want most— even more than great bodies.

First of all, it makes sense to me that a body would want a bit of extra padding when the average temperature is 35 degrees instead of 75 degrees. That doesn't mean it makes sense to me to gain 15 or 20 pounds of fat, or to eat a lot of fat just because it's cold out. It means I notice a subtle difference, and since I'm not deep in hysteria about how my body looks, I have the chance to consider that perhaps it's appropriate. Diet thinking, focused only on bullying the body shape and "weight" for immediate gratification, doesn't allow for such consideration.

Besides the need for warmth, I know another reason I gain some fat in winter is that my spring/summer activity level is dramatically higher. Come summer, I walk and bicycle everywhere, and rollerskate whenever I get the chance. In Seattle's long, wet winter, my stationary bike is pretty much the extent of my aerobic activity. I don't feel like walking or bicycling outdoors, and I don't have to—I don't "make" myself. That would ruin the happy relationship with physical activity that I relish.

Yet I keep eating like an athlete all winter; I won't deprive myself of food. Because my food intake is so high in carb and so low in fat, bodyfat is added so minimally and slowly that before the gain becomes visible to anyone except the two people (including me) who see me naked regularly, it's spring again—and my activity increases to create a definite demand for the full complement of fuel I eat.

Is my fat gain unhealthy? No, because we're talking about a jump from about 16 percent bodyfat to 18 percent (not, say, 27 percent to 33 percent). Also, it comes from excess carbohydrate calories—not excess fat, which easily and rapidly adds up as stored bodyfat, and leaves a nasty legacy on artery walls and blood cholesterol levels. And remember, the energy cost for converting and storing that carbohydrate reduces the actual amount being converted to a bare minimum.

How have I achieved this tranquillity about how much fat I have on my body? Knowledge of the scientific facts gives me power. Connection and commitment to my future keeps me caring for myself, instead of harming myself in repeated, doomed attempts to browbeat my body.

I would be irresponsible if I presented my relationship to eating and exercise as utopic. There are days I feel like a slug; when PMS convinces me that—after all this!—I am going to be a whale; when I would sooner nap than bike. I just don't buy into it anymore. I don't have to worry about a lot of things that don't matter, because I know what does matter. I don't have to engage in a lot of things that don't work, because I know they don't. It's about a million worlds away from where I used to be. It's where you can be too.

12

THE "FAT-LOSS/MUSCLE-GAIN" MOVEMENT: Words of Warning

Women, who once believed you couldn't be too thin or too rich, now equate thinness with weakness and sickness, and the muscled body with power.

In the 80s, the status outfit was the Power Suit. Today it's the anatomically corrected Power Body . . . Suddenly, to be merely slim, without muscle definition, is to be out of shape, a lightweight.

—*Allure*, March 1993

Idon't completely agree with this. The majority of women I meet and talk to—from teenage to middle age—still don't know who Linda Hamilton is and just want to be thin and lose "weight."

Yet, undeniably, there is a trend afoot. The more muscled, sculpted look for women is slowly, in selected circles, replacing the thin-at-any-costs ideal. I think this is particularly true of upwardly mobile, young urban professionals (or whatever they're called nowadays).

Is there a problem here? Just that it doesn't make any difference if diet thinking doesn't get addressed. In that case, it's just the latest hot trend headed for the diet-thinking junkpile.

IT DOESN'T ADDRESS DIET THINKING

Riding this wave is a rash of new books, programs, and media articles that might appear at first glance to be deceptively similar to some of the material in this book. Technically, some of them are. And you might be drawn into thinking, "Oh, here's something good! It's about losing fat and gaining muscle, so it's not diet thinking." But that's not necessarily true. It all depends on its purpose—and yours.

Remember, BodyFueling is about your *thinking*, not just trying to *do* the latest technically correct thing in an effort to fix your body. Informed choice is not just about information alone; it's also about perspective. You haven't gained a new perspective simply because you've replaced counting calories with counting fat grams and hours at the gym—in fact, the fat-loss/muscle-gain mentality can all too easily become a new, even more demanding kind of diet thinking, complete with new "control tools" to help you chase the new standard.

Even if the trend and its products didn't represent diet thinking, they don't help you address your own diet thinking. If you're still setting out to tweak and toggle your body into the "right" shape, all you get is a more accurate, precise way to do it. That's why, for example, I'd never provide the previous how-to chapters without the context of the rest of the book.

But with many of these new programs, that's essentially what you get. While some may present basically sound to-dos, they don't take you off the diet thinking merry-go-round. For one thing, from Greg Phillips' "ThinkLight! Lowfat Living Plan" to Susan Powter's "Stop the Insanity" program, these are still being delivered—and accepted—as diets and programs. They're new and ultra-improved: commendably, you eat more, ignore calories, and forget weight (usually). And, without question, all of that is, I'm glad to say, worlds apart from "eating less, exercising more, and losing weight."

But you still "do" them, you still "follow" them; you still fight (fat, diet companies, whatever) and focus on getting a lean body—as soon as possible. None of them present the holistic approach that I know is the only way out of diet thinking: inspiration, education, and tools for integration. And when

I say inspiration, I don't mean someone on a stage whipping you into a frenzy; I mean the type of ongoing, self-directed inquiry detailed in "Fueling Your Future." When I say education, I don't mean just "how to eat," but rather the complete background on how your body works. They are programs for how you don't look or feel (yet). Instead of being about weight, now they're about fat (or muscle). They're still not about your life.

IT'S NOT ENTIRELY ACCURATE

Further, some of what the "fat-loss/muscle-gain" faction has to say—especially through the media—is *not* scientifically sound. Misinformation and confusion are as rampant within this trend as they were with classic dieting. The media are massacring even the most informationally sound and well-intentioned concepts by pasting together sound bites without a context of understanding.

For example, the spotlight on weight-lifting is spawning a "more protein" push. This is a classic symptom of diet thinking's "one thing will do it" mentality. Instead of learning the whole picture, you continue operating under the assumption that there has to be One Right Way. Thus if one thing that's needed is protein, the next deduction is that protein is The Thing.

The March 1993 issue of *Allure* featured two articles on the subject—one called "Body Makeover" and another called "Body-Building Food." The latter carried the tag line: "As women seek stronger bodies, protein has been making a comeback." The diet of a "thin, health-conscious and fat-phobic" woman is described: bran muffin for breakfast, salad for lunch, and pasta for dinner. "What's wrong with this picture? She forgot the protein." Except it sounds like she also forgot the carbohydrate, based on the measly breakfast and virtually nonexistent lunch.

But this article doesn't address carbohydrate. Instead, the piece quotes an L.A. fitness trainer who says that women's bodies "are cannibalizing their own muscle for energy because their diets are so protein-poor." As you now know, however, that's not why muscle breaks down. Protein isn't energy food; muscle is "cannibalized" for use as energy when diets are poor in carbohydrate. (And yes, many women's diets are carbohydrate-poor.)

The article also displays a commonplace symptom of fat-and-muscle ignorance by including the hackneyed blooper "Replace body fat with muscle," which leads too many people to believe that fat can turn into muscle and vice versa.

In a true salute to diet thinking, the magazine's own editor-in-chief misunderstood the article's recommendations. In her Editor's Note, she summarizes: "All it takes is a low-fat, *high-protein* diet and two hours a day in the gym, and voilà, Linda Hamilton II." But *high* protein is not what the article said! In the end, its message is that a small amount of lean protein at each meal is ideal for muscle building, repair, and maintenance (although that conclusion is preceded by numerous distractions that isolate protein).

This editor tasted a bit of her own medicine: the kind of dangerous leap you can easily make reading an article like this one.

A NEW MAGIC PILL INSTEAD OF
A TOTAL EDUCATION

The above mishap occurred because neither editor nor writer has the full picture. They aren't educated. It's true that you need protein for certain things, but if you understood the human body, you'd already know that. You'd also know you need other things just as much as protein. You wouldn't be at the mercy of a magazine doling out a single, disembodied scrap of information.

Instead of education, a new magic pill is tossed into the raging sea of confusion. Though sufficient carbohydrate is what fuels muscle once it exists, suddenly protein replaces carbohydrate as The Answer. Though both weight training and aerobics are valuable, suddenly weight training replaces aerobics as The Answer. "Suddenly, aerobics classes seem as dated as Isadora Duncan dancing barefoot with scarves," said the "Body Makeover" article. Meanwhile, you read the headlines, think everything's changed (again!) and feel more confused than ever.

The way of eating that's ultimately proposed in "Body-Building Food"— if you get to the article's end—is fueling. They're talking about a 65 percent complex carbohydrate, 10 percent fat, 25 percent protein diet—roughly what I eat, what I recommend, and what disease prevention researchers point to. But it's presented here as "a special diet" for muscle building that "allows" for "some form of low-fat protein at every meal." *That's not special!* That's what the body needs—whether you're trying to build muscle or not.

Appropriate warnings about excess protein and toxicity; a statement from Linda Hamilton's trainer that he also kept her carbs up; the fact that most Americans are still far from a diet that's too low in protein; and the fact that you don't have to starve to build muscle all make the final paragraphs of these articles. But many people will never read that far.

Interestingly, while articles like these focus on women and their "new" interest in muscle, it's taken for granted that men have always wanted to build muscle. Once again, the educational needs and true desires of men get trampled underfoot. The male worship of protein is legendary; their "lots of it" could mean anything. And a number of men have confided to me that they felt bulldozed into muscle building by trainers who have a one-size-fits-all Mr. America in mind. Now women get to join this diet-thinking club. Hooray for progress.

All those men wanted was to be toned, fit, and lean—without it dominating their lives. They didn't want to perform surgery on their bodies; they wanted to eat and live. In fact, I think that's what most people want. Being exhorted to lose fat and gain muscle for its own sake, as a pursuit isolated from the benefits it brings to life, just lures them away from that desire.

WHY ARE YOU DOING IT?

The *Allure* article "Body Makeover" did ask an excellent question that I thought deserved more attention: "Do women want to look stronger, or be stronger?" This question underlines the difference between manipulating your body and fueling your life. You can "do" any "fat-loss/muscle-gain" program—and stay in that driven, ever-searching mind-set. But whether you're a sleek young muscle-seeker or a conventional, thinness-oriented dieter, whether you're wielding the scale or the calipers, chasing 110 pounds or 14 percent—you're on the same treadmill.

I want to *be* strong. I like the look that comes with it, no question about it. But being strong holds far more relevance to living my life than merely *looking* strong does. One will help me on hikes and bikes; with books and babies. The other will only help me in front of the mirror. Mastery is great, but if it's always limited to one thing—your body's looks—perhaps it's unhealthy. I like the idea of mastering my musculature—but I also want to master my strength, my health, my skating speed, the guitar . . .

Muscle is valuable, for numerous reasons I have described in other chapters.

Losing fat will mean a healthier body for many people. But without a life purpose or context, you are nearly as dominated by the correct information ("eat more," "lose fat, not weight") as you are by lies. Headlines screaming "Lose fat now!" aren't intended or received much differently than "Lose weight now!"

Straining to manufacture muscle while deeply embedded in the shortsightedness of diet thinking, or with the sole purpose of looking like someone else, is not fueling. "Applying protein" (or even a more well-rounded strategy) with that hopeful, even mildly hysterical vigil over your body has the earmarks of dieting. It might not cause as much physical harm as classic dieting (provided you do get accurate information and don't embellish it, as in, "If protein builds muscle, then tripling the U.S. RDA must build more" or "Maybe 10 hours a week of weight-lifting will work better than four"). But no matter how accurate you are, there's no relief in mind and spirit.

Once again, I direct you back to Chapter 1: "Fueling Your Future." The definition and dismantling of diet thinking is what sets BodyFueling apart from "fat-loss/muscle-gain" diets. And "Fueling Your Future" is your path to personal disengagement from diet thinking. To me, it's more important than anything else in this book.

13

SURRENDERING THE SUFFERING:
Why the Hardest Part May Be That It's Easy

Settling into a lifelong way of eating for optimum performance actually requires a willingness to have it be easy. Fueling your body is not a complicated, high-tech prospect. If you were expecting highly controlled, tightly wrapped meal plans, "forbidden" foods, demands for perfect-to-the-gram, exacting-to-the-bite self-surveillance, and a push for pills and powders, you're probably stunned. You may also be surprised that the simplicity and ease offered by the knowledge and perspective I've provided seems almost . . . unpleasant.

It may, in fact, be so simple and easy that it goes right over your head. It may seem too insubstantial, as if complication and difficulty equal substance. You may not trust the value of something that doesn't require you to suffer at least a little. You may be waiting for the other shoe to drop, the real blow. "Aha! I knew there must be something else to this."

This is a very common, very human condition. George Leonard's book *Mastery* explores human tendencies to keep ourselves and others as they are, whether good or bad—and how these tendencies often sabotage progress or mastery.

"This condition of equilibrium, this resistance to change, is called homeostasis . . . and it applies to psychological states and behavior as well as to physical functioning. . . . Although we might think our culture is mad for the new, the predominant function . . . is the survival of things as they are. The problem is, homeostasis works to keep things as they are even if they aren't very good."

Leonard cites numerous examples, such as families that create new problems when an old one—say, a parent's alcoholism—is resolved in order to perpetuate the state of uproar to which they are accustomed. "Organizations and cultures resist change and backslide when change does occur."

This not only serves to explain the cultural persistence of weight mania and diet thinking (despite lack of factual support for, and the failure of, every practice and process related to it). It also accounts for an individual phenomenon I've encountered with some regularity: the person who dismisses effective, pleasurable fueling in favor of the drudgery and inefficiency of diet thinking, choosing to remain stuck with what never worked.

If there is an addiction related to weight and fat, the real one may be the suffering associated with those issues. As Americans, we think it's got to be hard and has to be complicated. *I* cringed when I read this letter to the editor of my local newspaper regarding Ross Perot during the '92 election season: "I cringe when I hear his simplistic answers to fix problems." Why? What if it is simple—and problems go unfixed because people tinker with complex minutiae? As with our politics, that's the problem with the American approach to fitness.

That's one reason it's been so easy to miss the most fundamental and obvious of solutions—answers that have been there all along. We trample right over basic biology in our certain assumption that there must be something more, something beyond, something different.

And even as you wait in hope for The One Final Answer to overfat, deep down most people "know" they must suffer in exchange for improved health and fitness. In particular, when it comes to eating, you are sure you must deprive yourself to get what you want.

You think you must never eat anything you like; that's the only ticket to health and/or a super body. You think you must eat weird, gross food, and exercise two hours a day. You think you must sweat rivers, turn red, blue, or white, grow calluses the size of stones and twice as hard, pull muscles, tear ligaments and rip tendons. And if you're not exercising so much that you feel crunched for time and as if you are shortchanging other parts of your life, then you figure you're probably not doing enough.

This belief runs so deep that I've found some people almost patently reject anything that sidesteps all this. Remember, this is the culture that came up with "No pain, no gain." You adhere to it in relationships, business, and of course in its place of origin: sports. If it doesn't hurt, it's worthless. You don't trust it.

Are you willing to put aside suffering about food and weight? Are you willing to consider that it's almost laughably simple—not a big, dramatic, futuristic kind of answer? When it comes right down to it, are you willing to have this be easier than you ever thought possible—and are you willing to have it handled?

"WHAT DO YOU MEAN, DO I WANT TO HANDLE IT?"

That may sound like a crazy question—as crazy as it may sound to suggest we're a culture that welcomes, even worships, pain and suffering. "Of course I want to handle this!" you may cry. "It's been a pain in my fat rear all my life!" But let's be honest. We're talking about our humanness.

This—"weight," diet, eating—is a hot topic. If you handled it for life, and one day just began eating in a constructive, consistent way, and it came naturally, and it was the way you lived and not your new "program," what would you talk about?

Suffering buys you payoffs. You get sympathy. You get agreement from others. You get out of doing things. Show me a problem that is a constant complaint, and I'll show you a situation in which the angst is somewhere, somehow, providing at least as much payoff as cost.

I've had clients admit to it. One woman I worked with told me bluntly on a follow-up call, "You know, I don't know what it is. I used to love bread, when I thought it was wrong to eat it, but now that you've told me it's good, I don't want it anymore. I hated dieting, but now that you told me I don't have to, I don't want to eat. I don't snack like I'm supposed to." She paused. "I guess," she said thoughtfully, "I just really want to suffer with this. I thought I wanted to do what works, but I don't." A young (and totally gorgeous) bodybuilder admitted she just didn't want to stop weighing herself, even though she knew it was meaningless to everything else she wanted.

Others are more covert. A successful, wealthy mother of four incredibly prodigious children spoke frankly during the workshop about the all-consuming havoc this issue created in her life. She animatedly described how her family would avoid her in the morning after she'd been on the scale, how "gains" of 1 or 2 pounds turned her into a raving bitch for the remainder of the day, how she obsessed about her size 4 days as a teenager. She could recite the chronology of what she'd weighed every year since then. She told us how her daughter, at age seven, already said things like, "Mommy can't eat, because she's on a diet."

What she learned in the workshop gave every indication that the suffering could end. She understood—intellectually—how her daily abstinence from food until dinnertime contributed to the shape her body was in now, and that her shape could change only by doing the very thing she thought was forbidden: eating. She could see conceptually that the scale had nothing to do with what she was really after.

But after the workshop and a bit of one-on-one work, she dropped out of sight abruptly, without explanation. She stopped returning calls, except for one terse message: "I've decided this isn't for me right now. I don't want to continue talking. Thanks." At first I was stunned, but the more people I worked with, the more sense it made.

One company had a "weight-loss group" that met for lunch every week. They were interested in the concept of fueling for high performance, but it never got further than a concept. During my presentation, I saw eyes glazing over at the apparently incomprehensible thought that one could eat food and still be lean. I wondered whether the thought of not needing a weekly "weight-loss group" anymore was too disorienting to pursue. It could have become a soccer group, a dance group, a guitar group, or a walking group. But it had been a weight-loss group for years; maybe it always will be. It's familiar and comfortable.

Another way in which homeostasis rears its head is by seeing even the most universally loved aspects of fueling as dismal; forcing a positive reality to fit your negative expectations. No matter how good it is, you say it's hard—because you're wearing "hard" glasses. Through them, everything looks like a hassle. This is the paradigm effect again: All you can see is what you expect to see or already "know." If you come to fitness "knowing" it's going to be all sacrifice and torture, you may not be willing to accept any other answer.

An example: Dan looked at his breakfast fuel profile (3 servings [18 grams] of protein and 4 servings [60 grams] of carbohydrate—the equivalent of a cup of yogurt, two ounces of turkey, two slices of toast, and a bowl of cereal) and blustered, "That doesn't seem like very much food." I was startled; the opposite reaction is more common. "Oh? What do you eat for breakfast now?" I asked. "Uh—nothing," he replied sheepishly.

Another woman caught me off guard during a workshop when I was asking the group which would take more willpower: the typical "eat less and exercise more" or fueling's "eat enough, often enough, and exercise." (Usually, everyone agrees that the diet-thinking word "willpower" has a place only in an environment of trying to "stick to" something miserable—which fueling isn't.) In this particular class, this woman raised her hand and said, "Well, I think eating enough, often enough would take more willpower." When I asked her why, she said, somewhat indignantly, "Because it's too expensive! If I eat more, it will cost more."

The woman's reaction perfectly illustrated diet thinking to the group: She was making a statement that wasn't necessarily true, but treating it as if it was truth; and she was speaking generally with no frame of reference (eat more than what? cost more than what?), which is a good way to stay confused and powerless.

Even if it was more expensive—and I emphasized that it definitely didn't have to be—then wasn't her body worth it? If Popsters® cost more than Ruffles®, was it worth spending a few more cents to get 70 fewer grams of fat per bag?

Most of all, the willingness to see this in a new way has to be there. If you have an investment in how hard life is, you'll make everything hard. You are responsible for how you see things. If you can find problems with eating lots of food often, you could probably also come up with difficulties about winning $10 million in the lottery. "I have to go all the way to Anytown to pick up the money, and then I have to go to the bank." "Can you believe all the taxes they're taking?" "I suppose Aunt Martha will expect me to pay for her daughter's wedding now."

"IT'S PART OF ME"

In one-on-one training, I gain even deeper insight into what keeps people from taking on something wonderfully simple that could end the agony they've dragged along for so many years—the diets, the losses and gains, the erratic health, the emotional distress. More than one client has grappled with the question "Who would I be if I didn't have this as an issue?"

Sound odd? Think about it—parting with something you've always worried about, worked on, tussled with. It's part of you; it seems to identify you as who you are. Sometimes, it's hard to give up a part of you, even if it's something you hate.

Clients have also confessed that their resistance to simply beginning to fuel their bodies is a fear of looking sensational, fear of being vulnerable, and a way of thumbing a nose at a parent or spouse.

When you get down to it, fueling is easy. It's not about depriving or restricting. I am not ordering you to reduce eating, cut out meals or snacks, exercise four hours every day, or eat sprouts and tofu. I'm asking you to try three hearty, high-carbohydrate meals a day, and at least three snacks of bread, bagels, fruit, rolls, juice, cereal, or fat-free/sugar-free cookies, crackers, cake, or bars. If that presents more of a problem than "sticking to" a carrot and celery stick "regimen," maybe something else is going on.

IF YOU SAY YOU WANT TO AND YOU'RE NOT: LOOK AGAIN

Sometimes brilliant and successful people will balk at fueling even when they confess they always dreamed it would turn out that eating and enjoying food is the correct thing to do. People who have started companies, lectured to thousands of people, raised millions of dollars, or competed in world-class athletics become helpless when they need to manage getting a snack into their bodies at three in the afternoon.

When we compare their roster of herculean accomplishments to the minuscule task of conquering a daily snack, people can see for themselves that something else is going on. It's clear the logistics of eating a banana mid-afternoon are not insurmountable for a person of their stature. Then we get down to what is stopping them from closing the book on this issue. Over and over, we hit rock bottom at a basic attachment to "it has to be tough." If this is all it's going to take to get where they always wanted to be, then they're going to find a way to screw it up.

Your reaction to all this may be, "Not me. If I could have it all work, I would." Okay. Maybe so. But if you're planning to take this whole thing on, committed to having a life of happily fueling your precious body, looking and feeling awesome, and having nothing to do with dieting, "weight-watching," calorie counting, overaerobicizing, or being hungry, don't be too surprised if some kind of resistance crops up.

ACKNOWLEDGE YOURSELF

You've probably noticed that criticism is an easy habit. Natural, easy recognition of our accomplishments and excellence is more rare. Who hasn't responded to a compliment with a sheepish "Oh, this old thing?" We look in the mirror and notice what we're not—and in the body department, this is epidemic. So it is with fueling as well.

"Oh, I'm doing . . . okay," is the ludicrously familiar sigh I hear virtually every time we follow up with a client a few weeks after a workshop. After asking a few key questions, the person invariably reveals that they have eliminated enormous amounts of fat and/or sugar; that they are eating more frequently and noticing much more energy; that cooking has been much simpler, and the family likes it, that they have begun walking every other day and actually enjoy it—or, at least, don't mind it. Or any number of other things that make me want to laugh or cry when I think of their initial "I *guess* I'm doing *pretty* good."

I'm not talking about silly little things for which I pat them on the back just to make them feel nice. People make amazing changes in their eating, shopping, and cooking—in a rapid and painless way that would make any nutritionist's eyes bug out. But all they can see, hear, or talk about is what they haven't done.

It makes me sad. One of my favorite parts of my work is simply praising people for the great strides they have made, repeating back to them what they have told me, until they can hear that they have just reported a near-miracle. Mature and professional adults become little kids: "Really? I'm really doing well? That's really good?"

Some people simply refuse the acknowledgment, so determined are they to maintain victimhood. Mary-Jane, a mother and midwife whose family actually sounded to me like a paragon of healthy eating, insisted that they were still "bad" because they frequently ate "health-food treats"—fruit-juice sweetened, low-fat cookies and frozen desserts. "Well," I said, "if you are, then we are too—we eat those things all the time. Why are you so convinced that you cannot enjoy anything—even modified treats—and still be doing a good job?"

Every change you make is a big deal. For each, there are thousands of Americans being urged to do the same thing—and not doing it. So, as you begin to try fueling on for size, include acknowledgments for what you are doing. Replace "I blew it; I buttered my toast this morning" with "I had all-fruit jam every day for two weeks." Note that "I've eaten at least two

snacks every day this week" instead of "I keep missing my evening snack."
Pat yourself on the back for exercising more this month than you have in
years—instead of chastising yourself for missing yesterday's walk.

THINGS THAT ARE GOOD FOR YOU SHOULDN'T HURT

Be suspicious of your wariness of comfort. If fueling feels good, and you've
begun enjoying food, notice if your first thought is that you must be being
"bad."

It's a good idea to replace that worn-out "no pain, no gain" edict. It
doesn't make sense that things that are good for you will cause ongoing
suffering, denial, or deprivation. Satisfaction is a good sign, not a warning
bell; hysterical hunger is a signal to eat, not a triumph to relish. Feeling
good is good, feeling bad is bad.

Such common sense can hail a return to more sane living that carries over
to other areas as well. Why not?

14

GETTING YOUR PRIORITIES STRAIGHT: Channeling Your Concerns Constructively

FIRST THINGS FIRST

A young mother straps her baby securely in a child safety seat—the baby is clutching a big, greasy doughnut in his fist.

A man urges his friend not to drive home after having a few drinks—but scarcely notices the friend's all-night consumption of beer nuts and pigs-in-a-blanket.

A couple joins an activist group to stop the use of certain pesticides on apples—but regularly treats the kids to Chocolate Zingies, Fruit Tweezils, and Double Decadent Frozen Explosions for doing their homework.

A family goes to extraordinary lengths to move away from power lines they fear will cause illness—while still eating every other day at Burger Bob's.

My local health-food store will not carry any food with artificial anything, but they will carry foods that are "naturally" 80 to 100 percent fat.

A magazine article asks, "Is your diet your energy problem?" and proceeds to cover in-depth the perils of . . . iron deficiency.

"Your choice of diet can influence your long-term health prospects more than any other action you might take," former Surgeon General C. Everett Koop told us during his term. Yet I've encountered an almost reflexive insistence in our culture upon downplaying or dismissing your power to drastically reduce risks shown by scientific research to be the greatest and most preventable—and to devote inordinate amounts of time and energy to fearing and protesting superficial or microscopic concerns. Diet thinking, which is a breeding ground for mindlessness and illogical thinking, makes rational comparisons between risks difficult.

Yet if you cannot distinguish what's important, you cannot make informed choices. Therefore it's important to be fully informed about major risks, to put them in perspective, and base your choices on logical priorities. Just as understanding your body eliminates the worry, confusion, and fear about "eating right," so does understanding the relative relationship of risks to one another eliminate needless, wasteful worry about imagined threats. It also eliminates unwitting dismissal of very real threats.

UNJUSTIFIABLE COMPLACENCY

It's common to hear someone launch into a sanctimonious account of how "healthy" they eat. "Oh, yes," he or she will say, "I've cut out caffeine completely, and I never eat high-sodium foods. Everything I buy is organic and all-natural—no additives, pesticides, or preservatives. I eat lots of vegetables, drink carrot and wheatgrass juice every day—juiced myself, of course. And I always make sure to supplement with [list of vitamins, minerals, and herbs]."

The person described above is not doing anything bad. In fact, this person has taken many excellent steps toward improving health and having a nice clean machine. My only contention is what may have gotten displaced or neglected in the wake of such virtues. Often, further conversation will reveal that this person, dazzled by her own pristine lifestyle, has no clue that the fact that she only eats one meal a day—or often "doesn't have time" for breakfast, or eats lots of "natural" (and high-fat) "health" foods like sesame butter, tofu, granola, and avocado—is creating problems that in the short and long term will have far more impact on her health than preservatives or mineral deficiencies would.

This focus on secondary issues poses several problems. First, you get a false sense of security that you're eating or living healthily, when in fact you've only handled peripheral issues that don't necessarily make a dramatic difference in energy, appearance, or longevity. Second, you get frustrated when you don't see results from making these peripheral changes, because you were under the impression such changes *should* make a difference. Third, you spend a lot of time worrying about issues that are trivial—compared to some basic ones that you could handle easily and pleasurably, and that would yield tangible benefits.

VITAMINS, MINERALS, AND OTHER MICROCONCERNS

The most exciting research these days is being done on a particular group of vitamins . . .
—"Anti-Aging Diet: Eat Less, Live Longer,"
Self, September 1992

While vitamins and minerals are important, your body can't run on them. A vitamin pill without a meal is like gas additive without gasoline. A car absolutely needs water and oil, but can't run on those; it must have gasoline. Fuel is a bottom-line priority.

People tend to concern themselves with the micro while the macro suffers. And macro and micro are apt descriptions, because the nutrients on which I focus in this book are referred to in nutritional science as *macronutrients*— carbohydrate, protein, and fat. All can be used as fuel. Vitamins and minerals are called *micronutrients*.

This doesn't mean vitamins and minerals aren't important! We need vitamins and minerals to be healthy. But we need fuel just to stay alive, just to survive each moment. Your body is not fueled by vitamins and minerals.

Nor can vitamins correct the effects of poor fueling. No pill will make up for the greater damage being done if you frequently go for long periods of time without eating, eat a diet very high in fat, or eat very little food overall. The body is not a neat system of checks and balances in which one virtue can negate another poison. "To ignore diet and just use supplements is like putting on a seat belt and driving like a maniac," acknowledges vitamin researcher Paul Jacques of Tufts University ("1992 Health Guide," *U.S. News & World Report*, May 4, 1992).

In fact, vitamins and minerals are not only powerless to absolve inadequate fueling (or any body abuse); they cannot do their own "real jobs" effectively if the foundation isn't laid with the right fuel. Before you can see results from (or even use) a gas additive, you have to have gas in the car!

But when the body machine starts sputtering, too often you don't even look at the gas gauge. You fling the hood open and start fiddling with the thermocalibrated-electronic blahblah. Maybe it's that, and maybe it isn't. But without gas in the tank, how will you ever know? No gas, no go. It doesn't matter what else you do.

Taking vitamin and mineral supplements, lowering sodium intake, taking herbs, cutting caffeine, eliminating artificial sweeteners, or avoiding additives, preservatives, and pesticides—are all valuable personal choices. If you're well fueled most of the time, those steps will fine-tune what you're doing.

Whether it provides fuel for the body to run is certainly not the only standard by which food ought to be judged. But it is a standard, and it is a bottom-line one. You can do a lot of other neat stuff to your car, but if you don't fuel it, in the end it won't matter.

An important part of moving beyond diet thinking includes moving your focus away from the borderline issues that get blown out of proportion, and addressing instead what will have the most impact. Statistically speaking, some dietary issues demand more of your attention than others. So first things first: Get the proper fuel in your tank. Concern yourself with the wheels and the paint afterward.

FOR STARTERS: HEALTHY EATING MEANS *EATING*

There are things it's healthier not to eat (or at least not eat very much of), but that's only part of the picture. Too much is made of the "less" part, and little attention is given the many "mores" (like eating more carbohydrates, more often) that people would be relieved and thrilled to know about.

Somehow, America conceptualized "healthy eating" and put it in a tiny little box with sprouts spilling over the top and soy milk leaking out the bottom, which turned off most of the population to even thinking about what healthy eating might be, and relegated the rest to a sort of private club.

The number-one thing about eating that's healthy is *eating*! You need to eat in order to be eating healthy. You'd be amazed how many people overlook that fact, which you'd think would be more obvious than who's buried in Grant's Tomb. Eating one meal a day, even if it's the most natural and organic stuff in the world, is not efficient fueling.

Eliminating "bad" substances doesn't constitute healthy eating. Caffeine and sodium are favorites in terms of substances that make people feel "safer" when they cut them out—even though there is no evidence to support that.

Sometimes when I'm sipping a cup of coffee before a workshop begins, a participant will come up to me and say, "You're drinking coffee," as if expecting me to fall to my knees and beg for absolution. "Yes, I am," I agree calmly. Caffeine is not a fuel issue; moreover, it has been studied extensively over the past decade and in moderate doses (one or two cups a day) has not been shown to cause serious health problems. No association has been established between caffeine consumption and heart attacks, cancer, or birth defects. It can aggravate the painful symptoms of fibrocystic breast disease, but it does not cause it.

People overreact to sodium as well. "You didn't talk about salt," someone occasionally accuses at the end of a workshop. "That's right," I say, "because salt is not a fuel; no studies have ever proven that salt causes hypertension (high blood pressure), while fat has been strongly linked to that condition. And, if you're fueling as we've just discussed, you're likely to eat more fresh foods and more progressive brands when you do choose packaged foods, which naturally means less sodium."

WHAT KILLS (AND DOESN'T): GROUNDLESS OUTRAGE

Americans obsess endlessly about both real and perceived health-related issues: pesticides, power lines, air pollution, drunk drivers, water quality, fluoride, shark attack, hair spray, electromagnetism, nuclear power, asbestos, dyes, hazardous waste disposal—the list goes on and on.

Yet statistically none of those even come close to posing the risk that our diet does. The fact is that more than two-thirds of all American deaths result from only three conditions: heart disease, cancer, and stroke. All three, according to the U.S. Department of Health, the Surgeon General, and innumerable research studies, are preventable—and all are fat-related.

Diet, therefore, has been identified as a key source of the problem—and a key solution. American health and health care would have a different landscape if every person in the nation "fueled." Yet the average person doesn't apply this perspective to the health scares they worry about. They continue to eat their way to a statistically predictable death—as they agonize about the dye in the paper that wrapped their chicken-fried steak sandwich.

WHY IS FAT EXEMPT?

Cigarettes, alcohol, and fat are all linked by scientific, medical, and government authorities to the diseases ranking among the top 10 killers in the U.S. The research evidence against fat is no less voluminous or clear than that against the other two.

Yet abuse of food—specifically, continually eating foods linked by studies to those top killers—is still a minor concern compared to abuse of cigarettes, drugs, or alcohol. "Dietary indiscretions" have acquired a certain acceptability that has been revoked for the other three. It's passé today to hang out in bars and drink all night, and certainly to drive home afterward. Friends and bartenders alike consider themselves practically second-degree murderers if they allow a buddy or patron to leave soused—and in fact can be legally charged under certain circumstances.

Yet people don't feel remorse about serving, or allowing others to consume, high quantities of fat. Somehow, the public relations campaigns have not successfully connected the burger, butter, or dieting to overfat; or the overfat to the heart attacks and cancer—not with the authority of campaigns that have brought home the connection between the cigarette and lung cancer or the drink to smashed windshields. But there must be a way to bring immediacy and urgency to the result of destructive eating. Just because accidents can kill instantly while diet-related diseases may take a few decades doesn't make the latter any less inevitable.

RISK-REDUCTION RETROGRADE:
DATA IN DISARRAY

In response to a reader survey on modern health concerns, a cover article in *US Week* (*USA Today*'s Sunday supplement, with 33.5 million readers), focused on electromagnetic fields and, to a lesser degree, indoor pollution, pesticides, and AIDS, playing neatly into the utterly backward level of concern over health risks.

The cover alone was a monument to disproportionate outrage. Next to the huge headline, "Is My Electric Blanket Killing Me?" sit a mom and her child. Mom is clearly overfat, perhaps obese. Based on statistics, if anything is killing her it's her visible 40-some percent bodyfat level, and the food (or lack thereof) that sustains it. And how often does that child eat at fast-food restaurants and consume fatty, sugary "treats"?

But the article doesn't even ask. It ignores statistically significant risk factors. This not only reflects the misappropriation of public concern, but does the public a huge disservice by supporting minutiae-mania. As another example, the article quoted a 34-year-old nurse who has breast cancer: she said her only possible risk factors could have been smoking, early pregnancies, and a family history of cancer. She doesn't know if any other risk factors have been identified, and the article doesn't tell her that thousands of studies—population studies, cohort studies (of women over time), animal studies, randomized research—suggest that a high-fat diet is a risk factor for developing breast cancer (not to mention heart disease, which kills many more women each year than all cancers combined—a fact the article also fails to mention).

The piece did find room to report that one study disputes a fatty diet as being a cause of breast cancer. To dispute is not to disprove—especially in the case of one study up against such an enormous (and still mounting) body of literature suggesting a link. Even more importantly, the article didn't detail that this Harvard study of 89,494 nurses depended on the subjects' own assessments of their dietary fat level—a subject's opinion, for example, that she consumed a 32 percent fat diet. As I've demonstrated (and as have many others I have quoted), people do not evaluate their own diets effectively. Based on my experience with people who complain "I'm eating a no-fat diet and not getting results" but who turn out to be eating mounds of hidden fat, that study has zero credibility.

Other studies suggest that the specific fat levels studied in this one—25 percent and 32 percent, as opposed to 44 percent of calories—are insufficiently low to prevent breast cancer, identifying 20 percent of calories or less as the probable target for prevention.

In fact, the study's own author, Walter Willet, has carefully qualified the results by urging us not to intepret this as free license for fat consumption, that by all means a low-fat diet is still advisable. But this statement of his always appears at the end of reports on his study; most people don't read that far. The headline is never "A low-fat diet is still important, says study author, despite questions"—instead, it's always: "Is fat in the diet irrelevant to breast cancer?"

Environmental conditions do represent a risk factor for developing cancer—it's just a very tiny one, relatively. Such factors pale compared to the risks associated with eating the typical American diet and smoking cigarettes. R. Doll and R. Peto's "Proportions of Cancer Deaths Attributed to Various Factors" (*Journal of the National Cancer Institute*, vol. 66, no. 1193, 1981) attributes 30 percent of total cancer deaths to tobacco and 35 percent to diet. E. L. Wynder and G. B. Gori's "Contribution of the Environment to Cancer Incidence as Epidemiologic Exercise" (*Journal of the National Cancer Institute*, vol. 58, no. 825, 1977) estimate is even more aggressive, attributing to diet 40 percent of male and 60 percent of female cancer deaths.

That makes diet the single most threatening health risk—even more than smoking, which the public pretty universally acknowledges as a cancer risk.

Since people use the news media as their source of information and education, stories showing the total risk picture with the statistical rankings of each factor would give people the perspective they desperately need. It may be less titillating, it may sell fewer newspapers, but it is the responsible way to go. Articles on electric blankets and shavers divert attention from true risk factors—even sanction their dismissal—when there is no evidence that America's most pervasive, painful, and costly health problems can be solved by rerouting power lines or banning hair dryers.

Robert J. Scheuplein (Acting Director of the Office of Toxicological Sciences, Center for Food Safety and Applied Nutrition, Food and Drug Administration, Washington, D.C.) has written a pivotal report on risks and public perception. He succinctly defines the American phenomenon of misdirected priorities and emphatically articulates its dangers. He calls it "the outrage factor," as first defined by P. M. Sandman, a term that refers to the level of public outrage generated by statistically insignificant risks.

Notes Scheuplein, "Sandman . . . argues that peoples' concerns are often more a function of outrage than hazard. When risks are perceived to be voluntary, controllable by the individual, familiar . . . they tend to be minimized by the public. The experts conclude that people consistently underestimate the hazards of risk that are low-outrage and overestimate the hazards of risk that are high-outrage."

Scheuplein calls diet "a perfect illustration" of a low-outrage, high-risk factor. "While widely acknowledged in scientific literature and in several government reports, the risks from an improper diet, both from known and uncertain causes, have scarcely caused a ripple in the media or in the public consciousness."

Scheuplein—regarded as highly conservative by the scientific community—conducted a very detailed and technical analysis of more than 60 studies of food-related carcinogens and concluded that "the large attribution of the total cancer burden to two causes, cigarettes and diet, is widely accepted by experts as correct. . . . Carcinogens overwhelmingly originated from food itself and not from additives, pesticides or contaminants. . . . Even a modestly effective attempt to lessen the dietary risk of natural carcinogens would probably be enormously more useful to human health than regulatory efforts devoted to eliminating traces of pesticide residues or contaminants."

And what are those "natural carcinogens" (cancer-causing agents)? Scheuplein cites a recent Surgeon General's report on Nutrition and Health which concluded that a chief risk factor is the "disproportionate consumption of foods high in fats, often at the expense of foods high in complex carbohydrates and fiber."

AND THERE'S MORE . . .

There are literally hundreds of mixed-up outrage cases being "tried" every day by the media.

I remember seeing a cartoon, I think by Gary Larson, with two obese people sitting at a table, drinking alcohol, eating something big and greasy, and smoking cigarettes. The caption said something like, "Aren't you glad we don't eat apples with that Alar on them, Fred?"

Mark, a client who works as a water quality analyst for a major city near ours, relates this favorite story of his supervisor's telltale encounter with the outrage factor: "Dave" finally visited the home of a woman who had called the water department repeatedly over a several-week period, complaining that her doctor believed her "health problems" might be caused by poor water quality. When he knocked on the front door, it was opened by the woman herself—obese, holding a cigarette in one hand and a cocktail in the other. She led him to a sink piled high with dishes in dirty dish water.

At a drivers' safety course given by my auto insurance company several summers ago, the instructor asserted that the most dangerous thing Americans do is drive their cars. While accidents do take many lives, and even one is too many, it's clear that the most dangerous thing Americans do—if you look at the top causes of death in this country—is reckless eating. While 1 million die every year of cardiovascular disease alone, less than 40,000 die every year in automobile accidents (about 20,000 of those are drinking-related). Statistically speaking, you're safer on the freeway than you are at your kitchen table.

We live in a toxic world. We will be exposed to things. I'm not saying that's great, or that it isn't wise to avoid as many risky things as possible. But number one, fuel yourself (and your kids). You can slash your odds against falling prey to the most common and preventable risks, and make your body as tough and strong as possible to deal with all the rest. Don't fray your body by depriving it of what it needs, and then hope the sharp corners of the world don't pierce your thinning shields.

WHY DON'T I FEEL GOOD? LOOK AT YOUR PLATE

When you don't feel well, you may think it's your workplace atmosphere, artificial sweetener, or air pollution. Do you ever wonder if it's the fact that you didn't eat breakfast, had a candy bar for lunch, and a meatball sub at 10 P.M.? That you worked out at the gym for two hours after eating nothing but popcorn all day? That you had fettucine alfredo with a couple glasses of wine at lunch?

You think people don't do this stuff? I promise you, they do.

The nice thing about handling the basics first—fueling and seeing if that handles your low energy or stomachaches or headaches or whatever—is that you're not trying to find a needle in a haystack. You can rule out "no/little/poor fuel" as a problem and go from there. If fueling doesn't handle it, you'll know something else is up.

Also, handling the basics naturally leads you to the secondary concerns. When you put the basic fueling of your body into balance, you become aware of other sensations. You can feel how other things affect you. Robert didn't realize how lifeless diet soda made him feel until he began fueling. When you're in a constant state of low-grade breakdown, it's hard to identify what's going on. The general well-being you get from fueling provides a basis for comparison. You really know what it's like to feel great—so it's very obvious when you've done something to disrupt that well-being.

MAGIC PILL MANIA

Eating a carrot a day may significantly lower your risk of stroke and heart disease, according to a study by researchers at the Brigham and Women's Hospital at Harvard Medical School in Boston, Massachusetts.

—"Health News," *Mademoiselle*, October 1992

A corollary to the outrage factor is what I call magic pill mania. When Americans do set their sights on diet, the tendency seems to be to seek shortcuts—those things that will compensate for lack of responsibility and destructive behavior—rather than direct action. It's a tunnel vision approach that amounts to putting out fires that *you* started. And it's exhausting, because instead of simply removing the inflammatory material, you have to chase your body with a fire extinguisher forever.

"Even the most educated health-conscious consumer is likely to harbor a fantasy that somewhere, somehow—in the next television commercial or on the diet shelf at the supermarket—a panacea awaits," observed the *U.S. News & World Report* cover story on May 14, 1990, entitled "Getting Slim."

The recent attention on chromium as a mineral that helps make fat metabolism and muscle synthesis more efficient is a great example. While there is good evidence for chromium's promise, the people looking for magic pills don't see it as a possible complementary supplement to a proactively healthy way of living. It's "the new pill to take to speed up your metabolism to lose weight" while continuing to eat recklessly. And, of course, those marketing the stuff don't hesitate to take advantage of that mind-set.

You can see it in the media's definitions of "breakthrough"—products that allow us to keep abusing and not change anything. The constant search for high-tech "cures" keeps us from seeing the marvelously simple prevention right in front of us. The answer couldn't be right there in the basic biology we've understood for years—that would be too banal, too unscientific.

I saw this wacky item in *Self* in September 1991: "First oat bran, now celery? Rats who were given celery, in an amount equivalent to humans eating two large stalks a day, dramatically lowered their blood pressure and cholesterol levels. But don't stock up just yet, cautions William J. Elliott, M.D., Ph.D., at the University of Chicago School of Medicine: 'Celery contains salt. Eating too much of it can raise blood pressure. Our hope is to extract the beneficial chemical and administer it in a pill.' "

Perfect—take nature and engineer it one better to create a drug that will allow people to keep the lifestyle that causes high cholesterol and blood pressure, rather than find workable substitutes for saturated fat. Take a celery pill and keep downing that grease.

This type of one-directional research that seeks The Answer just creates a never-ending succession of Answers that serves only to further confuse. A October 1992 *Consumer Reports* article stated this well: "If Americans are uncertain about how to choose a nutritious diet, it may be partly due to the crosswinds of scientific debate. . . . A third of adults are confused by the reports which give dietary advice, according to an American Dietetic Association survey. It's little wonder. In the past year, we've been advised to: use oils sparingly, but load up on olive oil. Avoid being overweight, yet avoid 'yo-yo' dieting. Drink red wine because the French have fewer heart attacks, but refrain from alcohol because the French have more liver disease."

What it costs to keep researchers working to isolate solutions that allow Americans to continue abdicating responsibility for their lifestyle and health is a whole other story.

While they search for the holy grail of microsolutions—a pill, an exercise, a machine or contraption that will ensure protection against bodyfat and disease, no matter what you eat—there are simple things you can do to greatly improve your odds against having to deal with cardiovascular disease and many cancers. Diet provides the power to steer your own destiny in matters of disease. If you stop trying to do it with aspirin, red wine, fish oil, and oat bran, you could invest that energy and time in forging a path you'll be glad to walk for the rest of your life.

MAGIC FROM ABROAD: THE FRENCH STUDY

The incredible amount of hoopla generated by reports comparing the French diet to ours, pinpointing a supposed inconsistency in our incidence of disease compared to theirs, is a prime piece of evidence for magic pill madness.

"60 Minutes" stated that the French eat 30 percent more fat than Americans do, raising the question: "Why is the rate of death by heart disease 40 percent lower in France if they eat so much more fat?" Everyone was abuzz about the well-known high-fat French fare: "They eat so much cheese! And fatty birds!" You could just imagine researchers setting their hounds loose to isolate the key element, the magic Thing that made the French able to ingest unlimited amounts of fat, supposedly without ramifications.

For a while, we couldn't have a workshop without at least one person asking: "How come the French can gorge on fat and be so healthy, while we can't?" Some people were indignant that we weren't offering them the Magic Answer from France about how they could fry their food and live to tell about it.

But the *Berkeley Wellness Newsletter* set the facts straight in April 1992. The statement that the French eat 30 percent more fat than we do was false. They eat a 39 percent fat diet—exactly what the average American diet is made of. Heart disease rates there are lower, but it's stretching the truth quite a bit to say they have no ramifications: *Heart disease is the number one killer in France as well.* Furthermore, a closer look shows that the French have been consuming this high-fat diet only since the mid-1980s (such a diet is associated with prosperity). Americans have been consuming the same high-fat diet since 1923! The newsletter asserts that the high-fat diet will catch up with the French. We're just 60 years ahead of them.

Still, in the glow of hope for a Magic Answer, industries leapt in eagerly to peddle their angles. French cheese merchants claimed that the calcium in the cheese flushes out saturated fat from the body. (Wrong!) Wine merchants clamored that the phenomenon was due to the red wine that the French drink. (The *Berkeley Wellness Newsletter* noted that while moderate consumption of any alcohol, not just red wine, has been shown to lower risk of heart disease, in quantities greater than an ounce a day it leads to cirrhosis of the liver.)

For every new Magic Answer (and there are many others like the French example), there are always similarly solid, sensible explanations. The facts always end up pointing back to personal responsibility for self-care—largely diet-related—which the Magic Answer was attempting to avoid. By harping on the fad rather than the facts, the media keeps people hanging in hope, not bothering to create a basic lifestyle that works because one day there will be an answer. Space that could be devoted to educating people about body basics and how that translates into action is used up by the latest flash on what's hot in biotechnical gadgetry.

HORMONES

In March 1992, newspapers across the country featured coverage of new scientific breakthroughs on aging. The lead paragraphs of these stories all centered on discoveries related to hormones that may slow many characteristics of aging and may increase longevity. There is no long-term research yet on side effects of these hormones.

A *Seattle Times* article did cover health and fitness, identifying nutrition and exercise as the most important elements in making aging a much nicer prospect. If you fuel your body and exercise, you'll have a great head start. Then, if the time comes when you want to take hormone supplements, you'll be enhancing an already solid foundation, not trying to bolster a sagging, worn structure. Putting a "magic pill" into a poorly cared for, poorly conditioned body is no different than putting superb oil, anti-freeze, and wiper fluid in a beat-up car with no (or poor-quality) gasoline.

STUDY-ITIS

Unfortunately, the tendency of research and its media coverage is to promote what I call "study-itis"—a reluctance to commit to any conclusive recommendation until there is "enough" research evidence to support it (and "enough" is rarely, if ever, defined). Researching what's already documented is another symptom of this condition.

The cover story "Pumping Immunity" in the April 1993 issue of *Nutrition Action Newsletter* is an interview with five health authorities—professors, scientists, physicians—who discuss how immunity can be preserved and boosted using various dosages of different vitamins and minerals.

The piece begins with an anecdote from Jeffrey Blumberg, associate director of the USDA's Human Nutrition Research Center on Aging at Tufts University. He notes that "It was only about 30 years ago that people even discovered that nutrition affected immune response." The evidence he cited was "in studies of starving kids. When these children were given food, their immune systems improved." (Am I the only one to think it's crazy that any study was needed to tell us this?)

Later in the article, an immunology professor shares the story of a surgeon in England who prescribed for his cancer patients a special fat developed to feed malnourished patients intravenously. He thought it would help them "regain weight and muscle." Instead, this fat helped the patients' cancers spread, which supports recent findings that a low-fat diet may not only prevent cancers, but help cure them. Yet when asked, "Could the amount of fat in the typical American diet cause damage?" the professor responded, "Right now we don't have the answer."

Even *Nutrition Action Newsletter* itself—a publication which I recommend and almost always find extremely informative and incisive—has demonstrated study-itis: "We'd like to think that whole grains make people more energetic than refined grains or sugary cereals, but there are no good studies that prove it, as far as we know" (April 1993). Why in heaven's name would we need a study to prove that? Not only does ordinary biology illustrate that whole grains are processed differently than refined, but just about every BodyFueling workshop participant has acknowledged that whole grains sustain their energy much better than refined. Biology suggests it and human experience supports it. Needing a study to "prove" this makes no more sense than needing a study to prove that gasoline makes a Toyota perform better than cyanide does.

THE HEREDITY CRUTCH

The most important heredity is the environment you create.

My father's father died of stomach cancer, and all of his father's nine brothers and sisters died of some form of intestinal cancer. My mother's family was plagued by heart disease—cardiac arrests and high blood pressure down the line.

But am I scared of my "heredity" factor, the genetic threat that I will die of a heart attack or colon cancer? No—because I eat a 10 to 15 percent fat diet, I'm lean, and I'm cardiovascularly fit. Those who died on either side of my family were all overfat, all ate a diet rich in beef, eggs, whole-milk cheeses, and fried foods, and all were sedentary. I didn't inherit the thing that killed those family members: their lifestyle, values, and cooking habits.

Money that's now spent trying to document beyond a hair of a doubt whether people are fat because of their "bad genes" could be better spent on education. Heredity may be somewhat a factor in obesity as well as high blood cholesterol. Some people may be more predisposed than others to make, store, and save fat. But to emphasize the possibility of such a predisposition is too often to relieve people of responsibility. Even if such a predisposition exists, it will be made significant by poor fueling, which trains the body to become adept at what it is supposedly predisposed to do.

The fact is that what you have now learned to call "fueling" is an overfat or obese person's best bet for health and fitness. But that doesn't make them "different," because the same way of eating is also ideal for a fit person. And it's also ideal for a diabetic, and an athlete, and a person treating heart disease, or reversing it, or preventing it—or preventing any number of diseases.

It works for all people because it's based on how the human body is designed to use food as fuel. A slowed, clogged, overfat body resulting from direct denial of this design should not be considered a mystery requiring endless study! If the care and treatment of a machine doesn't take into account its basic needs and design, the machine will probably break down.

It all gets back to working the best you can with whatever you have. Obese people *may* be more likely to gain fat, but as I said earlier, I still have never worked with an obese person who was fueling his or her body appropriately. Never. I would like to see studies in which children of families determined to be "genetically" obese are from birth fed plentifully in ratio of 65 percent carb, 20 percent protein, and 15 percent fat. I have a very, very hard time believing they would become obese. They might not tend toward the exceptionally lean—but who knows?

The Carbohydrate Addict's Diet says, "Overweight runs in families." When I am at a buffet and I see an overfat mother, father, and children all piling danish and sausage on their plates, am I to believe the child is obese because he got Mom and Dad's genes? Even if he does have a genetic switch that the fates have thrown in favor of fat, does that mean he should throw all sensibility to the wind and stuff himself with fat and sugar?

It's the same with cholesterol. A small number people seem to have a difficult time managing it by diet alone, and only with the help of drugs does their blood cholesterol level seem to stabilize. But too many times I see people taking drugs to lower cholesterol—and eating fettucine alfredo for dinner. What's the point?

"IT'S OUT OF MY HANDS . . . ISN'T IT?"

You're not at the mercy of age and disease. Statistics and odds confirm it and my own observations have utterly convinced me. Just getting one's eating in order drastically tips the odds in one's favor.

Yet listen to people talk about heart disease and cancer—people who have it, who know others who have it, or who are commenting in general. The tone is matter-of-fact resignation. I hear: "Oh, well, you know, he was old," or "Well, these things happen—it's a real shame."

In *Recalled by Life*, Dr. Anthony Sattilaro's story about how he became cancer-free through diet, he said, "I had suffered from intestinal disorders for twenty years. . . . My intestines were obviously having trouble digesting the food I was eating. Rather than change the food, I took medication to suppress the symptoms . . . I never addressed the underlying causes. Ultimately, those causes brought on my own cancer. Because I did not understand this, I viewed my lot as capricious and my cancer as outside of me. I had nothing to do with it—other than the fact that it had struck me down. It was all bad luck."

HIGH HOPES FOR STAYING HEALTHY, LOW STANDARDS FOR HEALTH

Doubts about our power to stay healthy are often aided by dismally low standards of what "being healthy" really means. I think to many people, "health" means "not in intensive care right now." The father of a past co-worker of Robert's chain-smoked and lived on fried fast food. The guy could barely walk, Robert says, but when he died, the co-worker's wife commented, "It was so sudden—he was so healthy." Robert nearly fell over. He said it seemed like what she meant was, "He didn't have a cold."

Often in our workshops, after all the educating has been done, someone will pipe up, "But my Uncle Fred (or whoever) ate grease (smoked, drank, etc.) all his life and he's 95 now and still going." My answer is always the same. One, Uncle Fred may be breathing and have a pulse, but is he truly alive? Is Uncle Fred active, feeling and looking good, and enjoying life? In other words, we are talking about fueling not just to make it to a certain age, gasping and wheezing or on a stretcher—but to really live. Not just a long life, but a quality life. Two, if after all that abuse Uncle Fred is indeed doing what he loves to do—hiking, working, boating, or whatever—then he is the very rare exception. No matter how common people think it is to abuse yourself and "get away with it," the statistics show that it's not common. Currently, two out of every three people you know will die of cardiovascular disease or cancer. These illnesses are conclusively preventable, largely through diet. Period.

If you want to bank on having the luck of Uncle Fred, go right ahead; this is all about choice. But know that, even if Uncle Fred is living a life you'd want to live, your chances of doing the same while abdicating all responsibility and conscious thought about what goes into your body are not good. Chances are Uncle Fred is probably semicomatose by the TV most of the time.

These diseases don't "just happen." Contrary to popular belief, we are *not* passive victims of these diseases due to old age or heredity (except when we "inherit" poor lifestyles and habits). We are *not* helpless against strokes, heart attacks, and the most common and deadly cancers.

A NOTE ON THE FAT/CANCER LINK

Contributing to this sense that there's not much you can do is the fact that many scientists are still reluctant to come forward and declare that a fat body and/or diet are definite risks. While the link to heart disease is now widely considered indisputable, the link to cancer is not. Some say it is unquestionable; others will only say "studies suggest a link" and "more research is needed." Some say statistical correlations are not enough, because they don't prove cause and effect. (In that case, smoking doesn't cause lung cancer, either.)

HOW DOES FAT CAUSE CANCER?

This is not certain yet. Several theories about fat and cancer are presented by various publications, books, and reports. Fat may promote cancer by influencing the metabolic processes of normal cells, leaving them vulnerable to the development of malignancy brought on by other agents. Carcinogens which might not be effective otherwise are thus able to create abnormalities. Most recently, some research suggests that fat may act as a solvent that actually enhances the effects of certain carcinogens.

Fats can also upset the balance of our hormones, which has been linked to certain cancers, most notably breast cancer. Fat in the diet as well as an overfat or obese body seems to increase estrogen production, and increased estrogen levels have an established role in breast cancer (estrogen seems to feed tumor cells). One study showed that in women who switch to a diet where fat is 20 percent of calories, estrogen levels quickly drop by 10 percent. Besides, fatty acids also affect production of the hormone prolactin, which governs breast growth and milk production and influences the circulation of estrogens as well. Abnormally high levels of prolactin have been found in woman with breast tumors. Additionally, as far back as the 1940s, scientists were finding that mice fed a high-fat diet suffered more mammary tumors than mice on a low-fat diet. And overfat animals consistently develop more tumors than lean ones.

Finally, since a high-fiber diet has been linked by studies to lower incidence of cancers, especially intestinal ones, the fact that eliminated fatty foods are likely to be replaced by high-fiber complex carbohydrates may be a source of protection and prevention. (In fact, the assortment of literature I've reviewed, both lay and scientific, does seem unanimous in confirming a definite link between dietary fat and colorectal cancer.)

The Japanese have virtually no cancer of the breast, colon, or prostrate. Also, heart and artery diseases are rare among Japanese. Scientists now believe that the Japanese diet—exceptionally low in fat—is the key. Once they migrate to the United States and consume the high-fat diet that is from a worldview peculiar to the United States, Canada, and parts of Europe, their rates of cancer (and the other diseases that kill Americans) rise correspondingly. If you graphed the varying levels of fat in the diets of countries the world over, and then graphed the varying rates of breast, colorectal, and other cancers, the two graphs would mirror each other perfectly. (Not surprisingly, in this country the Seventh Day Adventists who follow a vegetarian regimen for religious reasons show a much lower rate of cancer and cardiovascular diseases than the rest of the general population.)

Two friends who each worked for four years at the East Coast's largest cancer research center told me privately that, given the voluminous collection of studies reinforcing the breast cancer/diet link, questioning it is playing with fire; there is no question in their minds about the connection. While I have spoken with health professionals who argued that "the case for a low-fat diet should be obvious to people," I don't think they realize how mixed the messages are. On breast cancer, for example:

▶ Dr. Susan Love, M.D., Director of Faulkner Breast Center in Boston and Assistant Clinical Professor in Surgery at Harvard Medical School, says in a 1992 *Mirabella* article that asked why more women than ever are getting breast cancer, "We don't have a clue."

▶ Epidemiologist Maureen Henderson, of Fred Hutchinson Cancer Research, said flatly of the breast cancer/fat connection in a January 1991 *Time* magazine article, "I'm sure of it."

▶ *Self*, October 1992: "The best way to beat breast cancer is to detect it early."

▶ An 18-page booklet from the National Cancer Institute lists seven risk factors for breast cancer. One is being a woman. Fat is not among them— nor is it mentioned anywhere else in the pamphlet. Saying that "the biggest risk factor for breast cancer is simply being a woman" is not only a maddening push for "early detection" when early prevention would be so much cheaper and less painful—it's also just not true. It's a technicality. You could get really clever and say that the biggest risk factor for dying is being alive, or that the biggest risk factor for totaling your car is owning one. But what's the point? Why waste time and money educating people about a risk factor that's such a given that it's meaningless? Women want and need to know what they can do, not be gripped by terror simply because they have breasts.

In fact, the same goes for men. Since the cancers that afflict them most also happen to be those most strongly linked to dietary fat (colorectal and prostate cancers, for example) it is unconscionable that our scientific community is inviting the public to believe that all the data amassed so far is coincidental. Populations with high-fat diets have strikingly high rates of prostate and intestinal as well as breast cancer (not to mention coronary diseases).

Meanwhile, the diet thinkers make a low-fat diet sound like a sentence in hell: *Health*, in its January/February 1993 issue, said, "Some women cut out fat. . . . For these women, fixing a meal can become a rigorous chore, and eating with friends nearly impossible." In January 1991, *Time* said, "Another concern [about funding cancer/fat studies] is that women participating in such trials would have trouble adhering to the drastic regimen." (I dare anyone to observe a day in my life and tell me honestly that the vast smorgasbord I relish is a "drastic regimen" and "rigorous chore.")

A public television feature on Dr. Dean Ornish's program to reverse heart disease quoted a doctor as saying, "It is impossible for most people to live on a 10 percent fat diet." He asserted that it makes one "constipated, depressed and neurotic about food."

The tug-of-war and lack of a clear position plays directly to the inability of people to perceive risks and priorities. What the research community calls "playing it safe" is probably playing with people's lives. Murmuring, "There may be a connection," in the face of so many studies showing a conclusive link is what finally leaves the anxious, overfat people in my workshop squinting, "But the fat connection is kind of iffy, isn't it?" People are listening hopefully for authoritative hesitance and clinging to the vague and ambiguous statements they hear.

How much must something be studied before the public can be told the link is certain? We'll all be dead before some things are "proven" to the satisfaction of some scientists. Since the evidence "suggesting" fat/cancer links is voluminous, and since a low-fat diet does indisputably protect against the disease that kills 12 times as many women as breast cancer does (breast cancer deaths are 42,000 women a year, heart disease more than 500,000 a year), why wait? If the verdict that it's also a cancer buffer finally comes in after "more research," you'll be ahead of the game.

The 33-year Baltimore Longitudinal Study on Aging is meticulously monitoring physiological changes that occur during the lifetimes of more than 1,000 healthy volunteers. The study has so far found that an 80-year-old healthy heart can work as well as a 20-year-old one. According to scientists, this is not only due to the occasional stroke of genetic good luck. *Like an auto engine's, the human heart's performance over a lifetime is a direct result of how well it's been cared for.* [Italics my emphasis.]
—Madeline Chinnici, in *Self* magazine, April 1991

15

EDUCATION:
The Ultimate Answer

As a physician, I have observed that diet and lifestyle are the most important factors in promoting health and preventing disease. Yet many Americans eat and drink their way into sickness or premature death. In a recent study by the American Dietetic Association, 25 percent of those surveyed said healthy eating "takes too much time." . . . The study also revealed that 38 percent of Americans think a healthy diet means giving up their favorite foods.

—LOUIS W. SULLIVAN, M.D., Secretary of Health
and Human Services, *Parade*, March 29, 1992

Many Americans are still confused, misinformed or apathetic about the connection between diet and health. . . . Misconceptions about dietary change seem to have deterred many Americans from taking steps to improve their diets. Consumers frequently tell researchers they don't want to give up the foods they like.

—*Consumer Reports*, October 1992

Adam Drewnowski, Ph.D., director of the human nutrition program at University of Michigan's School of Public Health,

263

counters, "We've been telling people 'just say no to fat; eat vegetables' for the past 20 years, and basically it's not working."
—*Glamour*, September 1992

N o, it's not working—and by now, you know I have quite a few ideas about why. I believe educators must reexamine *what* they've been telling people, and *how*. You can only blame the student for so long before the tactics of the teacher come into question. Therefore, my goal is not only to educate the public, but to stimulate critical thinking among other educators.

Diet thinking is not simply an outgrowth of lack of education—equally at fault is the reliance on misguided, ineffective education. More education is important; different education is an even bigger priority. What matters is not just the information we provide and how much, but in what manner we provide it.

Diet thinking hampers incisive, substantial education. Impotent education creates fertile ground for more diet thinking. It's a catch-22 whose loop must be closed now by updating the content, the context, and the extent of education about eating.

People not only don't know what their greatest threats are (feeding the "outrage factor" described in the previous chapter); they are also at a loss about how to effectively deal with them. The result is a great number of people who don't do anything, many more who do the wrong things, and some who are unhappy about doing the right things. How do you educate people and have them act on that information—gladly?

Statistics on American fat and sugar consumption, and on the epidemics of heart disease, cancer, stroke, and diabetes, show that simply launching the latest research findings into living rooms via the evening news doesn't necessarily move people. Education must be consciously designed for digestibility.

The major flaws in current education efforts match a number of the basic characteristics of diet thinking. Missing from education are clarity, specificity, consistency, choice, a baseline of science to explain the rules, a sense of priorities, and positive language. Underlying it all is a lack of understanding about what people are really doing, and how they interpret and feel about what they are told.

Still, it's not hopeless. I wasn't trained to be an expert in education or even in nutrition—but I have been able to reach people successfully and powerfully with the messages so many health professionals are eager to get across to Americans. I've done it by recognizing and moving beyond those diet-thinking glitches. Other educators and health professionals can do the same.

However, it will mean giving up the investment in "the way it's always been done," and the safe and easy route of blaming the listener for not grabbing the data tossed at them. They'll have to be willing to take a few pages from my book—the work of "a young person . . . who has studied the paradigm but never practiced in it. . . . knowledgeable about the paradigm but not captured by it . . . an outsider" (Joel Barker in *Future Edge*).

Remember the phrases Barker said are typically used at first to put such people down: " 'That's impossible.' 'We don't do things that way around here.' 'It's too radical a change for us.' . . . 'How dare you suggest that what we've been doing is wrong!' 'If you had been in this field as long as I have, you would understand that what you are suggesting is absolutely absurd!' " I expect to hear a few of these. However, as I execute my vision for more cohesive, comprehensive, positive, and powerful public health education, I also hope to find that the majority are more interested in what works than in being right about past methods.

BE MORE UPBEAT!

In *Mastery* George Leonard says of conventional education: "The operative words are too often *don't, no* and *wrong*. The fundamental learning is negative."

Negativity is certainly a feature of the education born of diet thinking. Advice is usually limited to the few aspects of change likely to be considered negative—even though those aspects aren't as important in the big scheme of things as those that are positive (like eating enough).

For example, a staple of nutrition advice is what to cut from your current intake. No wonder people don't want to hear any more. "Don't eat fat. Don't eat this. Cut back this. Reduce this." People want and need to know what they *can* eat, what they *can* do! Those who counsel overfat people constantly try to extract commitments about what they're not going to do, what they're going to stop doing. What about *starting* something?

What prevails in the little education that exists today is diet-thinking vocabulary that's so worn-out and tired it's become almost meaningless. Even supposedly positive buzzwords have become banal. "When they tell me to 'change my lifestyle,' " said one workshop participant, "all I can hear is, 'Eat better. Eat less. Eat right.' All I can see is endless changing—and yucky health food." Even the words "dietary recommendations" sound dry—as if, like a "diet," they are separate from real eating and real life. Why not say, "This is what fuels your body" instead of presenting eating like some bitter antidote?

People listen more attentively if the story is expanded to include all the positive facts and truths. "You mean maybe if I do scale back in this one area (fat intake), it will also be okay—even healthier—to scale up in other areas (like total food volume and frequency)?"

The tone is as negative as the words and their meaning. Current education efforts are as full of resignation as they are empty of biological facts and rationale. I think educators and experts would do well to examine the effectiveness of their own delivery instead of blaming the psychology of the overfat individual for recidivism that actually results from the biology of deprivation. If psychology plays a role, it's that of educational style—not a person's emotional reasons for the "eating too much," "unrealistic expectations," "not learning to deal with temptation," and "feeling deprived so you fall off your diet."

Example ("Fat Gauge," *Allure*, January 1993): Sports nutritionist Michelle Vivas "tells her clients to try to accept their shape and make the best of it." (You can practically hear the big, martyred sigh that goes with this "encouragement.")

Besides being a knot of "nots," current education is always focused on control. Educators make themselves responsible for "getting you to" do something. And they "know" you won't want to. They work on your eating instead of your life; they try to change you instead of giving you a choice; they give you rules instead of a scientific big picture; and they try to move you with negative threats about disease. It's against, not for; it's what you're not, instead of what you are.

In short, they do the same diet-thinking things to you that you do to yourself. Where do you think you learned it?

BE CLEAR AND SPECIFIC!

In her *Vogue* article "Let It Be Light," Mary Roach cogently summed up the problem of vague generalities in dietary recommendations: "No more than

30 percent of calories from fat, says the American Heart Association. We nod. We look at our plates. We scratch our heads. It's one of those things you hear over and over and never quite understand, like 'consumes forty-seven times its weight in stomach acid.' "

My clients echo the bewilderment. "You hear thirty percent fat, but what does that mean?" Jessie asked us plaintively, and was greeted by a chorus of agreement from the group. "Yeah, you hear 'high carb and low fat,' but how do you eat that way?"

While the experts fight among themselves about whether 10, 20, or 30 percent is best, people struggle to figure out what any of that means and what's really important. Then those same experts moan about how no one listens to their recommendations. Well, maybe they're the ones who aren't listening. I observe very little sensitivity to what people may or may not already know, what they want, and how they hear things.

Most articles I see on the subject of nutrition leave the reader with more questions than answers. It is not prudent to make broad, vague statements to the American public. Educators and health professionals must consider how something will be reported or interpreted—not only by the reader or listener but by the sound-bite-happy media they must use to disseminate their recommendations. For example, a statement as general as "diets aren't healthy" is interpreted by many as all-out permission to abdicate all concern about food and health.

Here's a perfect example of the tangled web we weave when we aren't specific. Joann Manson, an epidemiologist at Harvard School of Public Health, stated in the "Great Weight Debate" (*Health* magazine, February 1992): "I would prefer . . . not trying to get women to aim for real leanness, which is extremely difficult to achieve and can result in serious eating disorders."

First of all, what is "real" leanness? (As opposed to "fake" leanness?) What is "really" lean, or "too" lean? To one woman it will mean size 5, to me it means below 13 percent bodyfat, to another it will mean 110 pounds, to my grandmother it meant only two chins instead of four. Give people some numbers; don't leave it to their uninformed imaginations!

Second, only a handful of female athletes ever actually flirt with being "too" lean—that is, maintaining bodyfat lower than 13 percent. Few reading that article would likely be in any danger of being "too lean." Too hungry, yes. Too "thin" (but not necessarily lean) for the wrong reasons, perhaps. Too lean, no. The danger that the vast majority of readers will face is from being too fat.

Quotes like this inspire leaps of reasoning such as, "I guess I'm healthier if I'm fat." Some undeniably overfat woman is out there right now reaching for another handful of fries or giving her kids bacon-and-mayo sandwiches for lunch, saying, "See, it's not healthy to be real lean, anyway." I know—because I've heard them.

Third, at 16 to 17 percent bodyfat, am I "real lean"? I'm lean, it's true. Yet I'm not within a continent's length of an eating disorder. Was it "extremely difficult to achieve" my "real leanness"? I exercise a few hours a week and eat unlimited amounts of delicious carbohydrates, with small amounts of protein and fat.

Fourth, would Manson make a statement like that to her peer group? We need to hear the same things they do, know what they know—at least to a point. My client Terry's naturopath told her, "Everyone needs fat in the diet." This is technically true, but what does that mean to Terry? Does he know she took it as license to put extra butter on her toast, when her total dietary fat was already more than 35 percent of calories? Did he consider that she might need some context, a frame of reference in order to use his advice safely and productively?

What would be the harm in explaining to her, "Every body needs a few grams of essential fatty acid daily, but even if you added no fat whatsoever to your diet, you will no doubt meet that need by eating carbohydrate and protein food."

People are sick of receiving brusque orders without understanding their biological reasoning. They want to be trusted with the same background information that led to the recommendation. In my opinion, that's one of the keys to empowering them to use the recommendation. Why should they take responsibility for their body if they're not trusted with its full story?

Don't assume they can't understand; that's condescending. I would gladly submit virtually any of my clients for testing by an independent, objective educational authority, with confidence that they would exhibit accurate knowledge about how the body works that's unheard of for a lay person. Many of my contacts with supportive health-care professionals began with them calling to ask, "How many weeks are the BodyFueling classes my patient attended? I'm so impressed!" (The basic workshop is four hours total.)

At the same time, it's also important to bridge the gap between academia and Everyperson by translating anything remotely scientific into real-person-ese. I speak the language of a lay person because I am a lay person. I know how people listen because I know how I listen. I know what's missing because I know what confused me before. When "the experts" begin communicating specific, graphic, complete science to people, it's going to have to be user-friendly as well. Perhaps there is a need for more "lay liaisons" to the public—"average" people with sound scientific knowledge and a gift for effective and empathetic communication.

ACKNOWLEDGE AND ENCOURAGE!

Without specifics, even those who are already doing a good job of reducing their intake don't recognize it or feel validated. People who are actually doing well have no basis for knowing it. The hazy, general "eat better!" message leaves them despairing that anything will ever be good enough. They assume that no matter what they're doing, it's already wrong. Encouragement is as scarce as a framework of facts.

A human resources vice president approached me at the first break in a corporate workshop to talk about his love of beef. He went on and on about how he really enjoyed red meat and couldn't imagine giving it up, but he believed it made him a "bad eater." It turned out he was eating one burger a week.

I understand his assumption: It's what he's been scolded and browbeaten to believe. "Too much red meat is bad." But how much is too much? Most of what people read and hear doesn't say. Some may decide that one beef meal a day is conservative enough, while others who eat any red meat at all feel guilty. Diet thinking, coupled with the human propensity for self-doubt, rarely tips the assumptions in one's favor.

There are two ways we can respond to what a person is doing: Point out what's wrong and how it should be righted, or affirm what has already been accomplished and point out what else can be done and why. Why do educators so reflexively choose the former? Why do the health and nutrition professions keep hounding people to change, hammering them with rights and wrongs? People must be rewarded for every step, encouraged to relinquish their own whip and appreciate themselves. People are at least as good at cutting themselves off at the knees as anyone around them. They don't need our help with that!

RECOGNIZE THAT "SOME" IS BETTER THAN "NONE"!

Closely related to the praise-and-reassurance blind spot is the all-or-nothing syndrome. Education often leaves people with the impression that anything short of total perfection means you might as well live on hot fudge sundaes and corn chips. Consistency instead of perfection is not extensively touted.

Yet it works—almost like magic. It's like pushing a button. Tell someone, "Hamburger and cheesecake are no-nos if you want to be healthy," and they will probably have one or the other before they go to bed that night.

If we hold people up to a standard and say, "All or nothing," and they say, "Okay, nothing"—what's the good? If they did some, for a long time, wouldn't that be better than nothing, or all for just a few weeks? So why not let them know that "some" is okay? Most people can commit to "some, mostly." Few will commit to "all, always." No one can be permanently perfect, but most people can be relatively consistent forever.

And that works out just fine, because being consistent is all it takes. It's a fallacy—or an excuse not to begin—that if you don't do what's optimal every minute of every day, you've blown it and might as well forget it.

Put yourself in the place of some brave soul who has never exercised in his life, or not for many years, but has decided to "go healthy." This person is in the middle of making all kinds of changes (some clients come to us in an orgy of new-leaf-turning—quitting smoking, changing their eating, everything all at once). They are determined to make this work—but exercising six times a week, even four or five, is daunting.

Consider that they may not yet have experienced the turnaround in energy that fueling will eventually provide, so all they have to go on is the lackluster way they feel at the moment. And their busy life schedules loom before them. Now say, "Three times a week will barely do anything."

If they have been doing a little, they feel as if this effort—which for them is a monumental one—is totally insufficient. If they've been doing something twice a week, and they hear they are "losing fitness," they may lose interest. Is this how we reward people for their efforts—with unyielding "standards" to use for self-flagellation?

My father is an excellent example. A star swimmer and avid basketball player in his youth, at the age of 55 he has been inactive for many years. Lately, he's been eating nonfat cheeses, fruit instead of cake—and talking about walking and swimming again. Now, if my dad began to walk twice a week for 20 minutes at a time, I would be walking on air (if I could get any higher, now that he's quit smoking after 30 years!). If he walked just that much, I would shower him with genuine joy and appreciation. How do you think that would affect his desire to keep walking?

On the other hand, what if—hearing of his twice-weekly jaunts—I said, "That's nice, Dad, but you really need to do it three times a week, for 30 to 45 minutes, or you're still 'losing' fitness." First of all, can that even be true? When someone who hasn't walked further than to the fridge or the TV for 10 years begins to walk to the store, is he "losing"? And second, even if it were true, which response will eventually coax him to 30 minutes?

My client Kelly is another example. She said after the workshop, "Now I see that I can start out slow with exercise and that's okay. The program my club had me on was too much, so I had stopped going. Now I'm swimming, walking, and doing light weights—varying it. I'm not going crazy trying to get to a certain heart rate. I feel great." A trainer at her club had also told her that her horseback riding "didn't count." What does that mean? Perhaps he meant that it isn't aerobic, and thus won't be the most effective choice for fat burning. But that's where specificity again becomes important: If he'd explained exactly that, he would have been putting her in an informed position—not merely putting her down. He never bothered to find out what she wanted to accomplish.

The most important point here is that anything is better than nothing. You should feel good about whatever effort you put in. And feeling good about what you've already done invites you to keep going. When I'm doing well, I want to do more. If I constantly feel I've fallen short, I want to give up.

LESS "SHOULDS," MORE CHOICE: WHEN THE RIGHT INFORMATION IS IN THE WRONG CONTEXT

One of the distinguishing features of health education is that people aren't treated as if they truly have a choice, as if whatever they decide is really all right. Even those who are pushing the "right" information don't necessarily address this issue. I've mentioned informed choice in the context of the individual's approach to fitness. I think it's also important for educators to address its role in their approach to delivering information.

It's time we recognized that people just don't do things because they "should." Give someone a should (or shouldn't) and you can pretty much count on a rebellion. The magnetism of the forbidden is simple reverse psychology; you don't need a Ph.D. to figure it out. Just observe human behavior: You say don't, we say do. They say should, we say forget it. You say naughty, we do it anyway—and feel guilty on top of it. (Guilt doesn't so much alter your actions as change how you feel about them.)

One classic interpretation of the "should" is administered by professionals who believe that frightening people into "eating right" is a good tactic. But threats (like all "shoulds") don't leave people wanting to care for themselves; it makes them feel like they have to. "Scared" and "concerned" are *not* synonyms for "inspired." I have met and worked with plenty of people who confessed to being absolutely terrorized by thoughts of cancer or heart disease, but who were doing nothing about their eating.

The most potent combination in health education is complete and accurate background information, and a genuine choice about using it. Providing neutral, nonjudgmental information, then giving people the freedom to go ahead and do whatever they want, creates an inviting "space" to do the right thing. Say, "Fueling your body will be optimal. The more you do it, the better off you'll be. But it's your body, your life. Here are the facts, so you can make an informed choice," and they tend to choose wisely—*because they actually have a choice.*

Informed choice is one of the most powerful "secrets" of BodyFueling, but it needn't be a secret. All you have to do is provide information and let go of your imagined responsibility to "make them" use it. But it must be a genuine release, not a manipulation strategy such as "maybe if I act like it's okay if they don't, that will get them to do it."

Why do professionals insist on moratoriums and "no-nos" as the standard modus operandi for education? Fitness trainers and nutritionists who participate in BodyFueling sometimes come up to me afterward to chat conspiratorially about how "hard" it is to educate people. "Don't you hate it when people don't do what you tell them to?" one said, or "How do you get people to . . ." If you "hate it" when people don't listen, you're essentially saying it's not okay if they don't do everything you say.

I think most people want to do what works. We don't need to "get them" to do anything—we just need to inform them about how things work. If perchance someone doesn't want to do what works, they won't. No amount of coercion will make them. Instead of trying to drag people in a certain direction, simply hand them a road map, describe the journey, point them in a good direction, and leave them thinking about compelling personal reasons they might have for going that way.

"Richard" is one client whose story is testimony to the power of choice. An accomplished fast-track executive in his mid-thirties, Richard was stationed in Hong Kong as vice president of a rapidly growing international division of one of the world's largest companies. His account of the corporate culture there included what sounded like a caste system based on one's drinking ability. He didn't consider himself an alcoholic (and neither did I), but he was concerned about his consumption.

I never once, in the four days we spent during an executive retreat, told Richard he should or shouldn't do anything—including drink. I did, however, provide him with a strictly factual, biological account of the body's reaction to ethanol alcohol, the toxin in alcoholic beverages (see p. 68 on ethanol), and simply suggested that in the future he choose wisely based on those graphic facts and based on his life commitments and the need for an energetic, healthy body to fulfill them.

About a year later at a convention, we spoke to Richard's boss, the division's president, and learned that since our work with him, Richard has never touched another drink again. He discovered nonalcoholic beer. "And he's driving us all crazy telling us how many grams of fat are in everything we eat," added the president. "What did you do to him?" I didn't do anything to him. I treated him like the intelligent adult he is, provided him with the facts, and gave him an authentic choice. He did choose—and wisely.

I wonder how many drinking problems could be eliminated with this approach? Certainly in physical addiction there are other factors, but not all cases of abuse involve physical addiction. In those cases, treating people like adults who can choose, instead of like children or sick people, could give a new face to what we call "treatment" today. Too simple? Too low-tech? But could it hurt to try?

Informed choice is clearly important to people. One BodyFueling client, Patti, described the experience this way: "It felt like a course in logic, not 'how to eat.' I definitely have a sense of what I need to do if I want health and fitness—and I also know that if I don't do it, that's my choice. It's totally up to me."

Robin, another client, explained, "What's neat is I feel very responsible for my choices now. I either want to feel good and be healthy, or not. And I know exactly how to get there if I do. Somehow it put the responsibility back with me, but without guilt."

When you stop trying to will people to respond, you can work with them on finding their inspiration in their own lives. Remember, that's positive and long-term inspiration, not "don't-wants," and three-month goals.

Linda, my client and a message therapist, hit it squarely when she said, "You really impacted the way I look at this. 'Feeding my muscles so I can heal other peoples' muscles' is much more positive and powerful than 'I should be eating right.' "

TREAT PEOPLE LIKE ADULTS!

People sometimes behave like babies about their eating—I think because they've been treated that way. Listen next time you hear or read recommendations on nutrition. Does it come off with at least a tinge of "Naughty, naughty, naughty! You know better than that, now, don't you?"

When you baby people, you get babies. Educate people as though they are dense little children, and that's exactly what you'll get. Observing peoples' conditioned response to the subject of food, I often am reminded of Emma, the beautiful and captivating daughter of our friends John and Jashoda. I remember when Emma was about four, she had a cranky, early-morning habit of loudly insisting that she didn't want something—even after you agreed with her. She couldn't hear your agreement. "I don't want orange juice!" she would begin. You'd say "Okay, Emma, no orange juice." Louder: "But I don't *want* orange juice!" You repeat, "Got it, Emma. No orange juice." Now a screech: "But I don't **want** orange juice!"

I had a workshop participant do the exact same thing once. "Shelley" raised her hand to tell me she just wasn't going to "give up" fat. I said, "That's certainly up to you. If there's something you love, don't give it up." She responded, "Because I love to cook, and it's just impossible to cook anything good without oil." I said, "If you feel that way, then by all means cook the way you choose." "But I . . . ." She got louder and more shrill as I calmly repeated over and over that it was fine, she didn't have to. She couldn't hear me.

I've seen the most staid businesspeople resort to the terrible twos. One male executive at a small southwestern company declared indignantly, "You mean you want me to take snacks or lunch to the office? That's for housewives."

That's fine. If it's too much for him to stick a banana in his briefcase or drink a can of juice mid-morning to keep his energy up, and help reduce his ample, heart-attack belly roll, let him decline. It's his body. (Of course, it's also our insurance rate base—but that's another story.)

KNOW THAT PEOPLE DON'T KNOW!

After appearing on one network's evening news program, I contacted a competing network to see if they would like to cover the story of BodyFueling as well. The assistant producer was enthusiastic about the story and pursued it for some time, but eventually came back to me with a "no" from the producer, her boss: "She says that everyone knows all that already," adding, "She's really into fitness, and she already knows all that stuff."

Maybe she does (and maybe she doesn't). Even if she does, she is dead wrong if she believes people understand how their bodies work; that they have a statistically based sense of health priorities, a powerful sense of freedom about making choices, and a long-term purpose for self-care. She's not down in the trenches every day, listening to people's comments, questions, and language.

I cannot emphasize this enough, both for the educators and professionals who assume people know the basics (or figure they don't need to understand the scientific rationale for "dos and don'ts"), and for those individuals who are sure they "know" everything. I continue to be astonished and awed at the dismally subterranean depths of unconsciousness and lack of comprehension demonstrated to me during my work.

I think nutrition professionals and others who share my mission sometimes forget that we must start at square one. Immersed in their own advanced state of knowledge, "the experts" forget that most Americans know very little about food and nutrition—regardless of what they know about anything else. You cannot just lecture people to lower their fat and cholesterol!

I worked with one very high-powered executive who said a well-known lecturer on eating for a healthy heart had spoken at his company that year. "Henry" really enjoyed listening to this person, so I thought "that's nice." But about halfway into my presentation, Henry expressed total shock that peanut butter is loaded with fat. He didn't even know hard cheese is typically high in fat! He didn't know any of the simple facts we taught about the body and how it works.

Very often at our workshops I'm struck anew at all the faces looking up front, expectant and faintly puzzled, waiting. Successful, educated people in their thirties, forties, and fifties who have no clue. It's a bit like being a history teacher who is dismayed to find out that his about-to-graduate high school students don't know what continent Somalia is on or where the Middle East lies, or even what part of the country Wyoming occupies.

Every day I come home with some new diet-thinking collector's item I've overheard: "I hear that . . ." I hear it in the supermarket, in movie lines, in the mall.

Overheard at my health club: "If I feel hungry when I know I shouldn't be eating, I have salad or vegetable juice. It's really filling."

"Hey, this treadmill says I only burned 100 calories! What was the point?"

Three teenage girls leaving the stair machine area: "Let's go eat now." "I just want a salad." "I don't want anything. I don't want to ruin what I just did."

A gasping, sweating, overfat man leaning over to Robert from the cycle next to him: "You should be doing it harder. See? You're only burning 400 calories an hour, and I'm burning 600."

Listen to the questions people are still asking. In *Shape*, September 1991: "If I lift weights, will I weigh more?" and "I'm worried about gaining weight from dairy products." In *Parade*, April 12, 1992: "Can fat be converted to muscle through exercise?" "Am I losing weight when I sweat during exercise?"

Marc was pouring olive oil on his pasta every day and was boggled about why he wasn't losing "weight"—he was certain he ate a "no-fat" diet!

It doesn't matter who you are. It doesn't matter how educated you are in other ways. I've worked with Ivy League–educated businesspeople, and I've worked with unemployed mothers on general assistance. They believe exactly the same things about what you "should" and "shouldn't" do; they're making exactly the same mistakes. Diet thinking knows no socioeconomic boundaries. I've worked with Fortune 50 CEOs (men and women) who made no connection between not eating all day and not having any energy. It's easy to assume, "Oh, *they* know all that," but it's just not true.

Cultural brainwashing and incomplete education can corrupt the instincts and common sense of the most intelligent people. In the June 1992 issue of *Bicycling* magazine, Tom Seabourne, Ph.D, wrote an article about how he "discovered" that eating more frequently could help you lose "weight." He explained how he was confused during a cross-country bicycling race because he was losing muscle and gaining fat on three meals a day, even though their combined 8,000 calories should have fueled his 100 miles a day. So what's the first thing he tries to remedy the situation? Switching to *one* meal a day. What in the world sent this highly educated person in that direction?

He only stumbled onto eating more frequently when his daughter became diabetic and was "ordered" to eat snacks as well as meals. He ate as often as she did, just to support her, and immediately experienced speed, strength, endurance, and energy boosts. He adds, "I know the idea sounds outrageous." Why? Any biology textbook would have pointed him in that direction.

Finally, I've found that even people who have already experienced the inevitable results of poor diet still aren't educated about eating. It's bad enough when people aren't educated about how to prevent their health problems—but to have suffered the consequences and still not understand why (and what to do next) is abominable. Eating dinner with a family in which several members are diabetic, I was aghast that every carbohydrate on the table—potatoes, stuffing, fruit—was drenched in some kind of fat, from butter to whipped cream. There wasn't a single one I'd have wanted to put in my body (and I didn't). There was no bread. Moreover, the dinnertable conversation revolved around how "healthy" everything was—because it had no sugar in it! They even distinguished between the "good" yams (brown sugar) and the "bad" (no sugar). But both were drowning in butter.

How can people be diabetic and not know what fat does to a diabetic body? I'll tell you how. When my own father-in-law was diagnosed with diabetes, he was given an exchange diet to follow and a kit to test his blood sugar levels. He was left uneducated and confused. Had he not happened to have a son and daughter-in-law who are immersed in this, he would have been competely lost. He learned nothing about what exactly was happening inside him, how it could have been prevented, or what opportunities he still had to be healthy. Instead, he learned that he was "sick," and that eating this new way was his "treatment."

The joke is that the way diabetics are supposed to eat once diagnosed is how they needed to fuel their bodies before they got the disease. It's what every body needs! For many Americans, it takes a disease to jolt them into beginning to fuel—and even then they treat it like a "have-to" curse. My father-in-law felt he had to eat this way because he was "sick," when in fact it is essentially the way I eat, and the way a healthy human body is best fueled.

STARTING YOUNG

Because they've had some basic education about how to operate a car, people don't try to start their cars with a bobby pin. Basic information about how to operate the body should take precedence over that. Giving all children some simple nutritional and digestive biology would mean an entire generation could grow up without being mystified about the way their bodies work—and without doing a lot of dangerous and counterproductive things to manipulate their bodies in pursuit of goals that fundamentally cannot be achieved.

If parents don't get it handled and kids don't get it in school, kids grow up emulating whichever fuel-foolish habits the parents happen to be stuck with. Sometimes it's forced on them: Among the horrible, poignant stories clients have told me was one from a woman whose mother put her on the Air Force Diet when she was eight years old; she was allowed to eat only eggs and milk. At a wedding recently, one woman brought her overfat daughter a wedge of brie cheese the size of a large pie slice. The couple at our table urged their son to have a second cookie, even after he refused several times.

Then, when the teens or twenties hit, "thin" becomes a priority, and kids start adding their own control games to whatever nonsense they picked up at home. A mistrust of one's own needs and body signals sets in ("Should I still be hungry, even though I had a whole banana?") so that they eventually grow deaf to their own body's cries and whispers. And they grow up and their kids get to watch and start it all over again—unless we start giving kids the scoop early enough so they can choose what their life, their body, their health is going to be like.

I have stopped grocery shopping during times when I know I will see many parents and children. I'm too pained by the sight of heavy-lidded children sucking on candies and chocolates, and wide-eyed toddlers drinking in the sight of mom overloading the cart with protein and fat, possibly getting the only education they'll ever receive about what foods to buy. I want to cry when I see Grandpa lovingly kissing his grandson's head, stroking his clear skin, while he waits for his four pounds of bacon to be wrapped, or Mom giving her two little girls candy bars if they'll promise to be quiet.

Before we know it, they'll be wandering the aisles in a distant daze the way their parents are right now, or sitting in a workshop like mine: overfat, uncomfortable, and confused, wanting to know "What do they mean when they say 'thirty percent fat?' Can you really cook without oil? But don't we need a lot of protein? Isn't fresh produce bad for you because of the pesticide residues?"

Sure, they could go to the library, as I did, and begin studying up about human fuel requirements. Some might, if they get frustrated enough (as we did) with the less-than-stellar results produced by hand-me-down diet wisdom that's been the party line for ages. But people really have no reason to believe that this "everybody knows" diet advice could be mistaken. It's so branded into our consciousness as "the truth" that if it isn't working for you, you think something must simply be wrong with *you*.

We shouldn't have to go out of our way to get the information as adults. We could have been educated when we were children. Why did I leave school knowing more about Christopher Columbus than what to feed my body? If I had known at 10 what I know now, I could have saved myself years of suffering, hunger, guilt, muscle loss, and confusion. So, I assert, could most Americans.

I've worked with 12-year-olds who quickly grasped the fundamentals of human biology; they understand that their bodies run on food, and that without it they can't run very well. They can see there are foods that are ideal, those that are less so, and some that harm. Kids can and do think about their futures, and if we present fueling in terms of what they want, they'll *want* to do it. It's amazing what even children will do with their eating when they know the costs.

PRIORITIES IN EDUCATION

When the "outrage factor" penetrates education, we pay an enormous price. Inconsistency in what experts choose to emphasize—as well as in what the media chooses to report—is terribly off-putting to people straining to make some sense out of "healthy eating." And once again, a catch-22: Without a solid substructure of basic education, you don't have the knowledge to sift through, keep what's meaningful, and discard the insignificant. With no basic operating system, you're helpless to evaluate the selective add-ons.

Education as to what's important is as crucial as advice on what to do about what's important. The media, educators, and health professionals should immerse themselves in priorities (Chapter 14). Forget inconsequential tidbits that debate relative trivialities. Do what Ross Perot did. Pick three or four messages—the most statistically important—and hammer on them endlessly. After the 1992 Presidential election, everyone knew the total national debt was (then) $4.4 trillion.

Sometimes, the squeaky wheel that's getting the grease is not at all inconsequential, yet nonetheless doesn't justify precedence over other concerns that top the list statistically. With AIDS receiving the growing attention it has in recent years, safe sex has become a more important issue than ever; today, sex education (or getting some into schools) is a tremendous priority for many in the field of education.

There's uproar about distributing condoms to kids at schools and upping the ante on curriculum subject matter. People feel it is urgent to have children understand the risks of sexual activity and know how to protect themselves. Stars and sports figures implore the young to take care with their sexuality. After Bill Clinton was elected, Donna Shalala—his newly chosen head of the Department of Health and Human Services—declared that childhood immunization and a national AIDS strategy would be her priorities.

I find nothing wrong with all that by itself. Safe sex education is vital. But what about safe eating? Why not be logical about this? Whether you look at it economically or socially, there's no comparison: If you're concerned about keeping American health care costs down (Shalala's third priority) or saving lives, the numbers talk.

▶ 175,000 Americans have died of AIDS to date.

▶ 175,000 Americans die of heart disease every two months—of every year.

▶ More Americans die of cardiovascular disease every five days than die of AIDS in a year.

▶ More than 2,700 people die of cardiovascular disease/stroke every day—about a million a year. That's one life every 34 seconds.

▶ Heart disease alone was responsible for nearly half of all U.S. deaths in 1992.

▶ About 69 million Americans are afflicted with a cardiovascular disease; 6 million have coronary heart disease (1989 estimate, National Health and Nutrition Examination Survey).

▶ Cancer claimed approximately another fourth of the U.S. deaths in 1992, taking more than 500,000 lives.

▶ There were 1 million new cancer cases in 1992.

▶ About 300,000 coronary bypass procedures are performed each year at $40,000 apiece, for a total of $12 billion.

▶ Heart disease costs $47.9 billion annually (Health Care Financing Review, 1992).

▶ Total cardiovascular disease costs about $120 billion annually (1992).

▶ The total cost of cancer in 1990 was $104 billion, plus another $3–$4 billion for detection procedures.

(Statistics are those available as of January 1993.)

I understand that AIDS doesn't appear to be slowing down and these statistics may change over the next several years. But right now this is where it stands. You have infinitely greater odds of developing heart disease than AIDS. There's good incentive here—financial, if nothing else—to bring these facts out of their relative obscurity.

That money and energy could be spent educating kids in a new and positive way about how to eat to prevent heart disease, instead of treating, or struggling to find a cure for, something that is preventable.

On the radio a few months ago, I heard an educator speaking on the subject of sex education in schools: "They [the kids] don't think two years down the road. They're just thinking now." Precisely my point. But neither do adults—when they're unconsciously passing through their lips foods as sure to kill as cigarettes, trying not to think about their elderly parents, hoping distant heredity or luck or that fish oil capsule or oat bran muffin will take care of it.

That's why this sort of education in schools is every bit as critical as sex ed. Kids must know how to eat. Make no mistake: I think *both* are important and, ideally, both would be taught. I'm not at all against AIDS education, just *for* healthy eating education to get its fair share. Given the odds, if I had to choose, I'd want my kids knowing first how to eat, then how to use condoms.

In the area of women's health, too, there is a wide gap between truth and hysteria on the part of educators and the media (and subsequently, the public). It's bad enough that the vast majority of press coverage on breast cancer focuses on early *detection* "breakthroughs" as opposed to prevention, and seems determined to debunk the dietary link. (Many thousands of studies suggesting this link have already convinced some researchers beyond a reasonable doubt, but that link will surely be undeniable after $670 million worth of large-scale women's health studies, commissioned by the National Institutes of Health in early 1993, are complete.)

What's more incredible is that breast cancer, while an undeniable risk, is not only not a woman's biggest threat, it's not even close.

It would be a huge understatement to say cardiovascular disease kills more women than breast cancer does. If you compare American Heart Association and American Cancer Society statistics, you find that there are more female cardiovascular disease deaths than *all* cancer deaths for *both* sexes combined!

Not a single woman in any of my workshops has known that cardiovascular disease is the number one cause of female deaths in the United States, claiming more than 500,000 women's lives each year. About half of all heart attacks happen to women—a quarter of a million women die of them every year. More than half of all cardiovascular disease deaths (including high blood pressure and stroke) are women!

Education about these facts is desperately needed to help set the public's priorities straight and to quell the outrage factor. That means those who educate (as well as those who fund education) must get *their* facts and priorities straight. Those who choose to invest in and support the cause of education should take a close look at these numbers before they choose their projects.

CELEBRITIES' HEALTHY EATING WORKS (CHEW)

Despite the above numbers, celebrities seem to bestow their money and clout on outrage-factor causes. Actors, athletes, and other "stars" send a message with the causes they choose; people then see those causes not only as the "hip" or "cool" ones to support but may assume that those must also be the most serious.

I would love to see those who command attention from vast numbers of Americans contribute to eating education. Statistically, it's where their clout is most needed. If you want to make an impact, do it here. I propose a nonprofit organization where widely respected celebrities could donate their time (in public service announcements) and money (for production and air time) to promote fueling.

The fittest and healthiest of our celebrities obviously have something to say. The admirably well-preserved, attractive, and strong physiques of the following (ages are as of this writing) didn't come from starving any more than they came from a high-fat, junky diet: Madonna (35), Linda Hamilton (36), Demi Moore (30), Cher (47), Clint Eastwood (sixty something), Paul Newman (70), Harrison Ford (fifty something), Mark Harmon (41), Pam Dawber (41), Kevin Costner (38), Jack Palance (73) and his now-infamous one-armed pushups, Jack Lalanne (eighty something), Patrick Stewart (fifty something), Patrick Swayze (thirty something). Except for Madonna, all of the women above have had more than one child!

EDUCATORS AS EXAMPLES

Peg, a 45-year-old marathon runner and physical therapist, commented during a workshop that she "gave up on healthy eating" when she was 24 and a registered dietitian came to a school class to give a talk on how to eat: "She was enormously obese. I took one look and checked out. I didn't hear a word she said."

How many health professionals and "nutrition experts" are overfat and unhealthy? Are they not doing what they were taught and what they teach? Or are they not taught what's being recommended to every American via the government and media? Either, in my opinion, has serious implications.

A dietitian on a local evening "magazine" program has recommended sugary animal cookies in place of doughnuts, peanut butter in place of ham, and salted peanuts in place of potato chips. Another in a magazine wrote that cheese and peanut butter are the "healthiest" protein choices for children.

The R.D. (registered dietitian) certification is required for those in charge of institutional feeding. Why, when my friend's mother was in the hospital, was she eating mashed potatoes with butter and gravy, salisbury steak, and regular (sugared) jello with whipped cream? Why was the school cook in my recent workshop so thoroughly confused after working with a dietitian to help streamline the school's lunch fare?

When my husband asked the dietitian assigned to his father (when he was diagnosed as diabetic) whether rice syrup or barley malt were acceptable, she had never heard of either. When asked if fruit-juice sweetened cookies were all right, she said there is no such thing. And when he asked why certain brands of cereals we know to contain sugar or corn syrup were on the list, she said, "Well, those have only a little." What about all the unsweetened brands? And if "only a little" was okay, why did Dad leave her office terrified of sugar?

President Clinton pledges to tackle health-care issues with a vengeance— and at least once a week throughout his election campaign and early in his presidency was photographed "with the people" at fast-food restaurants where the fat content of most menu items and the carbohydrate-protein-fat ratio of most meals violate the government's own dietary recommendations.

It is nonsensical to be indignant about peoples' choices when your own don't measure up to the same standards. I agree that having achieved personal fitness cannot by itself qualify someone to teach others, but it should be included as a prerequisite.

You will often hear or read warnings that any nutrition professional you consult should have a degree or credentials. I understand the intent behind such warnings: You want to screen out quacks who peddle fairy tales, like some of those discussed in Chapter 6. On the other hand, I've met and worked with too many R.D.s, M.D.s, M.A.s, and Ph.D.s who were not practicing what they were preaching, and/or who were preaching diet thinking instead of pure fact and an empowering perspective. Too often, it's the blind leading the blind.

I think the criteria should be the person's sources and how current and verifiable their material is, whether their attitude and manner is empowering to you, and whether they represent what you want. As I've demonstrated, having letters after your name does not necessarily guarantee amnesty from diet thinking; often, in fact, it brings its own biases and institutional obligations.

I have had numerous professionals contact me whose business it is to treat eating disorders or obesity who themselves suffer from eating disorders or obesity. They often are attracted by something they see or hear in the BodyFueling approach that they haven't been able to capture themselves. Some have heard about it from their own former patients.

This culture worships letters after a name in much the same way we do numbers on the scale—blindly. One dietitian who had heard good things about BodyFueling's perspective called me, but ultimately declined to work with me because she couldn't see taking guidance from someone who didn't have the credentials she did. She was obese, struggling with what she called compulsive overeating, and counseling others on the same issue. I was lean, eating happily, and had by then hundreds of clients eating as health authorities are practically begging them to. And my clients were seeing it as fueling their lives, rather than dryly "following the health authorities' rules."

If you feel you must doublecheck any of my material because I am missing those two letters, I welcome and even encourage it. *My* caution is to rely on scientific texts and abstracts as much as possible. If you consult with an individual for your second opinion, watch for signs of diet thinking.

MAKE IT MASSIVE!

Once the context and content of healthy-eating education have been overhauled to be more effective, it's time to consider the size and scope of that effort. User-friendly education that challenges diet thinking works. But, in order for it to last, the whole environment must support it. "Spot education," as opposed to a wholesale transformation in culture, is spitting into the wind—building a house with no foundation. Without recognition of not only health problems but also the flaws in education that underlie them, there can be no true relief from the suffering of diet thinking.

I (and others) can teach people that weight doesn't matter, and show them all the logic and scientific reasoning—but if they go out into a world chanting "weightloss-weightloss-weightloss," they feel outnumbered. They *are* outnumbered. The newly educated fueler is still a minority in a world screaming, "Thin, skip it, resist it, count it, work it off." New information and ideas can knock you out of the groove. But without widespread enlightenment in every corner, you may be pulled back in almost effortlessly by the monstrous machine.

A March 1991 *Seventeen* article was a great example of what's needed. Titled "Why You Should Eat," it briefly touches upon many of the points I make throughout this book. Subheads include "Eating keeps you alive," "Eating makes you attractive," "Eating keeps you healthy—short-term," "Eating keeps you healthy—long-term." The piece explains why eating helps you lose fat, and acknowledges that this long-obscured fact is "strange, but true."

The piece also asserts that eating makes you smart, strong, and happy, is fun, keeps you from gorging on junk, impresses guys. "Not eating wrecks your ability to eat smart. . . . Choosing what to eat—and eating sensibly and well—proves that you're in charge of your life." Brilliant! It speaks directly to what's important to teens—in their language—and lets them know that eating will give them what they want. Articles like this are especially important for young women who are still forming impressions about their bodies and what to do with them. Even though they may have already absorbed some of the old poison, there's still time to reeducate.

If we don't, there is a generation of teenagers out there preparing to become our next generation of frustrated, frightened, desperate adults—the ones I see every week moving through the grocery store aisles in a glassy-eyed trance.

EDUCATION AS BUSINESS

Why wouldn't the health and diet industries leap for joy at this prospect and turn themselves into educators on fueling instead of food-restriction product pushers? Maybe they will, but one thing that will surely be considered is that it won't be a billion-dollar business with a lasting future. Education can be effective as a one-shot deal. If you're not selling foods and pills, there's no repeat business. That's fine if your goal is to educate people—it's not if your chief goal is to make money.

Many commercial diet companies now claim they are "educational." Then why not pure education? Why the diet and weighing and packaged food and supplements? I've talked with my clients who have been through all the commercial diet programs. They don't know a thing about what works or why. I saw the commercial "plan" given Jean, an already lean woman whose only problem was in her mind. It was barely enough daily carbohydrate to feed me for breakfast.

I probably don't even need to point out the industries that would lose out if everyone ate the way I do, but I will anyway: The diet/weight-loss industry ($33 billion, predicted in May 1990 by *U.S. News & World Report*, to be reaching $50 million by the mid-1990s, but thankfully not growing as quickly as expected). The beef industry. The fast-food industries (unless they could adapt rapidly and all become deliciously low-fat). Specialized medicine (think of heart surgeries, cancer treatment). Pharmaceutical companies (several people I know each spent hundreds of dollars on drugs prescribed for the colds and flu I never got last winter). If everyone ate like I do starting tomorrow—if even half the nation did—some of these industries might shrink or eventually disappear.

A whole new series of industries could revolve around the shift. A huge market of older people would be established—people who can and will do wild stuff that 65-year-olds currently aren't inclined to do. Instead of selling these people drugs and walkers and hospital beds, we could be selling them bicycles, vacation travel, and a host of new food products. People wouldn't die as young, so insurance payouts would decrease.

The effect on health care would be phenomenal. All available statistics show that the high cost of health care is not the fault of health care providers, government, or insurance companies. The diseases that most burden our system are *diseases that people bring upon themselves* by the choices they make. Now, sophisticated technology for diagnosing and treating preventable disorders is outstripping our ability to pay for it.

An enormous percentage of our health care dollars are spent on illnesses known to be caused by what people put into their bodies (fat, tobacco, alcohol, and drugs). The overall cost is even greater when you factor in lost economic productivity due to illness and early (preventable) death. If Americans stopped trashing themselves, we wouldn't need so many "crash shops" and expensive high-tech procedures to patch them up. Those endorsing a "right" to health care are promising that even if you drive recklessly and destroy your vehicle, the repairs will always be guaranteed, perhaps even free of charge. Whatever happened to changing the oil, keeping it clean, and, of course, fueling it with high-quality fuel? Perhaps "cure" is simply more dynamic, even romantic a notion than prevention.

HOW YOU SEE YOUR INTERNAL ENVIRONMENT IMPACTS YOUR EXTERNAL ENVIRONMENT

An interesting transformation paralleling that related to food, my body, and eating has been the way I see other aspects of my own health and well-being, and of the environment around me. It's not something I planned, but I welcome it. There's a heightened sense of appreciation for and concern about environments both internal and external.

For example, we use sunscreen zealously now—every day, summer and winter. It's a habit we don't even think about. Used to be you'd have to tie me down to get me to floss my teeth. Not anymore. It's all because BodyFueling is more about caring for your body—which is precious—than it is merely about "trying to eat right."

There's also a sharpened edge to our environmental commitment. We recycle more and more. We sold one car and use the remaining one as little as possible, preferring to walk, bicycle, or bus whenever we can. I don't find this shift at all surprising. In his book *Mastery*, author George Leonard suggests that "those people who feel good about themselves, who are in touch with nature and their own bodies, are more likely to use their energy for the good of this planet and its people than those who lead sedentary, unhealthy lives."

I certainly don't want to be a healthy, fit 110-year-old living on—or leaving my children—a garbage-strewn, polluted earth. I have a constantly conscious sense of how I want things to be, now and later.

If everyone fueled, not only would people be healthier, fitter, happier, and more satisfied, not only would health care and the food industry (and thus economics and possibly politics) be affected, but perhaps also recycling would increase, wasteful consumption might decrease, and people with a new and growing compassion for their own bodies might naturally begin to extend that respect to plants, animals, natural resources, and other human beings. I have no evidence that this would occur, but it's an exciting thought.

THE EDUCATED PATIENT

Having your whole body make sense to you makes you a better patient—when you are one, which may also be less often. You can be a participant, not a victim being treated or a body dropped off for repairs. You're able to give more complete and accurate information, understand what is happening and what your choices are, and ask intelligent questions.

When you know how your body's systems function and interact, your body's behavior may make sense more often—which is comforting. When the body is a total mystery, you feel helpless—and that's scary. Certainly, the human body can be unpredictable, even to those who have devoted their lives to studying it. But when you know at least the basics, the mysteries seem more fascinating than intimidating.

Doctors may not be accustomed to such participation; that doesn't fit the current paradigm of health care. But it will. Prevention is the future—and you are prevention. No doctor can make you prevent something.

What can? You know. Look back at Chapter 1, "Fueling Your Future."

It's not the misleading media or the bad ads or the stupid products that are to be feared; it's ignorance. We can't rely upon the media to shoulder the task of educating America. They are there to report the latest and the most interesting news, and it's the nature of our current media that they will frequently do so in brief, glib, out-of-context tidbits.

But no matter what kind of nonsense gets the spotlight, it won't present a problem if it's reaching an already-knowledgeable audience. I am no longer dominated by the conflicting information, because I am a tremendously informed consumer. I absorb what I know to be consistent with facts, and I ignore the rest.

The average American doesn't have this luxury. If you don't know your car, you can get screwed by the mechanic—you'll believe just about anything, and pay for it too. If you don't know your body, you're going to keep getting screwed—and paying for it—but the consequences will be more dire.

Misinformation will be stripped of its power when every one of us knows beyond a hair of a doubt what our bodies need—and when you care more about what it needs than what you want it to weigh (or look like next week). That is my vision. It will require a culture-wide breakthrough—which, ultimately, is what BodyFueling is all about.

EPILOGUE

At the second session of a two-part workshop just prior to the completion of this book, a woman raised her hand and asked to tell this story:

"After last week, I was so excited, I came home bouncing off the walls. I couldn't believe all this. I was so full of the information! My son's girlfriend was at my house, and she's on a diet, so I started pouring out what I learned. I told her about carbohydrate deprivation and muscle loss and all the reasons why weight doesn't count.

"I didn't think she was listening. She even argued with me a little. But the other day, when I saw her again, I said something about losing weight and she turned around and corrected me, 'No, you don't want to lose weight. You want to lose fat.' I was shocked."

I wasn't. Don't underestimate *your* power as an educator. There are 256 million Americans; that's a lot of educating to do. And you know there's a lot of diet thinking out there. One person sharing the facts with another can make a difference. I'd be honored if every BodyFueler did so with someone in their lives.

Good luck, and happy fueling.

INDEX

Made in the USA
San Bernardino, CA
08 November 2014